To Comfort Always

Oxford Medical Histories Series

This title from the Oxford Medical Histories series is designed to bring to a wide readership of clinical doctors and others from many backgrounds a comprehensive text setting out the essentials of the history of palliative medicine. Volumes in this series are written by medical experts and with doctors, in particular, in mind as the readership.

History describes the knowledge acquired over time by human beings. It is a form of storytelling, of organizing knowledge, of sorting, and giving impetus to information. The study of medical history, just like the history of other human endeavours, enables us to analyse our knowledge of the past in order to plan our journey forward and hence try to limit repetition of our mistakes—a sort of planned process of Natural Selection, described as being in the tradition of one of the most famous of medical historians, William Osler. Medical history also encourages and trains us to use an academic approach to our studies, which thereby should become more precise, more meaningful, and more productive. Medical history should be enjoyable too, since that is a powerful stimulus to move forward, a fun thing to do both individually and in groups.

The inspiring book that led to this series introduced us to clinical neurology, genetics, and the history of those with muscular dystrophy. Alan and Marcia Emery explored *The History of a Genetic Disease*, now often styled Meryon's disease rather than Duchenne Muscular Dystrophy. The first to describe a disease process is not necessarily the owner of the eponym but the Emerys are helping put that right for their subject, Edward Meryon. The second book in the series, on radiology, took us on a journey round a world of images.

Thus future volumes in this series of Oxford Medical Histories will continue the journey through the history of our bodies, of their relationship to our environment, of the joyful and the sad situations that envelope us from our individual beginnings to our ends. We should travel towards other aspects of our humanity, always leaving us with more questions than answers since each new discovery leads to more questions, exponential sets of issues for us to study, further thoughts and attempts to solve the big questions that surround our existence. Medicine is about people and so is history; the study of the combination of the duo can be very powerful.

Christopher Gardner-Thorpe, MD, FRCP, FACP
Series Advisor, Oxford Medical Histories

To Comfort Always
A history of palliative medicine since the nineteenth century

David Clark
Professor of Medical Sociology and
Wellcome Trust Investigator, School of Interdisciplinary
Studies, University of Glasgow, UK

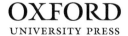

OXFORD
UNIVERSITY PRESS

OXFORD

UNIVERSITY PRESS

Great Clarendon Street, Oxford, OX2 6DP,
United Kingdom

Oxford University Press is a department of the University of Oxford.
It furthers the University's objective of excellence in research, scholarship,
and education by publishing worldwide. Oxford is a registered trade mark of
Oxford University Press in the UK and in certain other countries

First Edition published in 2016
Impression: 2

Published in the United States of America by Oxford University Press
198 Madison Avenue, New York, NY 10016, United States of America

British Library Cataloguing in Publication Data
Data available

Library of Congress Control Number: 2016937924

ISBN 978–0–19–967428–2

Printed and bound by
CPI Group (UK) Ltd, Croydon, CR0 4YY

Foreword

It is truly a privilege to be asked to write the foreword to *To Comfort Always*. Professor David Clark is already well known to those working in palliative care for his insights into the development of the modern hospice movement and particularly for his evaluation of the role of Dame Cicely Saunders in this over the course of the second half of the twentieth century. In '*To Comfort Always,*' David looks at a much wider span of history, covering a period of nearly two centuries. He rigorously examines developments in the meaning of a good or peaceful death (the original meaning of euthanasia) and developments in the delivery of palliative care across the world.

I have been fortunate to witness many of the developments in palliative medicine and end-of-life care in the United Kingdom over the past 40 years. My father, a GP in Oxford, helped to establish the Sir Michael Sobell Hospice when I was a medical student in the 1970s. During my training as a medical oncologist, Robert Twycross kindly encouraged me to spend time at the hospice, which was of enormous value to me. Later, when I was appointed Professor of Palliative Medicine at Guy's and St. Thomas', Cicely Saunders made my appointment conditional on going to Canada to learn from Eduardo Bruera, then in Edmonton, and from Balfour Mount in Montreal. I owe each of them a debt of gratitude, so I am delighted to see their prominent roles in *To Comfort Always*. During my time at Guy's and St Thomas' I was also fortunate to work alongside colleagues at Trinity Hospice in Clapham (The Hostel of God in Chapter 2) and at St Christopher's. I have learned a great deal from them.

To Comfort Always starts with an assessment of the role of nineteenth-century doctors in the care of the dying. As David Clark points out, this was a period of widespread industrialization, urbanization, and population growth in Europe. The causes of death were also changing from infection and disaster to cancer and tuberculosis, with dying therefore commonly becoming protracted. Religion still played an important role in Victorian attitudes to death—i.e. that it should occur at home preceded by farewells, devotions, and prayers. The nineteenth century was also marked by medical advances, which included the isolation of morphine and the invention of the hypodermic syringe.

However, although nineteenth-century doctors were often involved around the time of death (at least for more affluent patients), relatively few wrote about it. There were some notable exceptions, whose insights are illuminating. Although I had heard of Munk in the context of Munk's Roll at the Royal College of Physicians, I was not previously aware of his book *Euthanasia*, referring to an easeful death. These important early works demonstrate the evolution of thinking about medical care for the dying and are beautifully chronicled.

Equally fascinating is the assessment of the role of 'proto-hospices' in the late nineteenth and early twentieth centuries. Although I had been aware of a number of these homes for the terminally ill, I had not realized that they had been established with little knowledge of each other in France, Ireland, London, Sydney, New York, and elsewhere. Interestingly, they were all founded by women. A key feature was that they saw saving souls as a top priority and focused their attention on the respectable poor who were within a few months of death.

The advent of the National Health Service in the United Kingdom in 1948 represented a major shift from provision of healthcare by charities to the state. Interestingly, this led directly to the establishment of the Marie Curie Foundation, whose key aim was to deliver end-of-life care in locations other than hospitals. The early and mid 1950s also saw an important shift towards gathering evidence of the needs of patients approaching the end of life and to detailed studies by Cicely Saunders of the care given to such patients.

The later chapters of the book chart the emergence and growth of palliative care in the United Kingdom and around the world. This has not, of course, been confined to care delivered in hospices, but also includes hospital support teams, specialist nurses, and education programmes. The establishment of the Association of Palliative Medicine and its recognition as a specialty for medical training were both pivotal moments, which came about through the dedication of a small group of passionate clinicians. Subsequently, the World Health Organization, international congresses, and palliative care associations have helped to spread developments across the world.

Despite all of the progress of the last two centuries, much more remains to be done. We know that many patients even in countries with the most advanced palliative care provision are still not dying well. This is especially, but not exclusively true for those dying in hospitals. We can and we must do better. Clinicians, health service managers, and policy-makers all have roles to play in this.

I thoroughly recommend this book to anyone working in the fields of hospice care, palliative care, and/or end-of-life care—the definitions still cause difficulties! It will give insights to others as it has done for me. Learning from the past should help us all to consider how to do better in the future.

Professor Sir Mike Richards
Chief Inspector of Hospitals,
Care Quality Commission, UK
May 2016

Preface

This book is the first to chart in detail the history of palliative medicine, from its origins in the nineteenth century to its recognition and consolidation in the twentieth century, and onto the challenges it faces today. It draws on a large body of published and unpublished sources, interviews with key individuals in the field, and my accumulated knowledge as one who has been active in palliative care research and education since the late 1980s. I hope that *To Comfort Always* will be essential reading for specialists in palliative medicine everywhere, and of significant interest to other professionals and volunteers working in palliative care across different services and settings. In addition to exploring the challenges, achievements, and dilemmas faced by a new medical specialty in the late twentieth and early twenty-first centuries, the book also has several things to say about the care of the dying and those with advanced disease. Indeed, it is a book about a public health challenge, to which medicine as a whole should give high priority in the coming decades.

In 1987, the specialty of palliative medicine gained formal recognition in the United Kingdom—the first country in the world to accredit this new field of medical practice. The achievement however built on at least 100 years of developing experience in which modern medicine, albeit reluctantly at first, gave growing attention to the needs of people with advanced and incurable disease. One hundred years earlier, in 1887, the London-based physician William Munk had published his groundbreaking work on 'easeful death', setting out a case for the skilled and sympathetic care of the dying patient. Over the next half-century, other prominent physicians and surgeons—including Herbert Snow, William Osler, and Alfred Worcester—wrote eloquently on the same subject. However, in Britain, the influence of these pioneers was limited and care of the dying remained a neglected field of medicine. A mere handful of terminal care homes and hospices, isolated and undeveloped, showed any consistent interest in the problem of suffering at the end of life.

After World War II, interest in the terminal care of people with cancer began to increase. Evidence of poor care, late involvement, and fatalistic attitudes on the part of patients and professionals painted a depressing picture. Meanwhile, the medical writings of the time confirmed a sense of limited skills, few educational opportunities, and a lack of focused effort to improve terminal care. When Cicely Saunders published her first paper in 1958, the tide began to turn. Her extensive writing, teaching, and advocacy over the next decade galvanized support—from clinicians, charities, health administrators, and the wider public. By the late 1960s and the opening of St Christopher's Hospice in south London, a modern movement was getting underway in Britain that would quickly have an international influence. The implications for medicine were far-reaching. Hospices increased in numbers, and at the same time, the practices they embodied spread to other settings, in Britain and beyond, where the term 'palliative care' was often used to describe them.

By the late 1980s, three factors were conjoining to build a platform for the broad consolidation of the new field of activity in the United Kingdom: a medical association was formed to support its practitioners; a scientific journal was established; and recognition was given to palliative medicine as an area of specialization. Initially a subspecialty of general medicine on a seven-year 'novitiate', in due course palliative medicine successfully became a specialty in its own right.

A period of rapid expansion and diversification ensued. In the United Kingdom, the new palliative physicians were trained to practice in any setting. Many chose not to work in independent hospices, but to develop provision across the National Health Service; and in particular, in acute hospitals and in the community. Cancer charities made significant investment in new posts and services. Teaching programmes and research activity started to expand. In university medical schools, senior lecturers, and the first professors in palliative medicine began to appear. In turn, there was greater policy interest, special funds to support palliative care, and burgeoning enthusiasm for extending the model to people with all life-threatening conditions, regardless of diagnosis.

At the same time, there were controversies and dissensions. Both inside and outside the field, questions were being asked about the nature of the new specialty, and the wider role it might play. Was its focus only on the last days of life? Could it migrate 'upstream' to earlier stages of disease progression? What evidence existed for its efficacy? Could it be taken seriously by other specialities? Did it risk an over-concentration on pain and symptom management and consequent loss of focus on 'holistic' care? What role could the specialty play in contributing to controversial ethical issues about the 'right' to die, euthanasia, assisted dying, and end-of-life sedation?

Many of these questions led to debate in an international context. Palliative medicine specialists were now to be found meeting with colleagues from other countries. Collaborations of various types began to develop—in education, research, and in advocating for palliative care development at the national level. Across world regions and jurisdictions, associations were formed to promote palliative care development, often involving leading doctors from the specialty. Endorsement came from the World Health Organization, as well as from international medical associations in cognate fields.

By the early twenty-first century, palliative medicine had made huge strides. However, development around the world remained patchy and there was clear evidence of a tidal wave of global need in the coming decades resulting from an ageing population and a predicted rise in the annual number of deaths. Could palliative medicine provide the expertise and leadership that would be necessary in the face of such demands? This book addresses these issues.

Here are a few points to guide the reader. The book begins from a primarily British perspective, but takes on more international and global dimensions as the narrative unfolds. This is the history of a specialty that is still emergent in many parts of the world and to that extent it must be a work in progress. I seek to document that specialty's evolution from the nineteenth century, when doctors began giving sustained attention to the management of pain and its associated symptoms at the end of life. I try to show the ambivalent orientation of modern medicine to care when disease is no longer curable. In turn, I examine how a focus on the idea of palliative care gained ground, sought recognition, and translated into a burgeoning field with services and critical mass in many countries of the world. I have been fortunate to be able to draw on oral history interviews with a number of key palliative care activists to illustrate some of this. The focus of the book concentrates in the period 1887–1987. In the opening chapter, I stray into the earlier periods of the nineteenth century. In the later chapters, I have inevitably attended to issues from the end of the twentieth and beginning of the twenty-first centuries—but readers should note that I have not attempted a full review of developments in palliative care in these more recent decades. Please see other works by myself for specific commentaries on some of these issues.

'To comfort always' is a phrase sometimes attributed to Hippocrates and is closely associated with Dr Edward Livingston Trudeau, founder of an early American tuberculosis sanatorium. It seems a fitting title for this book and has much to commend it as a guide to care, not only at the end of life, but wherever human suffering occurs.

David Clark
Dalswinton, Dumfriesshire
November 2015

Acknowledgements

I am grateful to the several friends, scholars, students, and palliative care activists who, over many years, have influenced my thinking on the matters contained in this book. I make special mention of David Field, Tony Walter, Sam Ahmedzai, Bill Noble, Marcia Meldrum, Joy Buck, Michael Wright, Neil Small, Nic Hughes, Sara Denver, Mary O'Brien, Jane Seymour, Michelle Winslow, Kathleen Foley, Mary Callaway, David Praill, the late Cicely Saunders, the late Eric Wilkes, David Oliviere, Barbara Monroe, Margaret Jane, Lynne Hargreaves, Audrey Clowe, Stephen Connor, Isobel Broome, Clare Humphreys, Ruth Ashfield, Avril Jackson, Denise Brady, Kjell Erik Stroemskag, Tom Lynch, Derek Doyle, Orla Keegan, Javier Rocafort, Henk ten Have, Anne Grinyer, Anthony Greenwood, Lars Johann Materstvedt, Suresh Kumar, Robert Twycross, Reena George, Trgvye Willer, Philip Larkin, Bert Broeckaert, Jim Hallenbeck, Balfour Mount, Jim Cleary—and the Lego Palliateurs.

Carlos Centeno at the University of Navarra, where I am privileged to be a visiting professor in the Faculty of Medicine, has in particular been a huge source of deep inspiration and friendship to me over many years; he has always encouraged my interest in the history and 'intangibles' of the field of palliative care, as well as our collaborations in studying its current development.

The Wellcome Trust supported my early work on hospice and palliative care history with some key grants in the 1990s; and this book has been concluded during the period of a Wellcome Trust Investigator Award. I wish to thank everyone involved at the Trust for the support, enthusiasm, and endorsement that have been so crucial to this area of my work over an extended period. I am also indebted to my Wellcome Trust-funded colleagues at the University of Glasgow—Catriona Forrest, Hamilton Inbadas, Rachel Lucas and Shahaduz Zaman—along with Naomi Richards, Sandy Whitelaw, Clare Roques and Jackie Kandsberger for their collegiality, inspiration, and constant enthusiasm.

At various points I draw on oral history interviews collected from palliative care activists around the world. I thank all those who have contributed to the creation of this archive, which continues to grow as a document of record for hospice and palliative care development in many places. I have been pleased to see such approaches used in the work of others, who have written about the history of palliative care in other countries—Norway[1] and Poland,[2] for example.

I have also drawn on some archival sources, which I gratefully acknowledge here. Most of my work on the papers of Cicely Saunders, including their initial cataloguing, took place before they were consolidated at King's College London Archives; I am grateful to Chris Olver, who undertook this extensive work, for his help and assistance on a number of occasions, and for his ongoing interest in the life and work of Cicely Saunders. The extensive Saunders archive now available at King's College London is a rich treasure trove indeed. I am also grateful for access to material located in the Imperial College Healthcare NHS Trust Archives, The National Archives, and the archives of St Joseph's Hospice, Hackney.

Finally, I thank my wife, Fiona Graham—for the countless conversations, debates, and deconstructions we have enjoyed on the always-intriguing question of 'what is palliative medicine?'

Notes

1. **Strømskag KE** (2012). *Og nå skal jeg dø. Hospicebevegelsen og palliasjonens historie i Norge*. Oslo, Norway: PAX forlag.
2. **Janowicz A, Krakowiak P, Stolarczyk A** (2015). *In Solidarity: Hospice-Palliative Care in Poland*. Gdańsk, Poland: Fundacjahospicyjna.

Contents

Abbreviations *xvii*

1 Nineteenth-century doctors and care of the dying *1*
2 Homes for the terminally ill: 1885–1948 *33*
3 Interest and disinterest in the mid-twentieth century *59*
4 Cicely Saunders and her early associates: A kaleidoscope of effects *85*
5 Defining the clinical realm *117*
6 Specialty recognition and global development *149*
7 Palliative medicine: Historical record and challenges that remain *197*

Index *227*

Abbreviations

ABHPM	American Board of Hospice and Palliative Medicine		IHI	International Hospice Institute
ABMS	American Board of Medical Specialities		IoM	Institute of Medicine
ACGME	Accreditation Council of Graduate Medical Education		IOELC	International Observatory on End of Life Care
AMA	American Medical Association		JCHMT	Joint Committee on Higher Medical Training
APCA	African Palliative Care Association		LCP	Liverpool Care Pathway
APM	Association of Palliative Medicine		MRCP	Member of the Royal College of Physicians
BBC	British Broadcasting Company		NCI	National Cancer Institute
BMJ	British Medical Journal		NHS	National Health Service
CSCI	Continuous subcutaneous infusion		RACP	Royal Australasian College of Physicians
EAPC	European Association for Palliative Care		SCM	Student Christian Movement
IAHPC	International Association of Hospice and Palliative Care		SHO	Senior House Officer
			TB	Tuberculosis
IASP	International Association for the Study of Pain		US	United States
			UK	United Kingdom
			WHO	World Health Organization

Chapter 1

Nineteenth-century doctors and care of the dying

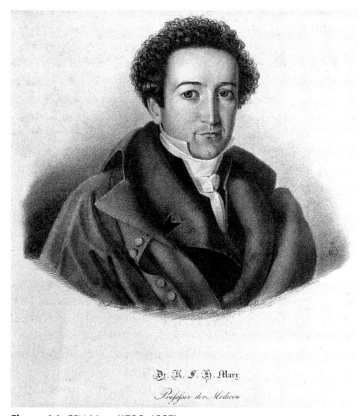

Dr. K. F. H. Marx

Professor der Medicin

Figure 1.1 CFH Marx (1796–1887)
Marx's thesis of 1826, presented at the University of Goettingen, explored the role of the doctor in producing 'euthanasia'—a peaceful death. It was not until the end of the nineteenth century that 'euthanasia' came to denote the deliberate ending of life or hastening of death by medical means. The carefully documented clinical observations of Marx were maintained in the writings of other nineteenth-century doctors, who succeeded in setting out some of the principles that were later to embody the practice of what came to be known as palliative medicine.
Reproduced from Wellcome Images, http://catalogue.wellcomelibrary.org/record=b1181192, Image ID: L0025130, Copyright © 2016 Wellcome Library, London.

Demographic change and the consequences for dying and death

By the late nineteenth century, the people of Europe and North America were living longer in societies of rapidly increasing size. A transformation of unprecedented proportions had brought widespread industrialization, urbanization, geographic mobility, the rise of scientific rationalities, political and ideological upheaval, and a growing questioning of religious values. The population of Europe had doubled during the course of the century, from 200 million to 400 million. Mortality rates were falling and the prospects of living into old age began to increase for many people. Nevertheless, with the benefits of longevity and the diminished threat of early death came particular consequences and repercussions. The predominant causes of death had started to shift—from sudden demise brought on by infection, disaster, and plague, to protracted dying associated with the emerging chronic diseases of the modern era, not least of which were cancer and tuberculosis. Whereas in Europe during the Middle Ages, the death that came too swiftly was something abhorrent and to be guarded against, now fears began to grow about lengthy dying and the suffering that it might entail.

The changing social world of the dying

Popular culture and Victorian fiction[1] presented idealized images of a slow and controlled farewell to the world, with family members gathered around the dying person's bedside and a sense of shared confidence in the imminent passage to a better world—the good death as a sign of coming salvation. However, by the later years of the century, concerns were emerging about the precise manner of dying, now coming to be seen not only as a social and cultural event, but also as a medical process. Strict rules existed for how to behave *after* a death occurred. Yet, there appeared to be less confidence in people's dispositions towards the act of dying. The changing personnel around the deathbed, a new secrecy about the imminence of death, as well as the desire to quell the threat of pain and suffering—all revealed a growing *anxiety* about the dying process. That in turn opened up a space for medical intervention, which first took hold towards the end of the nineteenth century, but was to have implications for more than a hundred years thereafter, indeed right up to the time of this book's writing in 2015.

For the French historian Phillipe Ariès, the nineteenth century was associated with the emergence of sentimental orientations to death that reflected major changes within the culture and structure of family life.[2,3] He argued that as the meaning of family relationships deepened and became more nuanced, so parting with a dying relative—and the subsequent grief follow-ing that loss—became increasingly emotional and expressive. A growing em-phasis fell on the personal pain of separation and on keeping the dead alive in memory, enhanced by new developments in photography that enabled care-fully staged post-mortem images to be captured and preserved for posterity. It also meant elaborate rituals of mourning and funeral observance, along with the emergence of the cult of the grave as a family resting place. Undoubtedly it led to new representations of the deathbed itself. The wider Romantic move-ment contributed to notions of the 'beautiful death', to *la mort de toi* ('thy death'), personified in the death of a loved one.

Ariès also describes how in the nineteenth century the rise of modern sci-ence brought challenges to religious authority, and specifically to the neces-sity of dying in the presence of the official representatives of formal religion. Medical men began to replace priests, clergy, and ministers at the bedsides of the dying. However, this created new dilemmas; for if the role of medicine was to focus on the technical preoccupations of attending to the relief of pain and the easing of physical distress, who was to address the fears of the dying, the distress of the bereaved, and the achievement of the 'good death'? Using this point of reference, we might see this as the period in which dying was drained of meaning by science and medicine, forcing its retreat from public, religious, and family dimensions into the sequestered spaces of hospitals and, ultimately, homes for the terminally ill. For Ariès, the mid-nineteenth cen-tury was also the origin of 'the lie' wherein the gravity of the dying person's situation was kept from them. Death was on the way to becoming something 'shameful and forbidden'.

Later historians and sociologists have questioned Ariès's linear conceptual-izations. There are assertions that he relies on superficial readings of material relating mainly to the upper and middle-class elite, and that the experiences of working-class families and communities are misrepresented, or obscured in his grand narrative. He is also accused of romanticizing a bygone era and somehow caricaturing death in the twentieth century as anonymous, re-pressed, and pathological. From the perspective of Ariès's critics, there was no golden age of grief that was subsequently 'ruined' by the scientific and medi-cal discourses of modernity.[4] As Julie-Marie Strange puts it, 'the Victorian culture of death is a myth of our own making'.[5] Perhaps it is better therefore to regard those living in the nineteenth century as no more and no less skilled than their forebears or successors in dealing with the experiences of dying, death, and bereavement.

The encounter with death is universal and as human beings we all know that we must die, but in every age and culture there are variations in how we experience our mortality—and our dying. There may be tendencies towards the framing of death as a uniquely personal experience for both the dying and the bereaved, and something requiring individualized adjustment. Other discourses put a strong emphasis on the place of death in society, its impact on social cohesion, and the legal, public, and policy consequences of dying and bereavement. In some contexts, discourses of religion may dominate; in others, the perspectives of science and humanism, even historical material-ism, may hold greater sway. Using this approach, historians have argued for understanding death through the cultural values that shape how we describe it, rather than seeking to uncover any particular 'truths' about how we experi-ence it. This is an important consideration for our focus here. There are incon-trovertible ways in which our ability to care for dying people has improved and become more sophisticated in the period since the late nineteenth cen-tury. Nevertheless, we should beware the assumption that this means there can be wholesale improvement on the way death was managed in the past. The shift of dying from the social, community, and family realm to become the preserve of specialists, professional carers, and service providers of vari-ous types should not mask the fact that death remains a profoundly social experience. Reforming the social component is a far more challenging goal than, for example, improving the technologies of pain relief. When death becomes a matter of public debate, dissension is not far away. As we shall see in Chapter 7 of this book, death in the contemporary world has become a *contested space*, in which the interventions of palliative medicine are only one set of forces at play—and one not always welcomed unequivocally. As we delve into the historical record, it becomes clear that since at least the late nineteenth century, medicine has had a problematic relationship with death that is still far from resolved.

Experiences at the bedside: Representations of the dying patient and the grieving family

There is a certain amount of scholarship on nineteenth-century care of the dying in Europe and North America, beginning with research on the cultural aspects of death, dying, and bereavement, particularly the experiences of elite groups in society. This has led to encouraging signs of further interest in these topics that has taken us into the lives not just of lettered and literate affluent families, but also alongside the end-of-life experiences of people in poor com-munities, and those in both rural and urban environments.

In Britain, our understanding of the Victorian culture of dying and the place of doctors and families within it derives from a small number of historical studies, each with a specific focus. Outstanding among these is the work of Pat

Jalland,[6] who not only surveys the characteristics of medical practice for those at the end of life, but also takes us to the bedsides of the dying—at least in upper middle-class families[7]—to show how the rituals and practices associated with dying and death were shaped by wider Victorian values and beliefs. Jalland shows how the role of religion is key. It circumscribed the cultural terrain of dying, emphasizing the need for unwavering faith, a sense of humility, and a readiness to submit to the will of God. By these means, the good death could be achieved. If this meant bearing prolonged agonies of physical suffering, then this itself was a spiritual test that might result in everlasting life. Protracted dying was also an opportunity to rekindle a lost Christian faith or indeed to give one's soul to Christ for the first time. Specifically, a powerful influence was brought to bear by the evangelical movement, which shaped Protestant dying around a script of atonement from sin, for which the final moments of life were a final opportunity to avoid everlasting torment. Such narratives found their way into widely distributed tracts, magazines, and memoirs. They were eagerly read and did much to influence popular beliefs about the appropriate manner of dying. As Jalland describes, these perceptions were echoed uncannily in the private correspondence, diaries, and deathbed memorials of middle and upper-class families in England, a finding made all the more powerful because these writings were often produced close to the time of the events and under the influence of intense emotion as death approached. The key difference that Jalland found between the two sets of texts—the public and the private—was that the latter were often remarkably frank about moral weaknesses, unpleasant symptoms, or 'unworthy' deathbed behaviour, elements usually expunged from the more widely published accounts.

What was clear, however, were the constituent elements of Victorian evangelical death: place, practice, and temporality. Death should occur at home, preceded by carefully orchestrated farewells, devotions, and prayers. The dying person should be awake, lucid, and able to seek forgiveness for past transgressions. Pain should be borne with fortitude and welcomed as a final test of fitness for heaven. Death in this manner was becoming an intensely private affair, a reaction against the public dying before a crowd that had been known in Britain and France in the eighteenth century and which persisted into the late nineteenth century for royalty and famous statesmen. Nevertheless, the evangelical good death also had its didactic elements and could be used as a stimulus to the devout and a cautionary example to the unbeliever, presuming at least a limited audience. For if the good death was not achieved, then eternal damnation might follow, and that was a message to promulgate beyond the deathbed itself.

Jalland demonstrates clearly that these idealizations of the good death were significantly eroded in the period from 1870 to 1914, as evangelical fervour waned within society. With the declining influence of religion, concern for the soul was less demonstrated, and this led to an increasing preoccupation with matters of pain and other symptoms. The balance was slowly swinging away from a primary concern with the state of the soul in the final days of life, towards a greater emphasis on the body that was free from physical suffering. Linked to this was a new evaluation of sudden death—once feared because it denied a chance of preparation for the next world, now at least cautiously welcomed as it obviated any fear of impending demise and a life taken away. Jalland sees this as the key condition, merely a short step away, which led to the practice of deliberately withholding knowledge of their fate from dying people. Out of this crucible of change, she points the way to the modern twentieth-century death, which attenuated the role of faith and amplified the importance of pain and symptom relief, while at the same time diminishing the role of the clergy and, to some extent, the family, replacing them with an increasing emphasis on the sayings and doings of doctors.

Julie-Marie Strange has contributed a perspective on working-class grief and mourning[8] in northern England over the period 1870–1914, precisely identified by Jalland as the time in which the foundations of the Victorian evangelical death began to shift. In acknowledging the paucity of historical research on this subject, Strange notes two points. First, the working classes left little correspondence or memoirs that might illuminate their experiences of dying and death, making this a challenging area for researchers. Second, she questions the assumption that grinding poverty, high mortality, and poor living conditions might have somehow created a sense of fatalism or resignation about death among poorer social groups, which perhaps made death less consequential for day-to-day life. Her focus is in a period when living standards were rising, attitudes to poverty were changing, mortality rates were declining, and access to medical care was increasing. Strange presents a rich picture of working-class attitudes and practices in the face of death. She shows how many accounts from the period reveal a sense of openness and pragmatism, in contrast to the growing veil of secrecy described by Jalland. However, when money was tight, it was common to prioritize subscriptions to the funeral club over payment for medical care. This was offset by a major investment of time and effort by family members and neighbours in informal networks of care for the sick and dying. Strange quotes Florence Bell's moving account of care among impoverished ironworkers in Middlesbrough, in the industrial north east of England:

> In one case, the husband, an ironworker, had been ill with rheumatic fever and pneumonia, the wife with consumption—both hopelessly ill; the husband died first, and the kindly neighbour . . . offered to take in the dying woman, who shrank from going to hospital. She took the invalid into her house and when the mother died, adopted the child.[9]

Strange found in her studies the pervasive influence of stories about attentive care and self-sacrifice. Families sought to hold onto their sick and dying members; they often equated hospitals with almshouses and places of stigma; and there was a belief that the care provided in such institutions would not match that available at home. However, at the same time, the protracted death, apparently idealized by wealthy families up until the 1870s, was feared as a further drain on limited resources. Illness brought unemployment, reduced income, and the need to expend more on the sick person, including medical bills. Death not only hurt the emotions, but also the family coffers. In such circumstances, the resilience and fortitude described by Strange is remarkable. Nor were there many options for the relief of pain and suffering, other than the use of alcohol, the companionship of close ones and, for those who could afford it, the prescription of morphine by the doctor. Strange observes that in contrast to the evangelical convictions of Jalland's early Victorians, the working classes of the later period seemed to favour an all-forgiving god of mercy. They casually overlooked obligations to a god of judgement, and thus left the deathbed free from last-minute conversions and prayers for the forgiveness of sin.[5]

To these observations can be added the work of D. P. Helm,[10] who sets out to understand the beliefs, motivations, and influences that shaped the care of the dying in the Victorian home, in an age immediately prior to the growth of hospitals and the subsequent shift of death from the home to the institutional setting. His focus is on data from three of England's rural counties (Gloucestershire, Herefordshire, and Worcestershire), and his attention is with families of the 'middling sort'—in other words, somewhere in-between those contexts described by Jalland and Strange. Helm shows how the key professional nexus in this regard was that of the clergy, nurses, and doctors, and he seeks to identify the currents of change that transformed care of the dying in the Victorian period. This study presents evidence from diaries, letters, novels, and the visual arts to suggest that family members' central role in the decision-making process, and in providing care, allowed them to draw on shared emotional and psychological support and derive comfort from religious beliefs held in common. The wider community of friends, neighbours, extended family, and the many middle-class women who undertook to visit the sick as a Christian duty, all provided further support to carers.

Throughout the nineteenth century, Christianity still provided the framework within which most people in British society understood death. Christian end-of-life care was focused on spiritual preparation and gave the dying respect and a dignity conferred by their perceived proximity to God. For the carers, Helm argues, the emphasis on preparedness provided them with a comforting role—for example, in praying and reading from scripture with the dying, when otherwise they could feel impotent in the face of untreatable bodily suffering. Contrary to suggestions that Christians disapproved of pain relief, the evidence from Helm's work suggests that analgesia was mostly welcomed once available, but when pain was encountered, Christian teachings about its purpose were drawn upon as a source of consolation and strength. Although doctors were becoming increasingly influential in end-of-life care through an increase in their professional status and an improving ability to provide effective pain management, Helm contends that they did not exercise the levels of authority and control over the domestic deathbed that they later came to assume in the hospital setting. These limitations on the doctor's influence can be observed in the process of negotiation through which diagnoses were arrived at, frequently involving recourse to second opinions, and through the constraints imposed by the lack of effective treatments. Finally, Helm challenges the persistent preconception that the Victorians were morbidly obsessed with death, suggesting instead that the Victorian response to death should be seen as both pragmatic and rational, given the prevalence of death in society and the changing nature of religious and medical practice.

We also have evidence of nineteenth-century homecare of dying people in the German context, gleaned from research that focused on the work of deaconesses associated with the diaconal centre at Kaiserswerth, near Düsseldorf. In the training of these deaconesses of Kaiserswerth, the nursing of the soul—caring for the spirit of the sick person—was given equal importance to care of the physical body. After finishing their training in the motherhouse, the deaconesses were sent to hospitals and into parishes and private care in many German cities. Their letters, written back to the motherhouse, offer insight into their experiences of caregiving in domestic settings. Karen Nolte[11] has provided an analysis of these experiences, which we can place alongside other depictions of nursing care of the terminally ill in Britain and America. This also gives insight into the forms of institutional care of the dying that were to develop from the late nineteenth century, and to which we turn in Chapter 2.

Sometimes, the mere presence of a nurse appeared to have had a soothing effect on the sick and their families. The Kaiserswerth sisters took care not only of the patients, but also of their family members. They cooked for husbands, children, and siblings, and provided personal and religious support for them. In administering pain relief, the nurses bore a great responsibility, which sometimes led to conflicts with the physician in charge. Some felt themselves better equipped than the attending physician to decide how much morphine a patient needed and at what time, while others seem to have administered morphine with considerable discretion. Nursing the soul became particularly significant once the doctors had no more to offer and the nurses could do little more with physical care. Nevertheless, even deeply held beliefs could be challenged by the severity of suffering. One particularly haunting report on the care of a woman with abdominal tumours appeared to trigger a crisis of faith, not only in the nurse, but also in the dying woman and her husband.

The Kaiserswerth nurses were expected to establish a professional distance between themselves and the patient's family. They were urged not to eat with the family, not to accept personal gifts, and to wear the required deaconess habit at all times. They were also expected to leave the family as soon as their care was no longer needed. In the event of death, the nurse was permitted to stay through to the funeral, but she had to travel back to the motherhouse or to her next location immediately afterwards. Nolte observes that, at times, the way the deaconesses dealt with the deaths of their patients appeared rather technical and pragmatic—for example, in letters to the directors in Kaiserswerth, they gave estimates on how long it might take for a patient to die so that they could then leave. During their training period, the sisters were prepared for the care of the terminally ill in a 'Course of Medicine', which covered in detail the special physical care requirements of the dying. The sisters were expected to stay with the dying person continuously and alleviate the process by regularly washing and drying, turning, and repositioning the patient. However, spiritual care predominated and, as Nolte reports, the medicine course handbook stated the following:

> The beautiful and sacred task of nursing not only in its seriousness, but also in its full meaning and importance is brought to bear at the bed of the dying. When the physician can help no longer, the love of the nurse is still working indefatigably, standing by the dying person with a caring hand and a gentle mind in the hour of strife and dissolution to bring him relief and consolation. She almost doubles her diligence and loyalty and her concern reaches even beyond the point when the decisive moment has passed.[11]

Emily Abel's work on end-of-life care in nineteenth-century America gives further context, detail and definition to this type of narrative.[12] Abel rejects the notion that doctors actively sought dominion over the dying process in these years, or that medicine eclipsed the role of families and religion at the deathbed. For Abel, the ability of medicine to control acute infectious disease was quickly offset by the rising tide of chronic conditions, within which the route to death could be protracted and unpredictable, and with unpleasant symptoms that were difficult to control. Patients were labelled 'incurable' (in the earlier period) or 'terminal' (somewhat later) and, by and large, 'devalued and avoided' by physicians and hospitals alike. Even though the American Medical Association (AMA) had drawn up a code as early as 1847 urging doctors not to abandon the incurably ill or those imminently dying, physicians were largely absent from the deathbed in this period. While medicine in the mid-nineteenth century made huge advances in the control of pain—using morphine and the newly invented hypodermic syringe—skills in relieving pain at the end of life lagged far behind those relating to pain relief after surgery. The AMA code also warned against making gloomy prognostications and this tended to foster a sense of false optimism, or even denial in doctors dealing with terminally ill patients. In this way, the stance of American medicine towards the dying could appear limited and detached. In 1873, America had only 120 hospitals, from which the dying were, in the main, actively excluded. Most people died at home, cared for by relatives who continued to view dying as a social and spiritual event that was largely the responsibility of the family. Nevertheless, death could also take place in the hospital, among strangers, and sometimes far from one's roots and origins.

So in the 'long' nineteenth century, the prevalent culture of dying in Europe and North America moved from an idealized and protracted process oriented around spiritual considerations, to one where the primary concerns shifted more to the relief of physical suffering than to matters of religious observance. While the comfortable circumstances of the middle and upper classes may have favoured easy access to a new cadre of physicians willing to intervene at the deathbed, for poorer families the material realities of suffering continued to be managed by relatives and neighbours, with limited practical resources to alleviate pain and distress. Against this contextual background, it is now time to move our focus to some of the key medical innovators of the period, to examine how medicine began to develop a discourse of care for the terminally ill in the nineteenth century, and in so doing, defined a set of parameters for intervention and conduct at the bedsides of the dying.

Emerging medical perspectives on care of the dying

Julie Rugg has observed that by the late eighteenth century, the doctor was becoming a common presence for both upper and middle-class families around the time of death[13] and this was a trend that continued as the nineteenth century advanced. As Lorna Jane Campbell notes, by the first half of the nineteenth century, attention was turning in earnest to the specific question of how best to care for the dying.[14] At first, doctors had little to offer, either in the way of curative intervention, or systematic modes of symptom relief. Their role may have been limited to a combination of self-styled imperiousness and well-honed bedside manner, coupled with the judicious use of laudanum and opium that had become commonplace in 'the anaesthetised age' of the eighteenth century.[15] As the nineteenth century progressed, however, medical men gained access to new technologies, and to the drugs that began to define the physician's place at the deathbed. In time they became active in collating and disseminating their practice in this regard, achieving a growing audience for their endeavours. It is possible to identify a small number of medical authors, frequently at the end of their professional career (although not always), who made a particular contribution to the question of caring for those imminently dying. It is hard to assess whether their practices were representative of the prevailing norms. Their approach was essentially a distillation of practical wisdom gained from experience and from the writings of their antecedents, and we must assume that they were at the forefront (rather than the rear-guard) of thinking for their time—with many others having less complete or informed practices. We should therefore beware of forming from these texts a more general representation of medical care for dying people in this period.

As early as 1802, Richard Reece, following medical practice in Chepstow and Cardiff, produced his expansive eight-volume work for a wide readership entitled *The Medical Guide, for the Use of Clergy, Heads of Families, and Seminaries and Junior Practitioners in Medicine; Comprising a Complete Dispensatory, and a Practical Treatise on the Distinguishing Symptoms, Causes, Prevention, Cure, and Palliation,*[16] a work that was still in print in its 17th edition in 1850, almost 30 years after his death. This is one of the earliest uses in medical writing of the term 'palliation', referring to the relief of symptoms and suffering. It is notable that Reece not only thought to include nonmedical persons in the readership of his book, but also gave prominence to care when cure was not possible. Yet, works of this kind were usually general texts that covered the entire spectrum of medical practice and were not in any sense specialist writing on the care of the dying. Those were much fewer in number.

Ninety years after Reece, in a lecture on the care of the dying first given to nurses at the Metropolitan Hospital in March 1892 that was then published two years later, Dr Oswald Browne remarked in his introduction on the paucity of literature available concerning his subject.[17] To the following half a dozen works, he acknowledged his great debt:

- Dr John Ferriar, *Medical Histories and Reflections* (1798)

- Sir Henry Halford, *Essays and Orations* (1842)

- Sir Benjamin Brodie, *Essays* (1865)

- Sir William Savory, *Lectures on Life and Death* (1863)

- Sir Dyce Duckworth, in the third volume of *Misericordia* (1885)

- Dr William Munk, *Euthanasia—or Medical Treatment in Aid of an Easy Death* (1887)

Such a bibliography, covering almost a century of medical writing, may seem slender indeed, although as we shall see in what follows it was not entirely complete, and at least a small number of other doctors in the period found time to lecture and to write about their knowledge and experience of caring for the dying. (The list is also notable in excluding the contribution of Florence Nightingale.[18]) Nevertheless, it provides at best only partial evidence to support the idea that from the eighteenth century onwards, medical practitioners were actively seeking to colonize the process of dying. Rather, we find in the collection the distilled wisdom of prominent medical men, moved at some point to comment on the care that should be afforded to the dying in their final hours and days—without any obvious sense that care at the deathbed was presenting some new opportunity for medicine or a new challenge to be overcome. Where this sense of opportunity is articulated, it is found buried in academic theses that had little wider influence for many years.

One such example, which we shall discuss in the next section, was the thesis of Hugh Noble, who was writing about the care of the dying in Edinburgh in the 1850s. There was also the thesis entitled *De Euthanasia Medica*[19] of Dr Carl Friedrich Heinrich Marx (1796–1887) (Figure 1.1), presented in Latin in 1826 at the University of Goettingen, which at that time was part of the Kingdom of Hanover. His work had some influence on German physicians, but did not reach a wider audience until 1952 when it was translated into English and published by Dr Walter Cane of Nassau County, New York.[20] Marx writes elegantly and comprehensively about the desired disposition of medicine to those who are dying and begins by asking what can be done to make the passing from life 'gentle and bearable'. He defines this as a science that controls the oppressing features of illness, relieves pain, and renders the supreme and inescapable hour a most peaceful one. He suggests that up until that time, the subject had not been thoroughly studied, and he is modest in the claims he makes for his own contribution. Nevertheless, he is also critical of those physicians who, when they find their treatments wanting, begin to lose interest in their patient, believing they are dealing with a disease, and not a human being. The nobler path, he asserts, is taken by some physicians, whom Marx observes in this wonderfully rousing passage:

> With no shining ray of hope remaining, consider it their more lofty duty to lay to peaceful rest a life they can no longer save. Accordingly they will extend their energy and their affection, they will follow each successive turn of events, they will apply

palliatives wherever they can, and with an all-caring heart they will put themselves in readiness for the great event, so that the last breath of passing may be light and not dreadful to those left behind.

He then lays out three principles to guide such an orientation. First, there is *foresight*: the watchful attendance of nurses and others, whom with skill take every opportunity to ensure the patient's comfort and the correct organization of the sickroom. Second, is the *avoidance of suffering*: this means eschewing dubious therapeutic and surgical measures, and focusing on eliminating or curbing pain, torment, and restlessness though sedative and analgesic medications. Third, is the pursuit of *higher comfort*: this should not be left only to the priest, but should capitalize on the known face of the physician, who endeavours to relieve agitation, bring confidence to the despairing, assure the doubtful, and assuage fear.

In all this, Marx is clear that 'euthanasia' is not about the physician bringing forward the moment of death, a practice he condemns: ' . . . least of all should he be permitted, prompted either by other people's requests or by his own sense of mercy, to end the patient's pitiful condition by purposely and deliberately hastening death'. In this context, Marx can still praise the use of narcotics, which 'if properly and cautiously administered, are the most salubrious medicines for the whole human race and particularly appropriate for euthanasia'. At the same time, practitioners must use them with care and be alert to untoward side effects, aware of how they can differ in every individual, and sensitive to their power to produce stupor at high doses. He singles out opium as the 'solace of phthisics' or the 'blessed anchor' for cholera.

According to Cane, Marx's thesis was later praised by Dr Heinrich Rohlfs (as a 'medical classic' in his work *Geschicte der deutschen Medizin,* published in 1880). Marx's short treatise contains many key elements in the nineteenth-century medical pursuit of euthanasia. That term would later in the century change its meaning significantly and, in so doing, serve to obscure the goals of care that Marx and others sought to identify for medicine when all therapeutic endeavour had become ineffective. As we shall see in subsequent chapters, his blueprint for euthanasia bears remarkable resemblance to later endeavours that came to be known as *palliative care*. It was not about actively seeking to end the life of the patient.

A paper by Mark Taubert and colleagues[21] investigated the occurrence of the word *palliative* within articles appearing in the *Provincial Medical and Surgical Journal* (later the *British Medical Journal*) in the first three years from its inception in 1840 (a dozen years before William Noble was submitting his thesis at Edinburgh). They found a smattering of references, some pejorative ('mere palliatives'), others implying a more purposive orientation to palliative treatments. Some concerned cases of cancer and some tuberculosis. None seemed to have been concerned with patients actively dying, but they do indicate that nineteenth-century doctors were distinguishing between clinical interventions that might have a curative intent, and those where the purpose might be to give comfort, alleviate suffering, and lift morale.

The final work on Browne's list for his 1892 lecture, Munk's *Euthanasia: Or, Medical Treatment in Aid of an Easy Death,* was already gaining significant attention among medical and nursing readers. For in Munk's 1887 work[22] we see something much more extensive, more rigorous, and more like a manual for end-of-life medical care that might be taken up and championed by others, and thereby have some wider influence on medical practice.

William Munk was born in 1816 and qualified in medicine in 1837, having attended medical schools in London and Holland.[23] He established a successful general practice in London, where he worked for over 60 years and became well known in the profession. He was not only a leading authority on smallpox, but also in his role as Harveian Librarian to the Royal College of Physicians, he single-handedly produced the Roll of the Royal College of Physicians of London 1518–1700.[24] Though a prolific medical biographer, he yielded a smaller output of clinical writings. In the present context, it is his *Euthanasia* book,[22] published when he was 71 years old and had spent more than 40 years in medical practice, for which he is most notable. This was a work that had an immediate impact in medicine and in nursing—on both sides of the Atlantic. For this reason, it is important to look at Munk in some detail.

Munk's reason for writing *Euthanasia* is not clear. It is against the tide of his other major publications, which were almost exclusively biographical.[25,26] As we shall see in Chapter 2, there was a cluster of people in the years immediately preceding the publication of *Euthanasia* whose religiously inspired commitment to caring for the dying resulted in the establishment of special homes for that purpose in London and elsewhere.[27] Yet Munk gives no indication that he is aware of, or engaged with, any of these people or their activities. The title of his work immediately gains the attention of the modern reader. But, as we have seen, at the time of Munk's writing, euthanasia still referred chiefly to the notion of a calm and peaceful death, the good death brought about with the assistance of the physician. It was not until the beginning of the twentieth century that the modern sense of euthanasia, understood as a deliberate medical intervention to end life, was fully articulated. Such it was described by Robert Saunby in his 1902 work on medical ethics as 'the doctrine that it is permissible for a medical practitioner to give a patient suffering from a mortal disease a poisonous dose of opium or other narcotic drug in order to terminate his sufferings'.[28] Munk, by contrast, uses the word euthanasia in its classical sense, to describe the goal of the physician in help-ing the sufferer to a more comfortable death. He is clear that care should be taken to avoid even the accidental premature death of the dying patient by the incautious administration of opium.[22] This sense of euthanasia had become widely understood in Victorian Britain and was also used to refer to the glori-ous deaths encountered through global exploration or other feats of heroism, and which did not involve the medical practitioner.

Munk's opening chapter covers four main aspects of dying. The first is to assert that the moment of death is not as dreadful or painful in reality as is often supposed. This was one of the contemporary arguments against delib-erate killing. Here as elsewhere, we see Munk drawing on the influence and arguments of earlier medical writers on his subject—specifically Sir Henry Halford, who had gained a significant reputation for his solicitous care of dying members of the upper classes in the late eighteenth and early nineteenth centuries,[15] but also the more recent influences of Sir Benjamin Brodie and Sir William Savory. He acknowledges that the process of dying may be painful, but maintains the distinction between the moment of death and the 'urgent symptoms of disease that precede and lead up to it'. There are some exceptions to this, where death is caused by disease of the heart and great vessels, as well as in cases of ileus, hydrophobia, tetanus, and cholera, in which 'some few do really suffer grievously in dying and expire in great bodily torture'.

The mental aspects of dying, the second phenomenon noted by Munk, echo the physical dimensions. That is, the moment of death is usually accompanied by calm, particularly if the physician, or the patient's friends, have helped to maintain an attitude of hope. The great shock of discovering that death is imminent usually gives way to a state of tranquillity, providing there has been sufficient time for the patient to adjust. Where the realization of death's imminence comes too close to the event itself, Munk notes, recovery from the shock is less likely, and this 'explains some at least of the harrowing scenes that occasionally mark the deathbed'. It is for this reason, he argues, that the dying person should be fully informed about their condition: 'An earlier in-timation to the dying person of the great change he is about to undergo is in all respects desirable.'

The third phenomenon Munk considers is the state of the intellect at the actual moment of death. This may vary from alert to delirious, but regardless of what state has been dominant during the process of dying, the transition to the moment of death is marked by a 'return of intelligence, that "lightening up before death" which has impressed and surprised mankind from the earliest ages'.

The content of Munk's first chapter is derived from his considerable experi-ence as a practising physician, and his assertions are supported by reference to previous authors, with whom he appears to always agree. A much shorter chapter follows, 'The Symptoms and Modes of Dying', in which Munk presents the variety and individuality of ways of dying, according to the nature and the site of the disease. A footnote informs the reader that he has not relied so much on his own experience in this part of the book, because 'Sir Thomas Watson, in his admirable lecture on the Different Modes of Dying,[29] has treated the whole subject so graphically that I shall follow him as closely as possible in what I have to adduce on this part of my subject'. Munk was a great admirer of Sir Thomas Watson[30] and saw him as the most important doctor in the land.

Munk's third chapter, 'The General and Medical Treatment of the Dying', opens with the proposition that much suffering is not 'naturally or necessarily incident to the act of dying', but is due to surrounding circumstances that can be changed or managed. These include the provision of appropriate bedding, physical position in the bed, fresh air in the room, and so on. In these observations and recommendations, Munk reveals the influence of Florence Nightingale's approach to nursing. Nightingale's *Notes on Nursing* (1859)[18] is cited three times: (1) regarding the desirable posture for a dying patient in bed; (2) the benefits of light bedclothes; and (3) the necessity to avoid whispered conversations in the sick room. The most important of the nursing considerations, according to Munk's account, is the provision of appropriate nourishment. He devotes seven pages to this, claiming that there is nothing of more importance in the management of the dying. The best *kind* of food depends on the nature of the disease and the likely prognosis. Where death results from 'slowly progressive exhaustion', as with cancer and some cases of consumption, then food should be more nourishing and given in relatively greater quantity. Sceptical of the value of beef tea and other meat extracts, favouring instead milk, cream, beaten eggs, and cereal, Munk also asserts that wine and spirits are of special use in the treatment of the dying. Alcohol passes readily into the blood, stimulating the heart and lungs, and promoting the circulation. It increases gastric secretion, stimulates peristalsis, and aids digestion. Ideally, alcohol and food should be given together, as they mutually influence one another. Champagne is the best choice, but it needs to be given more frequently than other wines or spirits. In all cases, the wishes of the patient are the most reliable guide to what should be given. Munk's approach to the use of opium is discussed in the next section of this chapter, entitled 'The question of pain relief'.

Munk's book closes with prescriptions for the regulation of the dying chamber, specific recommendations for managing death from disease associated with the heart, lungs, and brain, and symptomatic management of hiccup, restlessness, respiratory struggle, and various other phenomena. The final paragraph describes death from old age, which Munk claims is 'so gentle . . . that nature herself provides a perfect euthanasia'.

The majority of physicians in England and the United States in the 1870s and 1880s were opposed to the deliberate killing of a dying patient, which they saw as morally wrong, dangerous to individuals, and to society.[31] Munk, for his part, gives no indication that he is aware of any wider debate on the matter and does not engage with arguments for, or against this practice. His insistence on using the traditional and literal meaning of the word *euthanasia*, at a time when other meanings were beginning to be attached to it, may have been intended as a quiet, but forceful, statement of his position. As Nick Kemp suggests, perhaps overstating the case, 'one of the principal reasons why nineteenth-century physicians were not engaged in discussion about the physician-assisted suicide variety of 'euthanasia' was because they were directing their attention to issues of palliative care which would secure 'euthanasia' in the classical sense'.[32] (See the final section of this chapter, 'End of the century', for a discussion on the tendency of both practitioners and historians to make use of twentieth-century concepts—in particular the concept of palliative care—when seeking to explain nineteenth-century practices.)

In 1888, the year after its publication, *The Lancet* printed a glowing review of *Euthanasia,* calling it a 'treatise by a thoughtful and experienced physician' and supporting fully both Munk's aim in bringing the subject to the notice of the medical profession and his execution of important instruction in the medical management of the dying. 'We have not a fault to find with this treatise', the review concludes. 'It fulfils its purpose and we commend it to our readers'.[33] According to Jalland, *Euthanasia* 'remained the authoritative text on medical care of the dying for the next thirty years'.[6] Munk's work certainly influenced the writer of an article that appeared in an American journal three years later, entitled 'Some notes on how to nurse the dying'. It borrowed heavily from Munk and sought only to praise his contribution.

> When I first took charge of wards there was nothing I so much dreaded as attending death-beds and nursing the dying . . . I in vain enquired for any book to help me and, with the exception of a few sentences in various medical works, found nothing; until a short time ago I read a most interesting and suggestive book called 'Euthanasia' by Dr. Munk . . . and I thought that perhaps a few hints and some account of this book might be interesting to some of my fellow nurses . . . Where all is so excellent it is most difficult to make selections. I can only recommend the perusal of Dr Munk's book to those nurses who find the efficient nursing of the dying one of their most anxious and difficult duties . . .[34]

An earlier transatlantic review had appeared in 1888 by the celebrated Canadian physician William Osler. He is more muted in his praise for the book, simply approving its 'general and scientific interest' along with its 'many valuable suggestions to practitioners and sound advice as to the medical management of the dying'.[35] Osler's main purpose in writing seems to be to show how Munk's opinions accord with his own, particularly on the subject of death not being the torment it is commonly supposed to be.

Munk's text was authoritative, according to Jalland, because it drew widely on the practice and teaching of the previous generation of doctors and showed an essential continuity with their experience.[6] Yet, if *Euthanasia* was influential within a narrow circle of reviewers and practitioners, its influence did not last significantly beyond Munk's own generation. In 1914 a medical correspondent to *The Times* cites, on the subject of 'the pains of death', earlier works by Savory and Brodie in support of his arguments, rather than Munk.[36] By 1926, the American physician Arthur Macdonald was still calling for a scientific study of death that would enhance the sum of knowledge and enable 'a general picture of the dying time, based upon a sufficient number of observations and with instruments of precision where possible' so that fear of death would be diminished and pain eliminated.[37] Moreover, as late as 1935, the American physician Alfred Worcester[38] argued that the previous half-century had seen a deterioration in medical practice, rather than progress, in the art of caring for the dying, with no mention of Munk.

Munk brought together the best elements of past medical practice and summarized them for his contemporaries and immediate successors. At the same time, he focused on the most modern technologies and the best of caring practices that could be used to relieve suffering. Yet Munk's influence seems to have been narrowly circumscribed and later generations of doctors had to discover for themselves how best to care for the dying effectively, and with humanity. The early twentieth-century search for 'root cause and ultimate cure', in Patrick Wall's words, inhibited a therapeutic approach to the symptoms of dying. This was until the mid-century palliative care pioneers in the emerging hospice movement began to draw attention again to the need to give comfort in the absence of cure, recognizing that 'the immediate origins of misery and suffering need immediate attention while the search for long-term cure proceeds'.[39]

If Munk was the first to attempt a *comprehensive* documentation and codification of the issues in the medical care of the dying, Sir William Osler reported the first clinical study of the manner in which patients die in his 1906 lecture *Science and Immortality*—'Observations of 500 dying patients'.[40] Following postgraduate training in Europe, Osler returned to McGill University's faculty as a professor in 1874. He was appointed chair of clinical medicine at the University of Pennsylvania in Philadelphia in

1884. When he left Philadelphia in 1889, it was to take up the position as first physician-in-chief of the new Johns Hopkins Hospital in Baltimore, Maryland. Shortly afterwards, in 1893, Osler was instrumental in the creation of the Johns Hopkins University School of Medicine, and he became one of the school's first professors in medicine. In 1905, he was appointed to the Regius Chair of Medicine at Oxford, a position he held until his death in 1919. He pioneered the practice of bedside teaching, making rounds with a handful of students, demonstrating what one student referred to as his method of the incomparably thorough physical examination. Osler fundamentally changed medical teaching in North America, and his influence spread to medical schools across the globe.[41]

Shigeaki Hinohara[42] has explained in some detail Osler's concern for the dying and the bereaved, and how Osler displayed a level of personal interest and concern for his dying patients and their family members from his earliest years in the profession. In general, Osler considered death from disease as unnatural and likely to be accompanied by pain and suffering, but he regarded death from old age as almost always the easiest of deaths, accompanied as much by pleasure as pain. Across a lifetime of writing and lecturing, Osler declaimed often on issues of dying and death. In a piece delivered in 1897, he condemned nurses for intruding at the bedside of the dying, offending the wishes of patients who may desire to be alone and usurping the role of family members.[43] More controversially, in his valedictory address at Johns Hopkins Hospital, he endorsed Anthony Trollope's account in the novel *The Fixed Period* whereby men at the age of 60, after a year of contemplation, are dispatched peacefully with a dose of chloroform.[44] In general, Osler is known for his view that death is less discomforting and painful than generally assumed, and he demonstrated this in his analysis of the deaths of 486 patients at Johns Hopkins Hospital during the period of 1900–1904. A nurse interviewed the patient in his or her last moments of life and items were recorded by a chief nurse on a questionnaire, which was then countersigned by the patient's doctor. Osler reported the following:

> I have careful records of about five hundred death-beds, studied particularly with reference to the modes of death and the sensations of dying. The latter alone concerns us here. Ninety suffered bodily pain or distress of one form or another, eleven showed mental apprehension, two positive terror, one expressed spiritual exaltation, one bitter remorse. The majority gave no sign one way or the other; like their birth, was a sleep and a forgetting.[45]

Osler was also greatly interested in his own mortality and when his health deteriorated significantly in 1919, exacerbated by the losses of his two sons, the second in Flanders, he engaged actively with his own process of dying. He spent his last days in active goodbyes, in visits from loved ones, and maintained his intellectual endeavours to the last.[46]

Essentially, Osler took the view that the dying patient's comfort was paramount and that aggressive and useless medical interventions should not be allowed to interfere in the last days of life, when a sense of closure was essential. Yet, he could not fully endorse Munk's view that the deliberate ending of life, even in the interests of relieving suffering, should always be avoided. As we shall see in the conclusion to this chapter, he straddled a period and a debate that was critical in redefining the meaning of euthanasia.

The question of pain relief

Rosaleyne Rey, in her comprehensive history of pain, sets out an expansive view of the achievements of the nineteenth century in both the understanding of pain and in its management and relief.[47]

> In the 19th century, there were an increased number of break-throughs in the understanding of pain mechanism as well as a flowering of clinical disciplines and therapeutic innovations. These were such that the century was truly one of great discoveries in which the terrae incognitae were revealed in a decisive way allowing men to better understand and sometimes better relieve pain.

It was, of course, across these decades that the so-called 'death of pain' began to be envisaged. The successful public demonstration of surgical anaesthesia with ether in 1846 in Massachusetts General Hospital in Boston led to a revolution in how pain could be both treated and conceptualized. It also brought a growing sense of hubris about what scientific medicine could achieve. It now became accepted as morally valid to obliterate pain in surgery, and then in childbirth, and so pain came to be seen more as a disease in itself—a phenomenon with little redemptive value. Yet, as Martha Stoddard Holmes[48] suggests in her essay on Victorian doctors and pain relief, the triumph over one kind of pain may have created for doctors a sense of conflict, or even shame in relation to pain that could not be relieved, so much so that:

> ... after 1846, the landscape in which doctors imagined and treated pain was a terrain where the pain of the dying was increasingly out of place, at odds with medicine imagined as a field of technological cures and miracles ... Unlike a discrete surgical event, moreover, the pain of chronic or terminal illness had to be addressed over and over again.

Campbell takes the view that, beginning in the mid-nineteenth century, medicine was establishing how to integrate the use of the new pain-relieving drugs into the repertoire of practice, but was at the same time seeking to uphold notions of the 'good death'. This was a particular challenge in a context where there was religious and theological opposition to the use of these drugs, which were seen as unnatural and un-godly. However, as the century advanced and these methods became more widespread and visible to families and the public, they set in motion calls for the further extension of their use. This was not only to relieve suffering in the context of a 'natural death', but also to deliberately end a life so that suffering might be overcome, however 'unnatural' the death that resulted.[14] This transition involved considerable theological upheaval. As Lucy Bending has described, in the 1840s, debates about the understanding of pain were closely linked to beliefs about eternal damnation, but by the 1860s, the principle point of distinction was between those who found theological meaning and divine purpose in suffering, and those who did not.[49]

During the nineteenth century in Britain and North America, opium and opiates were freely and legally available across society for enjoyment or for domestic use in treating minor ailments.[50] Barbara Hodgson[51] presents a fascinating illustrated history of the use of morphine and laudanum in daily life, showing how they were present in mixtures sold to the public for coughs, colds, diarrhoea, infant teething, and a multitude of other problems. Medical practitioners could also be liberal in their use of such formulations in pursuit of euthanasia, understood in that classical sense of a calm and easy death. However, a science of pain relief was also emerging. As Rey explains, this was the period in which 'chemistry applied to medicine' was taking off. [47]

After the initial work of the French chemist Charles Louis Desrosne, Friedrich Sertürner, a native of Hanover, achieved the isolation of the soporific principle in opium in 1806 in Paderborn, Germany. He originally named the substance 'morphium', after the Greek god of dreams Morpheus and for its tendency to cause sleep. The drug was first marketed to the general public by Sertürner and Company in 1817 as an analgesic, and also as a treatment for opium and alcohol addiction. Commercial production began in Darmstadt, Germany, in 1827 by the pharmacy that became the pharmaceutical company Merck, with morphine sales being a large part of its early growth. After the invention of the hypodermic needle in 1857 by the English physician Alexander Wood, morphine use became more widespread and this mode of administration was widely believed to be less addictive to the patient.

From the mid-nineteenth century onwards, those of the middle and upper classes dying of cancer and tuberculosis were likely to receive copious quantities of opiates to relieve pain and suffering at the end of life. Others, if they could afford to buy them over the counter, would have had access to laudanum or tinctures of opium. This picture of the fairly abundant medical and public use of morphine began to change as the twentieth century approached. Moral concerns about such drugs and their various mixtures began to surface, and greater regulation of the use of opiates followed (such the 1914 Harrison

Narcotic Act in the United States).[52] A long-running era of drug restriction was ushered in, during which a lack of access to opiates and pain relief became a problem for medicine and healthcare. At the same time, medical attention to those dying of cancer was diluted by a shift in emphasis to the emergent possibilities of curing and containing the disease, offered by new developments in surgery, immunology, and endocrinology.[53] Therefore, the relief of pain at the end of life was intermittent and erratic in its progression across the decades of the nineteenth and early twentieth centuries, making a simple narrative of 'improvement' both inaccurate and over-optimistic. As Campbell also points out, it is important not to overstate the wider progress in pain relief that came about in the nineteenth century: 'It would be an over-simplification to read this period as a heroic moment in history, in which the adoption of certain types of techniques was related solely to a triumph over pain.'[14]

As scholarly research advances, more evidence is generated concerning nineteenth-century doctors who were inspired by the importance of pain relief at the end of life. These accounts ranged from eminent physicians and surgeons with royal patronage and senior hospital doctors not afraid to express their views in strong terms, to country practitioners, and even those still undergoing medical education. A hidden treasure of these writings has been analysed by Campbell, who devotes an extended discussion to the thesis of the Edinburgh medical student Hugh Noble, a work submitted for the degree of MD in 1854, before the author apparently slipped into medical obscurity. Its title was simply *Euthanasia*.[54] With the refreshing openness of youth, and unintimidated by the status of earlier medical authorities on care of the dying such as Sir Henry Halford[55] and Christoph Wilhelm Hufeland,[56], [57] Noble not only provides a wide commentary on the medical care of the dying patient, but addresses himself to the specific issue of pain relief at the end of life. Like Munk, Noble uses the term *euthanasia* to denote a peaceful and idealized death. But as Campbell shows, he also nudges his thinking towards a consideration of what the new approaches to pain relief might mean for medicine, if challenged to use them for the purpose of bringing about deliberate and *final* relief of suffering. Noble considers the question of when to treat the dying patient, how much to take his or her wishes into consideration, and how much information to proffer or withhold. Halfway through the thesis, he raises this fundamental question:

> In regard to the active measures which may be adopted with the incurable or moribund, it may be asked how far the practitioner may be justified in interfering with the purposes of modifying or changing the mode of death.[14]

His response was that the sanctity of life placed such an action beyond the limits of medical practice and therefore rendered it something that must be condemned. He went on to observe that when the hope of recovery had passed, the physician often turned away from the patient, forgetting that 'more may be done—that the time has come for restudying the case from a different point with a new object in view'.[14] If the physician was forbidden from actively ending the life of a patient, this did not mean that he must aggressively seek to prolong it.

Stoddard Holmes, also considering this new objective, quotes the English surgeon and physician William Dale, writing in *The Lancet* in 1871, who emphasizes the twin principles of telling the patient of his or her fate, and then using active means to relieve their pain.

> Opium is . . . our chief medicine for relieving pain and procuring sleep—our right hand in practice . . . suffering humanity owes much to its virtues, and the physician could ill spare it in his battle with disease and pain . . . On the near approach of death, where much pain is endured, after having, as in duty bound, made the patient sensible of his condition, I see no reason why he may not be kept constantly under the influence of opium . . .[58]

Writing in 1874, John Kent Spender, a surgeon and physician based in Bath and also described by Holmes, saw pain relief by the doctor as 'the grandest badge of his art'. He writes that one of the 'chief blessings of Opium is to help us in granting the boon of a comparatively painless death . . . we may, without extinguishing consciousness, take away the sharp edge of suffering, and make the departure from this world less full of terror'.[59]

William Munk had been clear to state that an important aspect of managing the process of dying is the correct use of opium for the relief of physical pain and for the 'feeling of exhaustion and sinking, the indescribable distress and anxiety' that can accompany dying. Although placed second in importance to the administration of stimulants, Munk gives even more space to precise and detailed recommendations about how to use opium to best effect. Opium in this context, writes Munk,[22] is 'worth all the *materia medica*', but 'its object and action must be clearly understood'. It is given both to relieve pain and to 'allay that sinking and anguish about the stomach and heart, which is so frequent in the dying, and is often worse to bear than pain, however severe'. It should be given freely and judiciously, not timidly and inadequately, or it will not achieve its purpose.

A similarly bold approach was taken by Herbert Snow, who worked at the London Cancer Hospital (later the Royal Marsden) as a surgeon from 1877 to his retirement in 1906. Like a handful of his contemporaries, Snow was interested in the administration of strong opiates for the relief of pain and 'exhaustion' in advanced cancer. An advocate of early surgical intervention for malignant disease, he also believed that cancer, in many instances, had a neurotic origin and he sought to treat it by inducing an 'opium habit' in his patients. By the 1890s, he was arguing that the conjunction of both mor-phine *and* cocaine could not only relieve the symptoms of advanced cancer, but could indeed slow the progression of the underlying disease. His 1896 paper, published in the *British Medical Journal* and entitled 'Opium and co-caine in the treatment of cancerous disease' argued that the two drugs had the power of 'inhibiting tissue metabolism' as well as 'sustaining the bodily powers under excessive and protracted strain'.[60] He presented a number of case histories in support of his argument, stating that morphine was effective in relieving pain, while cocaine had value in 'sustaining vitality'. Less than a year later, however, in a letter to the same journal, Snow complained that 'for reasons of hospital finance I have been reluctantly compelled to abandon this costly medicine [cocaine] for the majority of my hospital patients'.[61]

Snow may have been confused about some of the effects of his prescribing methods, but his importance from a modern perspective was in highlight-ing the role of opiates for symptom management in advanced cancer. It ap-pears that his ideas about combining morphine and cocaine crossed the road (Cale Street) from the Cancer Hospital to the Brompton Hospital. There, the therapeutic goal of his successors was significantly different. For Snow, the chief virtue of the combination was its apparent effect on the progression of cancerous disease, and he seems to have reserved the use of the opium pipe as the chief method for 'palliation' and symptom relief in advanced cancer. When the combination was first reported at the Brompton in the early twen-tieth century, its use was recommended for the relief of physical suffering and pain associated with tuberculosis. As we shall see in later chapters, the *Brompton Cocktail*, as it came to be known, had a special place in the history of twentieth-century hospice and palliative care. Its origins go back to Snow, and he in turn was part of a wider community of nineteenth-century doctors who were eager to capitalize on the pain-relieving properties of the opiates, especially to relieve pain in those imminently dying. As we are starting to see, the purposes of such drugs were beginning to vary in the minds of physicians. And so it was that debates about access to pain relief and the principles of its administration would echo long through the decades as new possibilities emerged and, in time, a wider philosophy of modern hospice and palliative care took hold.

End of the century

In August 1899, only a few months away from the end of the nineteenth cen-tury, an article appeared in the *Fortnightly Review* by Joseph Jacobs,[62] an

Australian living in Britain at that time and well known for his extensive work in the field of folklore.[63] He set out a provocative account of the nature of death in contemporary society, arguing that it had lost its terror, that the church had become more oriented to the present life rather than the life to come, and that the fear of death was being replaced by the joy of existence. He attributed this to public health improvements, increasing longevity, and to the fact that when death comes with more warnings, 'We are more willing to go, less eager to stay'.[63] This tendency, he argued, could be exacerbated by medical science, which protracts life at the cost of extra suffering, making death not only a relief to the sufferer, but also to those who remain. Jacobs asserted that 'on all sides death is losing its terrors. We are dying more frequently when our life's work is done, and it seems more natural to die'.

Such a position runs into problems at the level of medical practice. A starting point for the present work will be the contention that since the late nineteenth century there has been a diminishing importance given to the matter of life or existence *after* death. Instead, the focus for professional and social interest has become the process of dying itself. *How we die* now matters more than *the consequences of our dying*. It was this notion that the nineteenth-century doctors recognized. Those among them who showed an interest in the care of the dying set out to create an approach that could be taught to others and which might merit the interest of fellow professionals through lectures, journal articles, and medical textbooks. Even so, the goals of medicine at the end of life were often problematic to lay observers and commentators. In 1911, the year in which he won the Nobel Prize for literature, Maurice Maeterlinck, the Belgian playwright and essayist, also writing in the *Fortnightly Review,* claimed that 'all doctors consider it their first duty to protract as long as possible even the most excruciating convulsions of the most hopeless agony'.[64] This he attributed to medicine's compulsion to prolong life at all costs. Yet, he also conceded, 'they are slowly consenting, when there is no hope left, if not to deaden, at least to lull the last agonies', although he continued to criticize those who 'like misers, measure out drop by drop the clemency and peace which they grudge and which they ought to lavish'. Maeterlinck's ideas on the subject were further elaborated in a short book published the same year, simply entitled *Death*.[65] We know that William Osler took a close interest in these writings, as he had with the work of Munk. In a letter to the *Spectator* in 1911, Osler objected to Maeterlinck's hysterical scaremongering about the pains of death and the prolonged suffering associated with the deathbed. He reiterated the findings of his empirical study of the dying, while rejecting Maeterlinck's call for doctors to intervene to end life when suffering is intractable, and death is imminent.[35]

Stoddard Holmes and Helm both question the Foucauldian[66] notion that in the period described here the patient's narrative of suffering disappeared from medical discourse, in favour of the cataloguing and inscribing of signs and symptoms. Each sees plenty of evidence that nineteenth-century doctors sought ways to find meaning in pain, along with their patients and families, and they also strived to relieve suffering, even when death became inevitable. A similar view is found implicitly in the work of Jalland. What emerges from a review of the historiography and of some of the medical writings is that whether provincially based in family practice or working in the metropolitan hospital, there were nineteenth-century physicians and surgeons who gave their extended time and attention to the needs of dying patients and their families. These practitioners grappled with important questions: whether patients should know of their imminent demise; how to accompany them on the journey to death; how to relieve pain and suffering; and ways to give comfort to distressed and grieving relatives. The developing interest in these areas, however, seems to have found only a limited audience; pockets of enthusiasm here and there among like-minded practitioners, but not a critical mass capable of fostering transformational change. Instead, the gaze of medicine looked away—to the benefits that science and new knowledge might make in the control of disease, to the potential for new specialisms, and to the growing influence of the medical schools.

Also important, as notions of the evangelical 'good death' waned and there was increased attention given to dying in the absence of pain and suffering, was the emergence of the first publications to use *euthanasia* in a new sense—as medicalized killing or physician-assisted death. Kemp traces the origins of the modern euthanasia debate to the early 1870s and sees it essentially as a philosophical discussion, in which the profession of medicine played no part. It was sparked by the publication of a paper given to the Birmingham Philosophical Society by a schoolteacher named Samuel Williams that gave strong support to the idea of voluntary euthanasia.[67] It appears that despite the appearance of numerous articles and editorials in the medical press after 1873, medical practitioners did not take a prominent part in these discussions. Kemp argues that while such discussions did take place in the United States[68] from a fairly early stage, in Britain 'the concept of mercy-killing failed, quite manifestly, to make any impact with the medical profession until shortly before the turn of the twentieth century'.[32]

A common theme among writers on the care of the dying and the use of pain relief in the nineteenth century is how the rich discourse of care and practice developing at that time became forgotten by the early twentieth-century medical professionals. It was not until the groundbreaking work of later pioneers of hospice and palliative care got underway in the mid-twentieth century that these antecedents were recovered. There may well be some truth in this. Certainly, it is a view held among professionals in the field as well as historians. It is a position taken by the pain specialist Patrick Wall[69] in an editorial in 1986 and echoed by Cicely Saunders in her foreword to the first edition of the *Oxford Textbook of Palliative Medicine*, which appeared in 1993.[70] Perhaps this is an understandable viewpoint among clinicians eager to uncover a deeper heritage to their current goals and ambitions. It is a more surprising tendency among historians, such as Jalland and Strange, who appear keen to interpret nineteenth-century cultures and patterns of dying and care through a late-twentieth-century 'palliative care' lens. Strange, for example, speaks of 'models of palliative care in the late Victorian and Edwardian period'[5] while, disarmingly, Jalland states that 'the nineteenth century medical authorities were remarkably close to modern experts in their view on the use of opiates for the dying', a very curious remark, given it was not until the 1950s that clinicians began to understand that morphine could work orally.[6] There were undoubtedly attentive doctors and nurses in the nineteenth century who were solicitous about the needs of dying patients and their families. This is not in dispute. But to describe their practice as *palliative care* is misleading for, as we shall see, this was essentially a concept of the later twentieth century, when the term became widely adopted and came to take on specific meanings and definitions. That said, some of the phrases of Marx, Noble, and Munk would not look out of place in the early writings of Cicely Saunders, though we have no evidence that she read any of them.

Campbell makes it clear that the questions the Edinburgh medical student Hugh Noble raised in his MD thesis in 1854 remained key to the practice of medicine for the terminally ill for more than a century afterwards. If his work appears groundbreaking in some respects, its influence was negligible. It was not published for a wider readership and Noble himself was not heard of again. Stoddard Holmes takes the view that the other Victorian doctors writing about pain were also rather peripheral to mainstream medicine, even suggesting that their ideas and influence diminished as time went on.[48] It is tempting, therefore, to view William Munk, whose work of 1887 was so widely and positively received, as the *grandfather* of modern palliative medicine. Exactly 100 years after the publication of his classic work on care of the dying, the specialty of palliative medicine was recognized in the United Kingdom. Munk was surely among the first of his profession to lay out so extensively the art and science of end-of-life care—in a form and manner that would influence others, and which was extensively praised at the time.

As David Cannadine notes, the 'denial of death', so often attributed to the period after 1945, was probably underway even before 1914. In addition to citing Jacobs's 1899 article,[63] he points out that the English of this period were less acquainted with death than any generation since the Industrial Revolution, that the death rate had fallen markedly, that ostentatious mourning had been in decline for 30 years, and that dying was increasingly associated with old age. In the same period, death on the battlefield—at the time thought unlikely—was seen as glorious, noble, and romantic.[71] The Great War would change everything. Death and destruction on an industrial scale eclipsed the suffering of the domestic and hospital deathbed. However, it also promoted a cult of the dead that prevailed in the interwar years when Britain and other European countries went into a prolonged phase of public mourning and bereavement. The societal focus at this time was on collective loss and establishing memorials. This may well have served to sequestrate dying itself, which did indeed become a societal taboo and a matter about which it was difficult to speak. The interpretation goes a long way in explaining medicine's loss of traction in the same interwar period with regard to improvements in care for the dying. But as we shall see in Chapter 2, there were a few small institutions, founded in the late nineteenth century and focused explicitly on the care of the terminally ill, which continued into the next millennium, and in so doing kept alight a flame of interest in medical care when death was imminent. It is to these homes and hospices that we will now turn our attention.

Notes

1. **Holubetz M** (1986). Death-bed scenes in Victorian fiction. *English Studies,* 67(1):14–34.
2. **Ariès P** (1976). *Western Attitudes Towards Death: From the Middle Ages to the Present.* Baltimore and London: Johns Hopkins University Press.
3. **Ariès P** (1981). *The Hour of Our Death.* London, UK: Allen Lane.
4. **Walter T** (1993). Sociologists never die: British sociology and death. In: Clark D (ed.). *The Sociology of Death,* p. 286. Oxford, UK: Blackwell.
5. **Strange J-M** (2005). *Death, Grief, and Poverty in Britain, 1870–1914,* p. 20. Cambridge, UK: Cambridge University Press.
6. **Jalland P** (1996). *Death in the Victorian Family.* Oxford, UK: Oxford University Press.
7. **Strange J-M** (2000). Death and dying: Old themes and new directions. *Journal of Contemporary History,* 35(3):496.
8. **Strange J-M** (2002). 'She cried a very little': Death, grief, and mourning in working class culture. *Social History,* 27(2):143–61. See also note 5.
9. **Bell F** (1985 [1907]). *At the Works: A Study of a Manufacturing Town.* London, UK: Virago, as quoted in note 5.
10. **Helm DP** (2012). A sense of mercies: End of life care in the Victorian home. Unpublished master's thesis, Philosophy. University of Worcester, UK.

11. **Nolte K** (2009). Dying at home: Nursing of the critically and terminally ill in private care in Germany around 1900. *Nursing Inquiry*, 16(2):144–54.

12. **Abel EK** (2013). *The Inevitable Hour: A History of Caring for Patients in America.* Baltimore, MD: The Johns Hopkins University Press.

13. **Rugg J** (1999). From reason to regulation: 1760–1850. In: Jupp PC, Gittings C (eds.). *Death in England: An Illustrated History*, p. 203. Manchester, UK: Manchester University Press.

14. **Campbell LJ** (2003). Principle and practice: An analysis of nineteenth and twentieth century euthanasia debates (1854–1969). Unpublished PhD thesis. University of Edinburgh, UK.

15. **Porter R** (1989). Death and the doctors in Georgian England. In: Houlbrooke R (ed). *Death, Ritual, and Bereavement*, p. 91. New York, NY: Routledge, in association with the Social History Society of the United Kingdom.

16. **Reece R** (1802). *The Medical Guide, for the Use of Clergy, Heads of Families, and Seminaries and Junior Practitioners in Medicine; Comprising a Complete Dispensatory, and a Practical Treatise on the Distinguishing Symptoms, Causes, Prevention, Cure, and Palliation.* London, UK: Longman.

17. **Browne O** (1894). *On The Care of the Dying.* London, UK: George Allen.

18. **Nightingale F** (1859). *Notes on Nursing: What Is It, and What It Is Not.* London, UK: Harrison.

19. **Marx CFH** (1826). *De Euthanasia Medica.* Dietrich, Germany: Goettingen.

20. **Cane W** (1952). Medical euthanasia. A paper published in Latin in 1826, translated, and then reintroduced to the medical profession. *Journal of the History of Medicine and Allied Sciences*, 7(4):401–16.

21. **Taubert M, Fielding H, Mathews E, Frazer R** (2013). An exploration of the word 'palliative' in the 19th century: Searching the BMJ archives for clues. *BMJ Supportive and Palliative Care*, 3:26–30.

22. **Munk W** (1887). *Euthanasia: Or, Medical Treatment in Aid of an Easy Death.* London, UK: Longmans, Green and Co.

23. **Hughes N, Clark D** (2004). 'A thoughtful and experienced physician': William Munk and the care of the dying in late Victorian England. *Journal of Palliative Medicine*, 7(5):703–10.

24. **Davenport G, McDonald I, Moss-Gibbons C** (2001). *The Royal College of Physicians and Its Collections: An Illustrated History.* London: Royal College of Physicians.

25. **Munk W** (1861). *The Roll of the Royal College of Physicians of London 1518–1700.* London, UK: Royal College of Physicians.

26. **Munk W** (1895). *The Life of Sir Henry Halford.* London, UK: Royal College of Physicians.

27. **Humphreys C** (2001). 'Waiting for the last summons': The establishment of the first hospices in England 1878–1914. *Mortality*, 6(2):146–66.

28. **Saundby R** (1902). *Medical Ethics: A Guide to Professional Conduct*, p. 12. Bristol, UK: John Wright and Co.

29. **Watson T** (1855). *Lectures on the Principles and Practice of Physic.* Delivered at King's College, London. Philadelphia, PA: Blanchard and Lea.

30. Royal College of Physicians. Lives of the Fellows: Sir Thomas Watson. Available at http://munksroll.rcplondon.ac.uk/Biography/Details/4657, accessed 5 November 2013.

31. **Emanuel EJ** (1994). The history of euthanasia debates in the United States and Britain. *Annals of Internal Medicine*, 121(10):793–802.
32. **Kemp NDA** (2002). *Merciful Release: The History of the British Euthanasia Movement*. Manchester, UK: Manchester University Press.
33. Reviews and notices of books (1888). *Lancet*, 131, no. 3358 (7 January):21–2.
34. **Sumner A** (1890). Some notes on how to nurse the dying. *The Trained Nurse*, IV–V:17–21.
35. **Cushing H** (1940). *The Life of Sir William Osler*. Oxford, UK: Oxford University Press.
36. *The Times* (25 February 1914):10.
37. **Macdonald A** (1926). The study of death in man. Letter. *Lancet* (18 September):624.
38. **Worcester A** (1935). *The Care of the Aged, the Dying, and the Dead*. Springfield, IL: Charles C. Thomas.
39. **Wall P** (1986). Editorial. *Pain*, 25(5):1–4.
40. **Osler W** (1906). *Science and Immortality*. London, UK: Constable.
41. This paragraph draws heavily on The Osler Symposia. Available at http://www.osler-symposia.org/about-Sir-William-Osler.html, accessed 22 July 2015.
42. **Hinohara S** (1993). Sir William Osler's philosophy on death. *Annals of Internal Medicine*, 118(8):638–42.
43. **Osler W** (1905). Nurse and patient. In: *Aequanimitas with Other Addresses to Medical Students, Nurses, and Practitioners of Medicine*, 3rd ed., pp. 147–60. Philadelphia, PA: Blakiston.
44. **Osler W** (1905). Valedictory address at Johns Hopkins University. *Journal of the American Medical Association*, 44:706.
45. **Osler W** (1904). *Science and Immortality*, p. 18. New York, NY: Ravenside Press.
46. **Jones S** (1994). Sir William Osler's views on euthanasia. *Osler Library Newsletter*, 77:1–3.
47. **Rey R** (1995). *The History of Pain*. Cambridge, MA: Harvard University Press.
48. **Stoddard Holmes M** (2003). The grandest badge of his art: Three Victorian doctors, pain relief, and the art of medicine. In: Meldrum ML (ed.). *Opioids and Pain Relief: A Historical Perspective. Progress in Pain Research and Management*, vol. 25. Seattle, WA: IASP Press.
49. **Bending L** (2000). *The Representation of Bodily Pain in Late Nineteenth Century English Culture*. Oxford, UK: Oxford University Press.
50. **Seymour J, Clark D** (2005). The modern history of morphine use in cancer pain. *European Journal of Palliative Care*, 12(4):152–5.
51. **Hodgson B** (2001). *In the Arms of Morpheus. The Tragic History of Laudanum, Morphine, and Patent Medicines*. New York, NY: Firefly Books.
52. **Achilladelis B, Antonakis N** (2001). The dynamics of technological innovation: The case of the pharmaceutical industry. *Research Policy*, 30:535–88.
53. **Pinell P** (2002). Cancer. In: Cooter R, Pickstone J (eds.). *Medicine in the 20th Century*. Newark, NJ: Harwood Academic Publishers.
54. **Noble H** (1854). Euthanasia. Unpublished MD thesis. University of Edinburgh, UK.
55. **Halford H** (1842). *Essays and Orations Delivered at the Royal College of Physicians*. London, UK.
56. **Hufeland CW** (1842). *Three Cardinal Means of the Art of Healing*. New York, NY: W Radde.

57. **Hufeland CW** (1846). *On the Relations of the Physician to the Sick.* Oxford, UK: JH Parker.
58. **Dale W** (1871). On pain and some of the remedies for its relief. *Lancet* (13 May): 641–2; (20 May):679–80; (3 June):739–41; (17 June):816–817, quoted in [48].
59. **Spender JK** (1874). *Therapeutic Means for the Relief of Pain.* London, UK: Macmillan, quoted in note 48.
60. **Snow H** (1896). Opium and cocaine in the treatment of cancerous disease. *British Medical Journal* (September):718–19.
61. **Snow HL** (1897). The opium-cocaine treatment of malignant disease. *British Medical Journal* (April):1019.
62. **Jacobs J** (1899). The dying of death. *Fortnightly Review*, 72:264–9.
63. **Fine GA** (1987). Joseph Jacobs: A sociological folklorist. *Folklore*, 98(2):183–93.
64. **Maeterlinck M** (1911). Our idea of death. *Fortnightly Review*, 90:644.
65. **Maeterlinck M** (1911). *Death.* Translated by Alexander Teixeira de Mattos. London, UK: Methuen.
66. **Foucault M** (1973). *The Birth of the Clinic: An Archaeology of Medical Perception.* New York, NY: Vintage.
67. *Essays by Members of the Birmingham Speculative Club* (1870). London, UK: Williams and Norgate.
68. **Dowbiggin I** (2003). *A Merciful End. The Euthanasia Movement in Modern America.* Oxford, UK: Oxford University Press.
69. **Wall P** (1986). Editorial. *Pain*, 25(5):1–4.
70. **Saunders C** (1993). Foreword. In: Doyle D, Hanks GWC, Macdonald N (eds.). *Oxford Textbook of Palliative Medicine.* Oxford, UK: Oxford University Press.
71. **Cannadine D** (1981). War and death, grief and mourning in modern Britain. In: Whaley J (ed.). *Mirrors of Mortality. Studies in the Social History of Death.* London, UK: Europa Publications.

Chapter 2

Homes for the terminally ill: 1885–1948

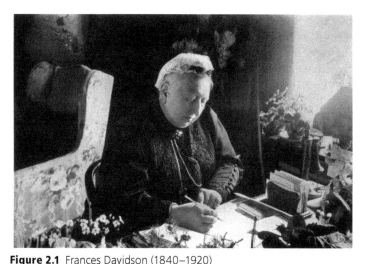

Figure 2.1 Frances Davidson (1840–1920)
Born in Scotland, Davidson established the first home in London to concentrate exclusively on the care of the dying. Known at first as *The Friedenheim*, it opened in 1885 and initially cared for people with tuberculosis, and later those with cancer. Later called St Columba's, it was one of a small wave of homes around the world that drew attention in the late nineteenth and early twentieth centuries to the importance of carefully organized institutional care for the dying. Reproduced by kind permission of David Clark.

Institutions taking precedence

The late nineteenth century saw many Western countries advance their ambitions to promote and secure public health, even in the face of continued epidemics of smallpox, cholera, and tuberculosis. There were innovations in disease prevention and health protection, and confidence was growing in the power of medical science to overcome the health problems that for centuries had seemed intractable. Populations and cities were growing in scale. Wealth was increasing, albeit along with attendant divisions and inequalities between the urban social classes, and these new fissures in society were replicated in the provision of and access to medicine and care. Institutions of one sort or another were widely seen as the overarching solution to the social problems of the day.

Hospitals, medical progress, and implications for the dying

In this context, there was a great upsurge in the building of hospitals, the new citadels of care and the sites of medical professionalization and academic respectability. Hospitals were reorganizing, becoming more specialized, and some were focusing on specific conditions. Many were reaping the benefits of new sources of private philanthropy and patronage. Confident, grand, and invested with the expanding prosperity of the age, the hospitals were edifices to medical progress and the treatment of disease. They were not, however, much concerned with the care of those nearing the end of life. Indeed, they were often actively resistant to dying patients, who were frequently turned away to seek comfort and solace elsewhere—in their own homes if they were fortunate, in the workhouse if they were not.[1] Even the tuberculosis sanatoria and cancer hospitals, purveyors of rehabilitation and cure, tried to exclude patients with little chance of recovery.[2]

Towards the end of the nineteenth century, however, small flickers of interest in the fate of dying patients became visible. As we have seen in Chapter 1, this was refelected in the growing awareness of some doctors and nurses, as well as a measure of public discussion. Despite the reluctance of the acute hospitals to admit dying patients, it was becoming more common for life to end in some form of institution, rather than in the home. In the United States after the Civil War, people increasingly died in hospitals[3] and, by the end of the nineteenth century, moribund patients were systematically transferred to special rooms for their last days and hours.[4] For the first time in history, special institutions were being established, often the work of religious orders or religiously motivated philanthropists, that were *uniquely* concerned with the care of dying people. Initially the influence of these 'hospices' and 'homes for the dying' appears to have been limited. They emerged in several countries throughout the later nineteenth and early twentieth centuries, but apparently made little impact on the wider environment of care for the dying. In the United States and Europe, they overlapped in mission and activity with homes for 'incurables'—those suffering from chronic conditions, for which the emerging science of modern medicine also had, as yet, little to offer.

Regardless of their limitations in scale, these places signified an important transition in which the dying were being repositioned behind the 'opaque veneer' of institutional care.[5] What was later called the *sequestration of the dying* was now getting underway. The needs of the dying were being recognized, but as persons to be hidden away from public space and, in particular, to be excluded from the day-to-day organization of the rapidly expanding public hospitals. Here were the first signs of how a new medical establishment was seeing death as failure. However, as Isobel Broome points out, while the major hospitals' indifference to the dying is well documented, until recently there has been little research into one of its consequences—the creation of a small number of charitable hospitals formed at this time to care for the dying and moribund. These hospitals, in contrast to other institutions, were actively seeking out such patients.[6] Pat Jalland's account of Victorian death and medical practice with the dying has nothing to say of them, despite the fact that she elucidates some key transitions in the orchestration of the good death in the period from 1885 to 1914. Nor did they merit much in the way of contemporary recognition or support: a commentator in the *Contemporary Review* of March 1891 wrote that 'there is not to be found any refuge, home or hospital but the workhouse for the man who is neither curable nor incurable, but actually dying'.[7] Therefore, it is welcome to note that in Britain two doctoral studies, by Clare Humphreys and Isobel Broome, take an in-depth insight into four of the homes for the dying that were established in London between 1885 and 1905. Coupled with the scholarship of Emily Abel in the United States, these are a rich source of detail and insight, not only into the institutional aspects and organization of these establishments, but also into some of the day-to-day clinical issues and experiences of the patients and families for whom they cared. These matters are the focus of this chapter. Table 2.1 is an indicative but not comprehensive list of homes of this type from around the world.

Religious foundations and the new homes for the dying

The role of women

A striking feature of this late nineteenth century 'turn' towards institutional care for the dying is that the various examples across countries and continents were often initiated by women—always religiously and charitably inspired—but

Table 2.1 A selection of nineteenth and early twentieth-century homes for the dying

L'Hospice des Dames du Calvaire:	
Lyons	1843
Paris	1874
St Etienne	1875
Hospice Desbassyns De Richemont, Pondicherry	1876
Our Lady's Hospice for the Dying, Dublin	1879
L'Hospice des Dames du Calvaire, Marseilles	1881
Friedenheim Home of Peace, London	1885
L'Hospice des Dames du Calvaire, Brussels	1886
Sacred Heart Hospice, Sydney	1890
L'Hospice des Dames du Calvaire, Rouen	1891
Hostel of God, London	1891
St Luke's House, London	1893
St Rose's Free Home for Incurable Cancer, New York	1896
The House of Calvary, New York	1899
St Joseph's Hospice, Hackney, London	1905

as far as we can tell, not linked to, or aware of each other's activities. At a time when women were largely excluded from medicine, their actions were rooted in a nineteenth-century religious culture that emphasized service in the world and was organized through nursing within religious orders, diaconal structures, and charitable groups and associations. The focus of such endeavours was often on saving lost souls from sin, caring for the 'deserving poor', and reaching into deprived communities to offer a glimpse of life beyond poverty, drunkenness, gambling, and other conditions inconsistent with a temperate and godly life.

The religious and charitable character of these first hospices and homes for the dying was deeply consequential for many decades afterwards, shaping narratives of care at the end of life and pervading the culture and orientation of professional practice. If the early homes had medical involvement, it was rarely a central or driving force. These were not the places where the leading writers on terminal care (as described in Chapter 1) were practising. Attending physicians offered help and support with the management of distressing symptoms, but the routine duties and daily care were the preoccupation of female nurses, many of whom were in religious orders. Safe passage to eternity was what they sought for their patients. The ideal of the *good death* continued to have strong religious components in this context and medicine was, most of the time, in an ancillary role to spiritual care.

Mary Aikenhead—Irish Sisters of Charity

Mary Aikenhead, born in 1787, in Cork, Ireland, became Sister Mary Augustine at age 25, and was established almost immediately as Superior of a new order, known as the Irish Sisters of Charity, the first of its kind in Ireland to be uncloistered. The order made plans to establish a hospital. Three of the sisters went to Paris to learn the work of the Notre Dame de la Pitié Hospital, and in 1834 in Ireland, they opened St Vincent's Hospital, Dublin. Following many years of chronic illness, Mary Aikenhead died at nearby Harold's Cross in 1858 having fulfilled her lifelong ambition. The convent where Mary Aikenhead spent her final years became Our Lady's Hospice for the Dying in 1879. This, and other services provided by the order, ministered to the needs of a highly impoverished population within Dublin, where mortality was high, and access to care and support extremely limited. As T. M. Healy writes: 'The cramped and often squalid conditions where birth, life and death all mingled, were a major reason for starting Our Lady's Hospice.'[8]

Its doors first opened with 27 beds under the guidance of Anna Gaynor, known as Mother Mary John, who quickly had to steer the establishment through a vile winter in which the sewers blocked up and an outbreak of smallpox struck the hospice itself. Over time the facilities were extended, more beds were added, and the hospice continued to consolidate its activities in the period up to 1914. The Sisters of Charity also developed other facilities to care for the dying as far away as Australia (1890), as well as in England (1905) and Scotland (1948). One of these, St Joseph's Hospice, Hackney, established at the beginning of the twentieth century in the impoverished East End of London, went on to have a particularly important place in the narrative of modern palliative care history, as we shall see later.

Jeanne Garnier—Les Dames du Calvaire

A young widow and bereaved mother, Jeanne Garnier, together with other women in similar circumstances, formed *L'Association des Dames du Calvaire* in Lyon, France, in 1842. The association opened a home for the dying the following year, which was characterized by 'a respectful familiarity, an attitude of prayer and calm in the face of death'.[9] Garnier died in 1853, but her influence led to the foundation of several other establishments for the care of the dying: in Paris and St Etienne (1874); Marseille (1881 and 1894); Brussels (1886); Rouen (1891); Bordeaux (1909)—La Maison Medicale, Notre Dame du Lac; as well as in Rueil Malmaison (1939); and Maison Jean XXIII at Freilingen (1966).[10] Reflecting a sense of religious calling to her endeavours,

Garnier remarked in a memoir towards the end of her life, 'J'ai fondée mon refuge avec cinquante francs; la providence a faire la reste'—I founded my refuge with 50 francs; providence did the rest.[11] Her name continued to be associated with palliative care services in France into the twenty-first century.

Frances Davidson—Friedenheim

Frances Davidson (Figure 2.1) founded the first home for the dying in Britain in 1885. Born in 1840 in Aberdeenshire, Scotland, she grew up in a middle-class home in a family of faith with an ethic of service. Little is known about her early adult life, but at some point after 1870 she was spending time in London and engaged in visiting the sick as part of the work of the Mildmay Mission. She is remarkably unacknowledged for her foundational work to secure institutional care for the dying in London.

The Mildmay Mission Hospital had its origins in the work of the Revd William Pennefeather and his team of Christian women, later known as deaconesses, who began visiting the sick of the East End during the cholera outbreak of 1866. The first Medical Mission Hospital opened in 1877 and moved to Hackney Road in 1892. The hospital was recognized for its training of nurses in 1883.[12] It appears that Frances Davidson, building on her association with the Mission and inspired by the needs of those dying of tuberculosis in particular, developed an idea *de novo* to create a 'home of peace' for the dying and, for reasons that remain unclear, she adopted the German name 'Friedenheim' to describe it.[6] Located at 133 Mildmay Road, Islington, near the Mission headquarters in Mildmay Park, she devoted all her energies to its cause, right up until her death in 1920 at the age of 80. Preference was given to those whose circumstances had been reduced by mortal illness and to those for whom the workhouse infirmary was a 'dreaded last resort'.[13] Admission was free, although there were private rooms for those who could afford to pay. The work continued under various names and in varying locations until the later decades of the twentieth century.

Rose Hawthorne—Servants of Relief of Incurable Cancer

In the United States, Rose Hawthorne (born in Lenox, Massachusetts, 1851) the daughter of Nathaniel Hawthorne, had experienced the death of a child and watched her friend, the poet Emma Lazarus, die of cancer. In 1891, both Rose and her husband, George Lathrop, converted to Catholicism. Five years later, they separated, and she devoted the rest of her life to the care of poor people with cancer.[2] After a three-month training course at the New York Cancer Hospital in the summer of 1896, she established premises at Scammel Street in the September of that year on New York's Lower East

Side, where she opened what is said to be the first home in America for the free care of 'incurable and impoverished victims of cancer'.[14] The work met with 'countless hardships and almost universal distrust', but was part of the efforts of an organized group of women known as the Servants of Relief of Incurable Cancer, formed with Alice Huber, the daughter of a Kentucky physician. Hawthorne used her literary connections and abilities to write and publish letters appealing for funds. Support was strong and she was able to move to better premises on Water Street in early 1897. Under the title Mother Alphonsa, she formed an order known as the Dominican Sisters of Hawthorne. Following the establishment of St Rose's Home for Incurables in Lower Manhattan, another home was founded at Rosary Hill, north of New York City, followed by others in Philadelphia, Pennsylvania; Fall River, Massachusetts; Atlanta, Georgia; St Paul, Minnesota; and Cleveland, Ohio. St Rose's Home, established in 1912 at Jackson Street in lower Manhattan, finally closed in 2009, leaving the sisters with four homes: in New York, Philadelphia, Atlanta, and in Kisumu, Kenya.[15]

Although unknown to each other, Mary Aikenhead, Jeanne Garnier, Frances Davidson, and Rose Hawthorne shared a common purpose in their concern for the care of the dying and, in particular, the dying poor. Directly and indirectly, they founded institutions which, in time, led to the development of other homes and hospices elsewhere, some of which still exist today and bear their names. They established base camp for what was to follow, and their achievements created some of the preconditions for modern hospice and palliative care development. The work of these women is a key precursor of hospice developments that took place in the next century and was a source of inspiration to hospice protagonists more than 100 years subsequently.

Terminal care homes in London

Two small institutions in London are known to have taken in dying persons of the 'respectable' poor from the mid-nineteenth century.[16] The Hospital of St John and St Elizabeth opened in 1856 and would accept dying patients, although for many years this was women and children only. It continued to operate as a Catholic hospital in the twenty-first century, with a modern hospice in its grounds in St John's Wood, London. St Peter's Home in Kilburn was founded in 1861 by Anglican sisters of the same order. Although we know little of the workings of these early endeavours, within a subsequent period of 30 years (1885–1905), four homes were founded in London that had the *specific* objective of providing a place of peace and comfort for the dying poor (a fifth contender was the Home of the Compassion of Jesus, established 1903, about which very little is known). As Clare Humphreys puts it, they were 'an institutional response to a domestic problem'[17] and relied heavily in their appeal on an ability to extract the moribund and the dying from the abject conditions in which they found themselves, in a London that was growing rapidly, and where social disadvantage sat cheek by jowl with wealth and privilege.

The Friedenheim

The Friedenheim was started in 1885. In what Broome describes as its 'experimental period', it was located in a small house at Mildmay Road, in Islington, where there were eight beds for patients. Its financing and management were solely the responsibility of Frances Davidson. A neighbouring building was acquired around 1891, but this only provided space for two more beds. When the leases on these accommodation expired the following year, the opportunity arose to move to larger premises. This was very much the work of Alfred T. Schofield, whose March 1891 article in the *Contemporary Review*[7] was in part a promotional device aimed at attracting funds to the Friedenheim. When the move came, it was to a more grand setting in Hampstead. The elegant villa on three floors was in its own grounds and benefitted from good air, in contrast to the smoke of Islington. In time, it would provide accommodation for up to 50 patients. The move also ushered in a new era of greater professionalism and scale, as were required in the running of a small hospital, rather than a modest 'home'. Photographs taken in the first decade of occupancy reveal an environment of comfort and taste. There were large well-appointed rooms with open fires and views to the garden. The furniture was of good quality and there were soft furnishings to bring comfort to patients and families. Over time, steady improvements were made to the available equipment and amenities. However, as World War I gathered momentum, there was unease. The German-sounding name of the hospital was attracting suspicion and criticism. With agreement from its patron, Queen Mary, the name was quickly changed to St Columba's Hospital, reflecting the Scottish origins of its foundress and avoiding the risk of xenophobic sentiment.

The Hampstead property was on a 50-year lease and when, by the late 1930s, efforts to extend, or to purchase met with no success, it was necessary again to find an alternative home for the hospital. The outbreak of World War II produced an extension to the lease, but when peace came, the hospital faced the challenge of the brave new world of the National Health Service (NHS). It was absorbed into the NHS under the auspices of the Paddington Group Management Committee, but it was not until 1957 that it moved to its final location, also in Hampstead, where it remained until closure in 1981.[6] In this later period, St Columba's appears to have been ill-fitted to the times and suffered an extended period of decline and uncertainty before it was eventually closed down. Nevertheless, Cicely Saunders made several visits there before she embarked upon a career in medicine, as she recalls here.

> When I was looking around as a social worker, I went to St Columba's and met Miss Howell, who was the matron. And I visited there two or three times. They had a fire in the wards, an open grate, which was why we built with a fire in our day rooms. Lord Amulree was one of their consultants, the geriatrician who was working at St Pancras and who visited us with his team when I was working at St Joseph's . . . I was really very interested in St Columba's . . . it was a nice place.[18]

Hostel of God

The Hostel of God was founded in Clapham as a result of an appeal in *The Times* on Christmas Day in 1891. It was by Colonel William Hoare, a distinguished local banker, written on behalf of Clara Maria, Mother Superior of the Anglican order St James's Servants of the Poor, then residing in Cornwall. The letter praised Alfred Schofield's *Contemporary Review* article and highlighted the need in London to care for those close to death, at a time when the only other institution of such a kind was the Friedenheim. Hoare donated £1 000, and a further £1 000 was raised by public subscription, enabling the home to open. Named after the Hotel-Dieu in Paris, it had 15 beds, and was run initially by the St James' sisters from 1892 to 1896, when the sisters of St Margaret's of East Grinstead took over. In 1900 new premises were acquired on Clapham Common, with facilities for 36 patients.[17] By 1933, it had 55 beds which, with the addition of St Michael's ward in 1953, brought the total to 75. Along with St Joseph's Hospice, but unlike its other nineteenth-century contemporaries, it made the transition to the modern era of palliative care.

In 1977, its management was transferred from the hands of the nuns to its council, which had been in place since the early 1900s. Henceforth, it operated as a secular independent organization, and in 1980, it adopted the name Trinity Hospice. In the same year, it saw the appointment of its first full-time medical director and the establishment of a homecare team. The hospice underwent significant refurbishment between 1978 and 1985, going on to expand its services in education and, in 1987, it opened a day centre to outpatients. In 2009, and now as the oldest operating hospice institution of its kind in Britain, an entirely new and purpose-built inpatient centre was added, offering patients private, en-suite rooms with balconies overlooking the gardens, family areas, counselling and bereavement rooms, as well as new medical facilities.

St Luke's Home for the Dying Poor

In 1893, St Luke's in Regents Park opened, founded by Dr Howard Barrett, the medical superintendent of the Methodist West London Mission. Although not run by a religious group, close contacts were maintained with the Mission and several of its sisters visited the home on a regular basis. Like the Friedenheim, it could claim comfortable amenities and facilities. With accommodation for 15 to 16 beds in four wards, as well as two isolation rooms, it also had cosy corners, plants, and easy chairs. In 1901, it moved to two converted houses in Hampstead. Despite major works on the site, it was relocated again when problems arose with the lease (which did not allow any other use but that of a domestic residence) and when neighbours complained that the home's presence prevented other properties in the street from being let. Closing in Hampstead in January 1902, it reopened in Pembridge Square before moving to nearby Hereford Road, Bayswater, in 1923. Barrett had retired in 1913, and from 1917 onward, St Luke's became a 'hospital for advanced cases'. The early religious influences began to wane and it became increasingly synonymous with a modern public hospital. With the inauguration of the NHS in 1948, its management was absorbed into St Mary's Teaching Group of Hospitals. Nevertheless, for a while at least it maintained its special character and its careful approach to the regular administration of pain relief. These qualities were what attracted Cicely Saunders to volunteer her services there in the 1950s, while working as a hospital almoner and on the point of embarking upon medical training. In 1974, the building was renovated and the hospital was renamed Hereford Lodge (thus avoiding the depressing connotations of 'advanced cases and dying'). It had 42 beds for pre-convalescence and terminal care. Hereford Lodge eventually closed in 1985, and its functions were reallocated to St Charles Hospital and the Paddington Community Hospital.[19]

St Joseph's Hospice

The Religious Sisters of Charity first came from Ireland to the East End of London in 1900, seeking to deliver their charism of service to the poor and dispossessed. Initially their focus was on the local Irish population, among whom poverty was endemic. They had been invited there by Father Peter Gallwey, an admirer of the work of Our Lady's Hospice in Dublin. Soon the home visits of the newly arrived sisters introduced them to those dying of tuberculosis, and to the need for a place of care modelled on that which had been successfully established at Harold's Cross. In 1904, an anonymous donor gifted them the Cambridge Lodge estate, consisting of a large property and two acres of land at Mare Street, Hackney. It was from there that they were able to establish the work of St Joseph's Hospice, which opened its doors on the night of 14 January 1905 to two patients—one a tram driver dying of consumption who was carried there by friends. By 1907, the hospice was staffed by eight Catholic sisters who worked as nurses, four part-time doctors, and two part-time chaplains, as well as domestic staff and untrained nurses. Now 25 beds were in constant use. A corrugated iron chapel was added in 1911, and this marked the start of a continuous process of building and re-building that continued for a hundred years. In 1922, three new wards with balconies were added; a flat roof allowed tubercular patients access to fresh air without the exertion of going into the garden. Care was free to the poor although contributions were welcome, and supporters could guarantee access to the hospice for themselves or a nominee. From 1923 onwards, the Ministry of Health recognized the hospice as a facility for those no longer eligible for a tuberculosis (TB) sanatorium, and this brought in a new stream of income. Further extensions and central heating facilities soon followed. The comple-ment of beds rose to 75. Adjacent land was bought in 1927 for a nursing home. In 1932, a new chapel joined the convent to the hospice and additional nurs-ing accommodation was included. However, as the economic depression of the period deepened, this was a time of great hardship, with a constant strain to make ends meet.

When World War II came and bombs fell on Hackney, the hospice was evacuated to the city of Bath, returning only when peace was established. There was war damage to make good, with the involved repair costs beyond all previous imaginings. Sister Mary Antonia, who moved to the hospice from Ireland as a young nun in 1947, recalls the careful approach to money that prevailed.

> The Sister in charge when I went there didn't want to be using money. I think she thought that the hospice couldn't afford it. She used to be a bit hesitant about asking the authorities for any increase in money or anything like that. But still we got by all right, because people were very generous with donations, even in those days. And I remember there was just one car outside, and that was the doctor's car, in my early days, when I went in '47.[20]

However, when the new developments were completed, the outcome exceeded all expectations. Our Lady's Wing was opened in the mid-1950s and provided a light, modern, and airy environment for the delivery of terminal care to patients. From its huge windows, the patients could look out onto the bustle of Mare Street. There were six bedded bays with a single room on each floor, as well as two day rooms. The new wing brought the complement of beds to 112. The whole idea had been the vision of Sister Mary Paula Gleeson, Matron and Superior at St Joseph's from 1954 to 1960, and then from 1976 to 1982. It was to this new facility that Cicely Saunders made visits as a medical student, and where she took on a full-time research position after qualifying in 1957.

St Joseph's was a hothouse for Saunders's thinking, as she began to make plans to establish her own hospice while she worked there continuously until 1965. St Joseph's continued to develop and in time to interact with St Christopher's Hospice, which opened in 1967, as well as with Our Lady's in Dublin. New facilities were added in Hackney in 1965. Gradually the original nineteenth-century buildings were all replaced. Homecare services were developed. By 1983, 25 nuns and a large group of lay doctors, nurses, ancillary workers, and volunteers were caring for 120 patients in their own homes and a further 112 in the hospice beds, which accommodated 600–700 admissions per year. Education programmes grew and purpose-built accommodation was provided to deliver them. By the new millennium, Our Lady's Wing came under the demolition hammer and was replaced with the Centenary Wing with twenty-first century facilities for the delivery of care to the terminally ill and dying.[21]

'Proto-hospices'

Grace Goldin termed these homes the 'proto-hospices'.[22] They paved the way for much future thinking and practice. Two out of the four that were founded survived through to the modern age of hospice and palliative care, and even the two that did not endure were both formative influences on the work of Cicely Saunders. Two were run directly by religious orders, while the other two had strong religious affiliations. There was also a marked denominational character to each of the homes (one Catholic, two Anglican, one Methodist), and this had a profound impact on the way in which the deathbed was managed. Above all, the religious, philanthropic, and moral concerns of the homes were inextricably interlinked.[17] Despite their denominational differences, each reflected the concerns of the Victorian church to recapture the hearts and souls of the poor and working classes, who were increasingly considered lost to the ways of Christianity. Such a starting point inevitably pervaded the mode of care delivered, and the ways in which it was described and presented to external audiences.

Religious influences in the homes

In this context, the patients' bodily suffering was regarded as important, but the management of the deathbed was determined primarily by spiritual objectives and the overriding aim was that of saving patients' souls. Most institutions placed a singular emphasis upon the importance of spiritual preparation. As Howard Barrett, the medical officer at St Luke's House, London, commented in one of his detailed annual reports: 'It is much if we can render the last weeks and months less destitute of comfort, less tortured by pain. It is far more if through any instrumentality of ours some become humble followers of Christ.'[17] Accepting that they could not offer any prospect of a bodily cure, the homes held out an alternative hope, what the sisters at St Joseph's Hospice called 'soul-cures', defined by them as the process of 'hardened sinners turning back to their Saviour in their last dying moments'. It was common within the homes for the patient to be perceived as made up of three separate, yet interrelated entities: body, mind, and soul. The soul was ultimately afforded precedence because it alone was immortal. As Barrett noted: 'At the last hour all externals, all mere clothing, fall off—there is nothing but God and the soul.'

Accordingly, attending to patients' bodily and mental concerns was felt to be a prerequisite for addressing the ultimate goal—their spiritual needs. In this, the homes formed part of a broader shift in thinking among late Victorian churches, which increasingly recognized that the ability to carry out spiritual ministration was dependent upon taking care of patients' physical concerns as well.[23] The chaplain at St Luke's described the relationship.

> How hard, how well nigh impossible it is to speak the comfortable words of Christ when the mind of both the sufferer and the minister are taken up with the untended needs of the body . . . Our teaching is maimed and undone unless the authority of the Gospel goes hand in hand with the infinite compassion and helpfulness of the Saviour.[24]

Ultimately pain and suffering were accepted as part of God's will. The Reverend Howard May, one of the visiting ministers to St Luke's, observed the following, rather dramatically:

> We must never look upon the pain and suffering in St Luke's *apart* from God; for however greatly we marvel at the sufferings which patients have to endure, the most wonderful thing is that Christ . . . is with them in the furnace.[25]

At St Joseph's, the sisters often referred to patients' pain as their 'cross', while the matron at St Luke's wrote: 'Pain, so hard sometimes to understand, has made our patient's realise as nothing else would, that they must make "their robes white in the blood of the Lamb" and thus through pain peace has come to them in the end.'[26] Similarly the sisters at the Hostel of God saw suffering as 'a token of love, and the one means, often and often, of drawing souls to the Fountain of Love'.[17]

At St Luke's House and St Joseph's Hospice, individual accounts of some of the patients who died in the home were recorded in annual reports and annals. Most of these accounts describe patients' dying experiences in the context of their wider spiritual history, investing the death with an added meaning and significance, linked to eternal destiny.

'Holy and happy deaths'

At St Joseph's Hospice, as Humphreys shows, every aspect of death and dying was deeply entrenched in the teachings of Catholicism. The sisters' accounts of patients were written purposively. Their principal objective was to recount the spiritual history of patients, before and after admission to the hospice, focusing in particular upon the place of their reconciliation or conversion to the Catholic faith. Most of the accounts describe patients who were only reconciled or converted after admission to the hospice. The importance of being able to die in a Catholic atmosphere, surrounded by the multitude of symbols and rituals of the Catholic church, was felt to be paramount in reconciling or converting patients and in helping them to achieve a 'happy death'. One female patient was

> very interested in the Holy pictures and statues about her in the ward. When she saw the Sacred Heart on the Communion morning, she made enquiries as to what they were receiving. She read the life of the Little Flower and was drawn specially to her because she died of TB. She asked to be taken to the Chapel on Holy Thursday. She was instructed and received into the Church and made her first Holy Communion on the Feast of the Sacred Heart. That evening she passed peacefully away.[17]

> Reproduced with permission from Humphreys C. 'Waiting for the last summons': The establishment of the first hospices in England 1878–1914. *Mortality*, Volume 6, Issue 2, pp. 146–166, Copyright © 2001 Taylor and Francis.

Ritual mediations were a particularly significant feature of the 'holy' death. Reception of the sacraments, saying prayers and aspirations, reciting the rosary, kissing a crucifix, attending Mass, and being anointed were regular observances. The sacraments were particularly important in imparting a 'soul-saving'[27] grace to recipients and helped to fortify them for death. 'Holy and happy deaths' were considered edifying to others, especially non-Catholic relatives. Once the patient was actually dying, Holy Viaticum (the last communion) and Extreme Unction (the last anointing) were administered, and the 'prayers for the dying' could begin.[28]

The 'respectable Christian death'

In the same way, descriptions of patients in the annual reports for St Luke's House reflect the influence of Methodism. The accounts by Howard Barrett about St Luke's House, ostensibly written as a way of generating public interest in the home, were also a reflection of an underlying nonconformist ideology and were attempts to prescribe what happened there. Varied in content and incorporating a number of different elements; moral, spiritual, humorous, social, and pathological, they show examples of patience, fortitude, courage, and cheer in the face of deep physical suffering. A large number also refer to the patient's moral character and this had an influential bearing upon the way in which death was viewed in the home.

Death at St Luke's House had a specific moral condition attached to it. In 1897, Howard Barrett described suffering as 'the one thing which brings all men together on a level'.[29] There was a clear discrepancy, however, between the acceptance of this maxim at a theoretical level and its practical implications within the home. The annual reports emphasized that only the 'respectable' or 'deserving' poor were eligible for admission. Barrett wrote that 'the unworthy poor must be treated and provided for differently'—in institutions provided by the Poor Law.[30] He had no qualms about dismissing a patient whose moral character he felt to be unsuitable.

The patients' spiritual condition was also believed to have a profound effect upon their manner of death. The stories written by the Visiting Sisters at St Luke's dealt primarily with the spiritual aspects of patients' lives. Most emphasized the place of faith within the patients' biography, and the way in which this influenced their attitude towards both their physical condition, and the approach of death. Many of the patients in these stories underwent conversion because of being at St Luke's. Faith in Jesus Christ as one's personal Lord and Saviour was felt to be more important than the denominational route through which it was acquired. According to Barrett, 'a dying man doesn't want an "ism" he wants Christ, broadly and simply presented'.[17] Patients who found faith in Jesus were described under the broader heading of 'Christians', rather than being identified with a specific denomination. Outward manifestations of faith were also less important; what mattered was being 'able to rejoice in the assurance of sins forgiven'. One of the Visiting Sisters neatly captured the dual nature of the 're-spectable Christian death' in her account of a female patient at the home in 1907.

> When it dawned on her she had a mortal illness and it was not just sufficient to have led a respectable life she gave herself to prayer and turned the face of her soul towards God.[17]

Spiritual passivity and ecumenical leanings

Broome paints a somewhat different picture at the Friedenheim. Here there was less concern about deathbed conversion and an absence of some of the proselytizing fervour and missionary zeal found elsewhere. Moreover, no specific religious barriers were placed in front of patients wishing to gain entry to the hospital. While there were multiple biblical texts to be found on the walls,

the messages contained in them were less likely to shape the interactions between staff and patients. As founder Frances Davidson wrote in 1910, 'I leave
them now to do most of my talking . . . But the texts speak and I have the assurance and the evidence that God's work does not return unto Him void'.[6]

Despite these endeavours in the goal of triumphal, happy, holy, and
Christian death, 'bad deaths' could undoubtedly occur. The reports and
annals of the homes all contain occasional examples where spiritual intervention and solicitude failed. A patient at St Luke's, dying from cancer, was
unable to swallow when he was admitted. The annual report described him
as 'doubly unfortunate, for he seems quite inaccessible to religious influences,
there is no "Faith" in him at all, as far as can be gathered, to bring him a ray
of comfort or light in the darkness'.[31] At St Joseph's, patients who refused to
be reconciled or converted to the Catholic faith were looked upon with disap-
probation by the sisters. One Irish woman, a lapsed Catholic described by the
annalist as 'not a very consoling case', was admitted to the hospice on New
Year's Eve.

> [She] could not be induced to go to Confession on the appointed day. She got sud-
> denly bad one morning and [the sisters] hastily sending for the priest made prepa-
> rations for anointing and in a state of fearful anxiety fearing he would be too late
> endeavoured to help her and dispose her soul for the reception of the Sacraments
> without much apparent effect. She was quite conscious but paid little heed to what
> the priest said and did. She couldn't get Holy Communion and he could only pray to
> the end that the Lord's mercy would be felt in that poor soul.[32]

Clinical culture in the homes

If the institutional history and character of the terminal care homes has over
time become more clearly understood, we are less assured in our knowledge
of the particular role of medicine within them. Several points stand out. The
homes do not appear to have been the locus of medical practice for those
doctors who at the time were writing about 'euthanasia', and the medical
care of the dying. Conversely, those doctors who did work in the homes were
largely disinclined to write about their experiences for a wider medical audience. Nor do the homes appear to have established any strong academic links
with the emerging teaching hospitals, at least in the early days. With religious
thinking and practice clearly dominating day-to-day care in the homes, what
is there to know about the specifically medical aspects of what was taking
place there? Most of the historical records provide details of the organization and staffing aspects of medical care. There is also significant detail recorded on admissions, types of patients, and their diseases and rates of death.
Nevertheless, we are poorly served by accounts of medical intervention, the

types of treatments used, and the detail of pain and symptom management. This came much later, in the mid-twentieth century, when as we shall see in Chapter 3, further significant changes began to happen.

In the London homes, there was mainly a reliance on visiting physicians, although the Hostel of God did employ a salaried medical officer and St Luke's had a designated medical superintendent. These senior physicians exercised authority over all admissions, something that was taken care of by the Mother Rectrice at St Joseph's. At St Luke's, three criteria influenced admissions. First, patients must be of the respectable poor; this meant those of the working and middle classes, who had fallen in their fortunes and for whom previous receipt of parish relief was a strong contraindication to admission. Patients must also be from London, where the need was considered greatest; so those from the surrounding countryside were discouraged. Finally, patients must be imminently dying; this was not an establishment for the infirm and incurable who might continue for protracted periods, despite their debilitations.[22] In a similar vein, services at the Friedenheim were only for those in the last stages of illness, who had also been rejected by the general hospitals, and found themselves of insufficient means and friendless.[6]

At the Friedenheim, many patients were referred from the London teaching hospitals; a fact which Frances Davidson took as evidence of the high regard in which the establishment was held.[6] With this in mind, it is difficult to explain why the homes gained little in the way of wider recognition until the 1950s, since they appear from the outset to have fitted in with the London medical scene and to have provided a useful and well-regarded service. At St Joseph's, the patients were mainly identified by the nuns through their work in the local area of Hackney. There was also some evidence that the 'proto-hospices' helped each other with cross referrals when bed space was limited.[6]

The vast majority of patients in the homes were suffering from phthisis (later known as pulmonary tuberculosis). Tuberculosis was the leading cause of death in Britain in the nineteenth century, and in Ireland mortality rates continued to rise into the next century, while falling elsewhere. In Dublin, between 1891 and 1900, 34.5 per cent of a population of 10 000 died from the disease. Often protracted in its course, TB was accompanied by painful and debilitating symptoms. At Our Lady's Hospice, Dublin, between 1895 and 1910, the proportion of patients with TB was between 68 per cent and 74 per cent. By contrast, cancer patients were in the minority and only started to increase proportionally from the 1920s onwards.

There are also indications that even in the terminal care homes, those with external cancers were less welcome. At Our Lady's, this was attributed in the early years of the twentieth century to a lack of facilities. However, there is evidence that the sheer repugnance occasioned by some patients' symptoms made them unacceptable to the nursing staff. At St Luke's, Barrett comments on one man whose 'malady gave rise to an odour so awful that none but the doctors could bear it, and *they* did not enjoy it. He was, of course, isolated, but the ward maids declined and nurses hesitated to enter his room, and if the chaplain entered with some qualm, he came out with worse'.[22]

At the Friedenheim, the orientation at first was specifically to TB patients and this continued over time, possibly because they were also easier to nurse than cancer patients. The early medical reports at the Friedenheim also distinguish between admissions for simple, complex, and acute pulmonary phthisis, as well as tuberculosis of the vertebrae, abdominal organs, glands, sternum, and knee joints.[6] It was not until after Frances Davidson's death in 1920 that the council of the home provided arrangements to extend care to those with cancer.

Broome provides a helpful summary of inpatient facilities in four of the London homes at the beginning of the twentieth century.[6] In 1905, bed numbers were as follows:

- Friedenheim (42)
- St Luke's House (35)
- Hostel of God (28)
- St Joseph's Hospice (12)

The patients were not of particularly advanced age. Most of the homes made it clear that they were not offering services for the elderly infirm, though from time to time they each reported problems of 'long stay' patients—seen by Barrett as a 'misappropriation of funds'.[6] Dr Percy Lush, medical director at the Friedenheim, 1892–1918, described the problem thus in 1904:

> Every care is taken to admit only dying patients—that is, as we interpret it, such as are not expected to live more than two or three months—and thus relieve the General Hospitals and allow them to admit more patients. This is not yet generally understood; hence we receive a great many applications on behalf of the sadly large class of chronic incurables, which we are obliged to decline. For it will be at once recognised that every patient who occupies a bed for, say, twelve months is preventing the admission of three or four really dying ones.[6]

At the Friedenheim in 1899, 85 per cent of the patients were under age 50, with 50 per cent between 21 and 40 years old.[6] The Friedenheim also served an extraordinary range of nationalities from some 20 different countries. Approximately 75 per cent of all admissions across the homes ended in death.[17]

When St Joseph's opened in 1905, four local doctors gave their services to its patients: Dr Berdoe, Dr Cahill, Dr Ross, and Dr Parsons. By 1911, the annual report was expressing 'deep gratitude to the eminent honorary physicians who devote their time and professional knowledge to alleviate the sufferings of the poor patients'.[21] Sir Alfred Pearce Gould, who died in 1922, was a visiting doctor at St Luke's. Dean of the Faculty of Medicine at the University of London, 1912–1916, he had a particular interest in cancer and participated in trial treatments for these patients, and for those with tuberculosis.[13]

The annual reports of the Friedenheim also contain entries praising the visiting doctors. Broome speculates that the distinguished physicians and surgeons who are listed as honorary consultants, particularly after the establishment moved to improved premises in Hampstead, may well have been more a sign of prestige for the home than evidence of their direct involvement in clinical matters on a day-to-day basis.[6] The employed medical officers, by contrast, were seeing patients on a daily, or twice-daily basis.

It is difficult to gain a measure of the type of medical care being delivered in the homes; still more so to establish the extent to which it was influenced by the writings of Munk and others. As Broome writes, 'There is no direct evidence of the extent to which the Friedenheim's medical officers recognised this evolution in medical theory of care for the dying',[6] and certainly there were no references to these writers in the annual reports produced by the homes. Notable among the medical officers at the Friedenheim were Percy Lush, John Clark Wilson, and Norman Sprott, who served between 1892 and 1948. This assured medical coverage for over 60 years from just three men, and they were committed not only to direct care of the patients, but also to the management of the Friedenheim's affairs through its executive council.

Lush's obituary in 1919 praised his consideration and politeness to the patients and his devotion to the creation of a homely environment. His registrar and locum, Clark Wilson, succeeded him—Edinburgh-trained and an elder of the Church of Scotland. The two undoubtedly forged a strong influence on medical care at the Friedenheim in its early decades, which was at the same time suffused with religious sentiment and values. Their reports give insight into their clinical work. We see evidence of tailoring medication to need: 'For many, indeed the great majority, a frequent change of medicine is called for to relieve the distressing symptoms as they arise', and there was a boldness in prescribing, in one case up to eight grains of morphia per day to control pain. Oxygen, although expensive, was widely used, and was the only thing that gave relief to some patients. Alcohol was forbidden at the Friedenheim, but patients were indulged towards the end of life. And clean dressings were liberally used; as Lush noted, 'it is no uncommon thing to use a pound of cotton wool, *inter alia*, upon one patient in a day'.[6]

Tuberculosis of the lung was described by Barrett as 'the despair of the Hospitals and of the District Nursing agencies'. By contrast, Barrett himself adopted a positive attitude to these patients: 'You may be veritably dying and yet not always in bed.'[22] There was a small garden, where patients could sit on sunny days; day trips out and drives though the park; then followed by a special tea. A group of visitors came regularly to give the patients comfort, support, and interest. Some patients confided their worries to the visitors—on occasions these were about their families at home, who had been left in extreme poverty; while in St Luke's, the patients themselves could feel guilty about being treated with a measure of luxury inconsistent with their life outside.

In 1949, Dr Norman Sprott parted company with previous practice among his colleagues in the terminal care homes and published an article about his work.[33] Although appearing at a time when other stirrings of interest in terminal care were in evidence (which we will explore in Chapter 3), he gives a good indication of regular practice at the Friedenheim, by this time St Columba's Hospital, and by extension, the practices at other homes for the terminally ill in that era. His focus is clear.

> At this stage, cure of the disease is out of the question and what is needed is medical, nursing and spiritual care. From the patients' point of view, kindness, encouragement and bodily comfort are much more important than frequent medical examinations, scientific investigations and useless attempts or pretences to cure. A friendly, homely atmosphere, both of which prevail at St Columba's, are all important.[6]

Sprott goes on to acknowledge that some measure of investigation into the 'clinical material' at St Columba's might repay investment, but states that this lies beyond the reach of the facility, and so his account is based on clinical and empirical experience rather than a 'strictly scientific' approach. Nevertheless, his experience was substantial—caring for some 200 patients with advanced cancer each year, compared to two to three for the average general practitioner. Patients coming to St Columba's often arrived with advanced disease and metastases present in the lungs, abdominal viscera, skin, and skeleton. The primary growth may have been removed by surgery, in Sprott's view making the case easier to manage, and occasioning less distress for the patient. He gives a comprehensive list of problems and complications that can occur in these patients and makes it clear that 'what is required is the relief of symptoms'.[33]

Some of this relief was delivered through simple measures such as diet, fluids, and comfort. Anxiety and insomnia might require the use of phenobarbitone and soluble hypnotics. Pain is the symptom demanding the greatest attention. Here he makes the important statement: 'Drugs should be freely given, the amount and frequency depending on the patients' symptoms and often on their wishes rather than on any preconceived idea of what should be necessary.'[33] Patients were often started on aspirin and codeine phosphate, and then graduated to morphia by injection, using one-and-a-half grammes or more. When morphia caused vomiting, the more expensive diamorphine was substituted. Very rarely had drug addiction been a problem and all doses of 'dangerous drugs' were carefully checked and recorded. Sprott also noted the potential (though he had little personal experience) of intrathecal injections, nerve blocks, and laminectomy.

Sprott devotes a whole section of his paper to 'treatment of the mind', which he regarded as of equal importance to physical treatment. At the core of this should be a relationship of trust between the doctor, patient, and nursing staff; with no place for deceit and falsehood: 'Most of the patients want to know the truth, though frequently their friends are most unwilling that it should be revealed to them.'[33] He concluded his piece with an emphasis on social activities and distractions, on the importance of a homely atmosphere, on limiting the size of such hospitals to around 50 beds, and on situating them where communication channels were good, rather than in the depths of the countryside.

Possibilities of wider influence

Sprott's paper contained no references, but as we shall see in Chapter 3, it appeared at a time when others were also beginning to come forward with medical commentary on such matters. He gives us a rare insight into the medical and nursing care that prevailed in the terminal care homes up to the mid-twentieth century. Broome argues that Sprott's paper marks a significant shift from earlier writings on terminal care, even from those of Alfred Worcester, the American physician, whose work on the care of the aged, the dying, and the dead had appeared in 1935.[34] Whereas Worcester (who was 80 years old when his book was published) writes in a style akin to nineteenth-century physicians, emphasizing oral hygiene, nutrition, the use of opiates, and 'watchful waiting', by contrast Sprott discusses disease processes and the matching of specific drug regimes to symptoms. There are hints here of a more medically robust stance on the part of Sprott, and one that might stimulate wider thinking in the profession. We shall see evidence of that in Chapter 3.

Worcester too merits further consideration. He lived a long and active life and his key later work remained in print for many years after its first appearance in 1935. Although he was not associated with the American homes for the dying, his ideas and thinking did, by contrast, influence the mainstream. He was a family doctor who championed the importance of nursing care and established the Waltham Training School for Nurses in 1885, as well as holding a chair at Harvard Medical School. His book bemoaned the lack of interest in the care of older people and is often seen as a forerunner to the modern field of geriatrics. Described by one admirer as having a 'nineteenth century essence' with an awareness of the 'new needs of the twentieth century',[35] the work was an 'early inspiration' to Cicely Saunders when she first read it in 1951, at a time when she had little material to feed her growing appetite for works on terminal care.[36] In due course, it led to Worcester being hailed as an indirect pioneer of palliative care.[37] Worcester's short work is packed full of the kind of practical wisdom that seems to have prevailed in the terminal care homes. He describes how to recognize the signs of approaching death. He refers to the 'process of dying', its associated symptoms, the role of fluids, and the problem of restlessness. He attends to the environment of the dying person's room, to the need for light and for ventilation. He endorses the liberal use of opiates and considers morphine to have 'no rival'. He also deals with the role of faith and religion, with visions and hallucinations and with the question of uncertainty. Moreover, he refers to the works of Osler, Munk, and other nineteenth-century commentators on the care of the dying and he regrets the lack of progress since their publication.

> Many doctors nowadays, when the death of their patient becomes imminent, seem to believe that it is quite proper to leave the dying in the care of the nurses and sorrowing relatives. This shifting of responsibility is unpardonable. And one of its bad results is that as less professional interest is taken in such service, less and less is known about it.[34]

Accounts of patient cases in the terminal care homes from the late nineteenth century reveal that something *was* known and that it had the power to influence others, if only the right mechanisms for dissemination could be found. It might well be that the strong religious orientations of the homes were a barrier to wider influence. Worcester, for example, seems careful not to labour the significance of religious elements in care of the dying ('this subject is generally conceded to belong to the clergyman rather than the physician').

Nevertheless, in the specialist homes, religious and denominational underpinnings played a large part in determining their organization, atmosphere, patterns of care, and attitudes towards death and dying. To varying degrees across the homes, tending to bodily suffering was a precursor to the more important goal of fulfilling a patient's spiritual needs. The provision of the 'soul-cure', although manifested in different ways in each of the homes, was central to the management of the deathbed. Humphreys has shown how the early London hospices and homes for the dying had three sets of concerns: religious, philanthropic, and moral.[17] Such institutions placed a strong emphasis on the cure of the soul, even when the life of the body was diminishing.

They drew on charitable endeavours and were often motivated to give succour to the poor and disadvantaged. They were not, however, places in which the medical or nursing care of the dying was of marked sophistication, and it is difficult to gain a detailed picture of the patterns of medical care that prevailed, particularly in the earlier period, with the exception of Sprott's article. Although rooted in religious and philanthropic concerns that would diminish as the twentieth century advanced, the early homes for the dying represent a vital prologue to the subsequent period of development that followed in the decades after World War II. Part of the shift was also associated with the decline in the incidence of tuberculosis and the growing visibility of patients with cancer. Sister Francis Rose O'Flynn spent many years at Our Lady's Hospice until she died in 2011, and for a time she was Superior General of the Religious Sisters of Charity. Speaking in 2004, she describes the context in Dublin some 50 years earlier.

> Now what happened here really, in Our Lady's Hospice, was that when it was built in 1879 the main purpose was to care for the dying, to give them care and comfort in the last days of their life. And by the mid nineteen forties or early nineteen fifties going into the early fifties, the infections that were really prevalent at that time, mostly tuberculosis and other kind of infections, they were pretty well eradicated by antibiotics and other types of therapy like that. So that the type of patient that was really in the hospice, most of them were either cured or they were sent home, or they went out to a sanatorium. So that this was a very big establishment, there were over a hundred beds and there were a lot of vacant beds, and a lot of people then that came in after that were elderly. Now they were varied, there was no specific category of patient admitted to hospital. They were all very ill, not necessarily terminally ill. And that really, I think changed in a sense, the whole emphasis of hospice. They were all very ill . . . because all the time there were cancer patients admitted but they weren't getting special cancer care until the seventies.[38]

By such routes, some of the homes, like St Joseph's and the Hostel of God in London, and Our Lady's in Dublin, made the transition into the new era of hospice and palliative care as a specialized area of activity. It is on this growing specialization that we now focus our attention.

Notes

1. **Abel-Smith B** (1964). *The Hospitals 1800–1948*. London, UK: Heinemann.
2. **Abel EK** (2013). *The Inevitable Hour: A History of Caring for Patients in America*, p. 68. Baltimore, MD: The Johns Hopkins University Press.
3. **Corr CA, Nabe CM, Corr DM** (2009). *Death and Dying, Life and Living*, 6th ed., p. 189. Belmont, CA: Wadsworth.
4. **Rosenberg CE** (1987). *The Care of Strangers: The Rise of America's Hospital System*. New York, NY: Basic Books.

5. **Wood WR, Williamson JB** (2003). Historical changes in the meaning of death in the western tradition. In: Bryant CD (ed.). *Handbook of Death and Dying*, vol. 1, p. 16. Thousand Oaks, CA: Sage Publications.

6. **Broome HI** (2011). *Neither curable nor incurable but actually dying*. Unpublished PhD thesis. University of Southampton, UK.

7. **Schofield AT** (1891). A home for the dying. *Contemporary Review* (March):423–7.

8. **Healy TM** (2004). *125 Years of Caring in Dublin; Our Lady's Hospice, Harold's Cross 1879–2004*. Dublin, Ireland: A and A Farmer.

9. **Bouillat JMJ** (n.d.). *Les Contemporains—An Early Twentieth Century Essay on the Life and Work of Jeanne Garnier*. [Place and publisher unknown.]

10. **Moulin P** (2000). Les soins palliatifs en France: Un movement paradoxal de medicalization du mourir contemporain. *Cahiers Internationale de Sociologie*, 108:125–59.

11. **Clark D** (2000). Palliative care history: a ritual process. *European Journal of Palliative Care* 7(2):50–5.

12. The National Archives. Records of the Mildmay Mission Hospital. Available at http://www.nationalarchives.gov.uk/a2a/records.aspx?cat=387-mm&cid=0#0, accessed 17 December 2013.

13. **Humphreys C** (1999). 'Undying spirits': Religion, medicine, and institutional care of the dying 1878–1938, p. 48. Unpublished PhD thesis. University of Sheffield, UK.

14. **Sister Mary Eucharia** (1965) The apostolate of Rose Hawthorne. *Sacred Heart Messenger*:46–9.

15. St. Rose's home in Manhattan to close (2009). *Catholic New York* (26 February). Available at http://cny.org/stories/St-Roses-Home-in-Manhattan-to-Close,2608?content_source&category_id&search_filter&event_mode&event_ts_from&list_type&order_by&order_sort&content_class&sub_type=stories&town_id, accessed 21 March 2015.

16. **Lewis MJ** (2007). *Medicine and Care of the Dying: A Modern History*. Oxford, UK: Oxford University Press.

17. **Humphreys C** (2001). 'Waiting for the last summons': The establishment of the first hospices in England 1878–1914. *Mortality*, 6(2):146–66.

18. Hospice History Project: Cicely Saunders interview with Neil Small, 10 July 1996.

19. Lost hospitals of London (n.d.) Available at http://ezitis.myzen.co.uk/herefordlodge.html, accessed 21 March 2015.

20. Hospice History Project: Sister Mary Antonia interview with David Clark, 28 November 1995.

21. **Winslow M, Clark D** (2005). *St Joseph's Hospice Hackney: A Century of Caring in the East End of London*. Lancaster, UK: Observatory Publications.

22. **Goldin G** (1981). A proto-hospice at the turn of the century: St Luke's House, London, from 1893 to 1923. *Journal of the History of Medicine and Allied Sciences*, 36 4:383–415.

23. **Williams CP** (1982). Healing and evangelism: The place of medicine in later Victorian Protestant missionary thinking. In: **Sheils WJ** (ed.). *The Church and Healing*, p. 285. Oxford, UK: Basil Blackwell.

24. St Luke's House Annual Report (1900), p. 19. Available from Imperial College Healthcare NHS Trust Archives at http://discovery.nationalarchives.gov.uk/details/a?_ref=1591, accessed 17 November 2015.

25. St Luke's House Annual Report (1905), p. 32. Available from Imperial College Healthcare NHS Trust Archives at http://discovery.nationalarchives.gov.uk/details/a?_ref=1591, accessed 17 November 2015.

26. St Luke's House Annual Report (1899), p. 30. Available from Imperial College Healthcare NHS Trust Archives at http://discovery.nationalarchives.gov.uk/details/a?_ref=1591, accessed 17 November 2015.

27. **Wilberforce W** (n.d.). St Joseph's Hospice, Mare Street, Hackney. *The Catholic Weekly*:2.

28. St Joseph Hospice Annals, 1909–1915. St Joseph's Hospice Archives, Mare Street, Hackney, London, UK.

29. St Luke's House Annual Report (1897), pp. 13–14. St Joseph's Hospice Archives, Mare Street, Hackney, London, UK. Available from Imperial College Healthcare NHS Trust Archives at http://discovery.nationalarchives.gov.uk/details/a?_ref=1591, accessed 17 November 2015.

30. St Luke's House Annual Report (1895), p. 4. Available from Imperial College Healthcare NHS Trust Archives at http://discovery.nationalarchives.gov.uk/details/a?_ref=1591, accessed 17 November 2015.

31. St Luke's House Annual Report (1913), p. 23. Available from Imperial College Healthcare NHS Trust Archives at http://discovery.nationalarchives.gov.uk/details/a?_ref=1591, accessed 17 November 2015.

32. Notes for Annals of St Joseph's Hospice, 1905–1909, pp. 29–30. St Joseph's Hospice Archives, Mare Street, Hackney, London, UK.

33. **Sprott N** (1949). Dying of cancer. *The Medical Press* (Feb. 16):187–91.

34. **Worcester A** (1935). *The Care of the Aged, the Dying, and the Dead*. Springfiled, IL: Charles C. Thomas.

35. **Freeman JT** (1988). Dr Alfred Worcester: Early exponent of modern geriatrics. *Bulletin of the New York Academy of Medicine*, 64(3):246–51.

36. **Saunders C** (1992). Letter [on re: Alfred Worcester]. *The American Journal of Hospice and Palliative Care* (July/August):2.

37. **Kerr D** (1992). Alfred Worcester: A pioneer in palliative care. *American Journal of Hospice and Palliative Care*, 9(3):13–14, 36–8.

38. Hospice History Project. Sister Francis Rose O'Flynn interview with David Clark, 28 July 2004.

Chapter 3

Interest and disinterest in the mid-twentieth century

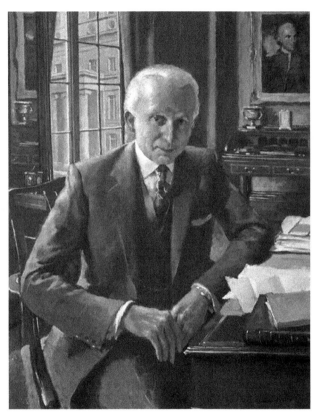

Figure 3.1 Ronald Raven (1904–91)
A London-based surgeon and former army officer, Raven chaired the joint committee of the Marie Curie Memorial and the Queen's Institute of District Nursing, which in 1952 published its extensive report on the social and medical conditions of people being nursed at home with cancer. The report stimulated Marie Curie to establish homes for the dying and a night nursing service for the terminally ill. Raven went on to edit a six-volume series on *Cancer*, published in 1960, for which he invited Cicely Saunders to contribute a chapter on the management of patients in the terminal stage. In 1975 he also edited a collection entitled *The Dying Patient*, to which Professor Eric Wilkes was a contributor. Reproduced by kind permission of the Royal Crown Derby Museum Trust. Copyright © 2016 the artist's estate/Bridgeman Images.

The creation of the welfare state

At the time of its establishment in Britain in 1948, the National Health Service (NHS) was unique. Offering free medical care to the entire population, it was a comprehensive system of universal entitlement based on collective provision of healthcare within a market economy.[1] It was to replace charity, dependency, and moralism with a new ethic of social citizenship.[2] The creation of the NHS signalled the final phase in the evolution of the voluntary hospital movement, which had first got underway 200 years earlier. As Charles Webster[3] has shown, the voluntary hospitals had continued to expand in the twentieth century, from 783 hospitals in England and Wales in 1911, to 1 255 by 1938, accounting for more than half of all acute services. Nevertheless, they faced growing problems of financial viability and were increasingly reliant upon patient fees. Their development had been piecemeal and administratively complex, and there was a sense that the new scientific and technical knowledge in medicine was outpacing improvements in services. As financial and administrative strictures tightened, the work of the voluntary hospitals was matched increasingly by the responsibilities of local authorities—for maternal and child welfare, district nursing, midwifery, tuberculosis aftercare, and for the care of those with mental illness and physical disabilities. The voluntary hospital legacy would continue to make its influence felt, however, even as the new system of health and welfare took hold.

From the outset, the organization of the NHS was a matter of immense complexity. The major problem, according to Webster, was 'to convert a defective and ramshackle collection of inherited medical services into a modern health service appropriate to the needs and expectations of the second part of the twentieth century'.[3] Underpinning this was an intensely modernizing ethic that entailed a deep ideological suspicion of charity and made cure and rehabilitation its clinical goals. As various commentators have observed, Aneurin Bevan captured this in stark fashion when, as Minister of Health in the postwar Labour government led by Clement Atlee, he introduced the NHS bill to the British Parliament. He stated he would 'rather be kept alive in the efficient if cold altruism of a large hospital than expire in a gush of sympathy in a small one'.[4] With such priorities, there was to be little attention paid to medicine's 'failures'—those in their last illness, whose time was short.

From cradle to grave?

In the early years of the NHS, we see no strategic or operational guidance on terminal care and no systematic commitment to the subject as a clinical issue. The UK welfare state was seeking to vouchsafe care 'from the cradle to the grave', yet at the beginning it paid scant attention to care at the end of life, focusing instead on addressing the widespread acute and chronic health problems of a society grappling with postwar social and economic reconstruction.

Fortunately, two major reports written during the 1950s provide evidence on the care of dying people, and upon the actual and potential organization of terminal care services. Although both emanated from outside the portals of the NHS, they painted a picture of need at that time, and they contributed to a modest shift in medical discourse on terminal care. Slowly, *anecdote* gave way to *evidence* as an orienting theme in care for the dying. The provision of such care remained the primary concern of charitable organizations, but by the early 1960s, a new discourse was emerging. It did so, however, against a background of policy neglect and clinical disinterest, which was slow to dissipate. The period from 1948 to 1967, therefore, displays some marked innovations in thinking and practice relating to terminal care, but also some obdurate continuities with the past. It is this combination of innovation and tradition, oddly located within the fissures of the modern welfare state, which provided the conditions of possibility for later hospice and palliative care expansion.

Upon these rather fragile foundations, the groundbreaking and deeply consequential work of Dr Cicely Saunders was gradually established, from the appearance of her first publication on terminal care in 1958 (written while still a medical student) to the opening of St Christopher's Hospice a decade later.[5] Led by her efforts, a particular view of 'modern' terminal care began to emerge from the late 1950s, which eventually had the power to consolidate into a strategy for action, initially at arm's length from the NHS, but eventually with wide-ranging effect. Moreover, as we shall see in Chapter 4, there was far more to Saunders's achievements, as she first helped define a new field of care and then promulgated it locally, nationally, and internationally.

Concerns about how and why to care for the dying had slowly developed in the first 20 years of the NHS. There were divided views within medicine about the legitimacy of care at the end of life as an area for specialization. Older doctors clung to a paternalist viewpoint, in which their primary role was that of the comprehending and sympathetic friend to the dying. The first wave of doctors who trained wholly within the NHS, however, produced some who later made care of the dying a specialized clinical, research, and teaching endeavour. Between these lay a not insubstantial body of medical opinion that lent at least some support to changes in the law on euthanasia, now seen as the deliberate ending of life by medical means. The proponents of hospice care and the supporters of legalized euthanasia were usually at loggerheads. Further tensions emerged in the debate about how much attention should be given to the dying elderly in general, as opposed to those of any age dying of cancer. This was resolved through further specialization, which undoubtedly led to geriatrics and terminal care becoming separate from one another as areas of expertise. Finally, a narrative appeared, in which those who did champion the cause of terminal cancer care found themselves struggling in the face of a more deep-seated resistance to the notion that medical, religious, and social care of the dying deserved any special recognition on the part of either the practitioners or policymakers.

Social conditions for the dying in 1950s Britain

The two major reports in question, compiled at the beginning and end of the 1950s, cast light on the social conditions for those dying in Britain during that decade and also served as powerful rhetoric for change. The first was prepared by a joint committee of the Marie Curie Memorial and the Queen's Institute of District Nursing, and was chaired by the surgeon Ronald Raven (Figure 3.1).[6] The Marie Curie Memorial was established in 1948 and held among its objectives the promotion of welfare and relief for cancer patients. A joint committee of the Memorial and of the Queen's Institute first met in 1950 with the purpose of investigating the needs of domiciliary cancer sufferers and its report was published two years later. Dr H. L. Glyn Hughes prepared the second report at the request of the Calouste Gulbenkian Foundation, based on enquiries carried out between November 1957 and December 1958.[7] It contained a description of current provision for the care of the dying, together with recommendations for development.

Concerning patients with cancer nursed at home

The joint committee's objective was to undertake a national survey of patients with cancer living in their own homes, with special reference to their circumstances and needs. It adopted a method that involved sending questionnaires to district nurses across the country from February to August 1951, and 179 of the 193 local health authorities that were approached cooperated in the survey. Nearly 70 per cent of the patients were aged 60 years or over, and more than 24 per cent were 75 years or over. It was among these older people that some of the gravest social problems were found, as the descriptions of different patients bear out.

> Illness very far advanced when friends called a doctor, and who lived in extreme squalor, resisting any attempt to wash or care for her.

> Alone in a bed-sitting room, seldom visited by her married children, relying on the goodness of neighbours . . . receiving very little nourishment.

Or, more graphically still, this account.

> House was dirty as she was too ill to clean it, and her clothing filthy with neglect and discharge from the ulcer . . . gave food to her pets which she needed herself.[6]

There were numerous examples of delays in seeking treatment, or even of the refusal to be treated. A high proportion of patients were considered gravely ill at the time of the survey, and district nurses often believed they had been called in at too late a stage of the illness. More than half of the patients were reportedly bedridden. The nurses also described the mental suffering of their patients.

> He does not become depressed by the very acute pain, but becomes very despondent and loses faith in every possible way as he feels he is gradually worsening, and that no-one is taking any interest . . .[6]

The survey placed a strong emphasis on the physical conditions in which the patients lived. Almost a third had only one room in which to live, less than half had running water, and almost 40 per cent had no accessible lavatory.[6]

The report concluded with a series of recommendations, including the need for more residential and convalescent homes; the importance of better information for cancer sufferers; and greater provision of night nursing, home-help services, and equipment. Some patients, the report indicated, were unaware of the provisions of the NHS Act, or of their eligibility with the National Assistance Board.

Stunned by the results, the Marie Curie Memorial alone was galvanized into action and, within a year of the report's publication, it had begun opening new homes for terminally ill cancer patients. Hill of Tarvit, established in Cupar, Fife, in east Scotland was the first, in December 1952. The property was leased from the National Trust for Scotland and contained an array of antiques and fine furnishings. Over the next 12 years, nine more Marie Curie Homes opened, from Tiverton in Devon in 1953, to Solihull in the west Midlands in 1965. They were each housed in converted buildings, including a preparatory school, a railwaymen's convalescent home, a police orphanage, and a handful of lavish mansions. In 1958, provision was further extended by the addition of a night nursing service; and by the early 1960s, 24 authorities in the provinces and 15 London district nursing areas were being served by over 200 Marie Curie nurses.[8] There is no evidence, however, of any systematic response to the report from elsewhere within the public health and welfare system.

'Peace at the Last'

The second report was prepared by Brigadier H. L. Glyn Hughes. A former army doctor, he had been the first allied medical officer to enter the Belsen concentration camp at the end of World War II. Like the joint committee, he gave considerable attention to the social conditions of the terminally ill, but his report was more wide-ranging, and devoted greater prominence to matters of policy and service organization.[7] His focus was on the terminal care of those with a life expectancy no greater than 12 months, and particularly in the very last stages of life. He began by highlighting the fact that while numerous enquiries and reports existed on the medical and social problems of the aged and the chronic sick, none had given adequate attention to the problem of terminal care. A particular aspect of his enquiry was concerned with 'the extent to which the Welfare State has made adequate provision to deal with this problem both now and in the future'.[7] Against the background of the Joint Cancer Survey Committee's findings, Glyn Hughes was concerned with the unanswered questions of where and by whom the elderly terminally ill would be cared for.

The Glyn Hughes survey sought information from every medical officer of health in the United Kingdom; in addition, the senior administrative medical officers who were responsible for hospital services throughout the regional hospital boards provided a range of statistical data on the use of hospitals for terminal care. Many voluntary organizations, religious orders, and other groups were also consulted, and 300 site visits were made. The National Council of Social Service provided information on 150 of its local councils. Finally, a survey was conducted of over 600 family doctors.

The report showed that two-fifths of all deaths in 1956 occurred in NHS hospitals, with under half taking place in the home. Almost 46 000 cancer deaths (approximately one-third of the total) took place at home, and it was considered that many of these would have required continuous medical and nursing care. Similar needs were thought to be in evidence among some of the 121 000 who died at home from diseases of the circulatory system. Overall, Glyn Hughes estimated that some 270 000 people in need of 'skilled terminal care' died each year outside of NHS hospitals.

The report's conclusions were prescient and acknowledged that 'for a long time to come there will remain a need to make use of accommodation outside the NHS, both in voluntary and profit-making establishments'.[7] By the former, he referred to homes for the dying run by charitable organizations and religious orders, of which (as we have seen) only a small number existed. By the latter, he made reference to the much larger number of nursing homes, which would increasingly come into private ownership. Neither group, in his view, could be given a clean bill of health. His comments were chastening. In the homes for the dying, although 'love and devotion' were in evidence from the staff, there were poor staff–patient ratios, a paucity of fully trained nurses, austere conditions, a lack of comfort, and an air of financial constraint. Among the nursing homes, a large proportion were deemed 'quite unsuited to provide the terminal care of patients who, in their last stages, require the most skilled nursing attention; in fact, in many of them the conditions are bad, in some cases amounting to actual neglect when measured by standards that can reasonably be expected'.[7]

While dying at home was seen as the preferred option for most patients, Glyn Hughes stressed the importance of calculating the total number of inpatient beds that would be needed for terminal care. He was eager to stress the value of special terminal care beds within the curtilage of hospitals for the acute sick. At the same time, he considered that the independent homes for the dying should develop closer links with hospital services to reduce their isolation.

The report quickly had a wider impact and some major medical journals now began to take an interest, as in this review of the report in *The Lancet*:

> We must attack the problem on every side: hospital services must be improved and extended, staff in residential homes increased, and voluntary as well as profit-making institutions helped in return for an approved standard of care.[9]

At the same time, *The Lancet's* reviewer recognized some impediments: the limits to hospital expansion; the inadequate supply of trained district nurses; and a lack of home help. The journal did however endorse Glyn Hughes's radical suggestion that payment be made to women for the full-time care of their dependent relatives.

Bookends

Like bookends at the start of the 1950s and the 1960s, these two reports highlighted the deficiencies of terminal care in the welfare state of Britain at the time. The joint committee had drawn attention to the abject social and economic conditions of many elderly people suffering with advanced cancer. Glyn Hughes had revealed the absence of a serious policy commitment to terminal care provision; indeed, his recommendations highlighted the need for voluntary and for-profit organizations to work in conjunction with the NHS to achieve the necessary results.

Both reports had alluded to a perceived underlying change in family values likely to have a bearing on the situation. Neither was categorical on whether or not families had become less willing to look after their sick and dependent members—although Glyn Hughes reports that this was widely perceived by general practitioners to be a consequence of the introduction of the NHS. Rather, a picture emerges of families struggling to balance a range of pressures and responsibilities. So the joint committee refers to the problems of relatives who have to earn their living during the day and may suffer from fatigue and undue stress from night-sitting over a prolonged period.[6] Meanwhile, Glyn

Hughes concluded that in a period when large sections of the population were moving to new towns and suburban estates, 'with the much smaller family of today the provision of help by relatives will get less and the requirement of institutional care at the end will increase'.[7]

Coupled with mounting demographic evidence, the reports argued for terminal care to become a priority for the NHS. By 1951, more than 10 per cent of the population was over 65, compared to less than 5 per cent in 1901. It was also an era that marked a shift from a high mortality rate associated with infectious disease towards a greater awareness of chronic illness and the long-term effects of disabling conditions.

On their own, these reports were not sufficient to create a sea change in policy. They did, however, stimulate, and were in turn strengthened by, a growing clinical interest in questions of terminal care that slowly drew attention to the needs of those in the final stages of life. As this interest manifested itself in published research and commentary, so it served to promote the conditions that would allow further fundamental developments to take place, and for the needs identified in the reports to be addressed.

Clinical discussions: From anecdote to a semblance of evidence

In August 1948, just one month after the foundation of the NHS, *The Practitioner* journal devoted a series of papers to the question of care for the dying. It was introduced by Lord Horder, the Physician in Ordinary to the King, who captured the overall tone of the collection in a combination of aphorisms and proverbs about death, coupled with simple descriptions of particular cases and warnings against the danger of prolonging the act of dying, in the name of extending life.[10] A key paper in this important issue of *The Practitioner* was by W. Norman Leak, a physician from Winsford in Cheshire, who was a regular writer for medical journals on a range of topics over several decades and later a council member of the British Medical Association. His piece here was on the care of the dying patient. It begins with the wider social context. A 'paradoxical and awkward situation' had been reached, in which death was commonly occurring at advanced age (when dying is said to take longer) and where medical and nursing skills were contriving to prolong life. At the same time 'relatives are not available or willing' to undertake care at home. The tone on matters of policy was fatalistic: 'However desirable it may seem to some that all old people should obtain the best skill and care in their dying moments, it seems pretty clear that this will remain an ideal for a long time to come.'[11] On questions of clinical care, the individual practitioner's personal beliefs, attitudes, and morality seemed to be the chief elements in the armamentarium.

> If he thinks that death is the end of all things and the sooner it is over the better for all concerned, then obviously a few doses of morphine or, even more rapid, no morphine at all, is all that is required. If, however, he is one who believes that kindness and goodness have absolute values and that there is some existence beyond the grave, his treatment will be much more individual and discriminating.[11]

Leak deals with nursing care under the headings of 'incontinence', 'the bowels', and 'care of the mouth'. A section on 'the relatives' offers advice on the emotional situations that can occur. Its tone is blunt and provocative: 'It is wise to put the brake on somehow, usually by giving one or two something definite to do, and by giving the ringleaders a good dose of a barbiturate with a cup of tea.' Medical treatment 'can almost be written in one word—morphine', although it may require the doctor to attend twice daily to deliver the injections if no trained nurse is available. The anecdotal tone is captured fully in the conclusion: 'What has been written has not been culled from books but is the result of experience, often gained by fumbling with no one more experienced at hand to guide me . . .'

There is no emphasis in this collection of papers upon clinical innovation in the care of the dying. There is, however, a sense that some of the personal attributes that the general practitioner brings to the care of dying patients may be lost—'dismissed as mere tosh'—by the younger generation of doctors and eroded by the growing tendency for patients to be cared for in 'the clean efficiency of the large hospital', rather than the 'less exacting routine of a local cottage hospital'. There is a sense here of modern mid-twentieth-century medicine having no space for the personal involvement of doctors, however paternalistic, in the care of their dying patients; yet, at the same time, having nothing with which to replace that involvement. Interestingly, Leak's paper contains not a single reference of any kind to a published source or study on the subject of the care of the dying, and it appears ignorant of the work already discussed here of the nineteenth-century writers, and of Alfred Worcester.

A general practitioner in the Scottish Highlands, Dr John Berkeley, who was just starting out in the mid-1950s, provides a fascinating personal insight into some of the challenges faced in caring for patients at home with advanced disease at that time.

> I can very, very clearly remember, within the first year or two of going into practice, a lady with advanced cervical carcinoma dying at home. And we were giving quite large doses of morphine. I mean they seemed *lethal* doses to us in those days. Now, looking back with hindsight, I think we were giving adequate doses but not frequently enough, and they were intermittent. And my feeling of *utter helplessness*, of

trying to help, not only this woman, but her husband and her daughters, and feeling that I had not got the skills at that time (and this was about two years into practice), to actually deal with this situation. It made quite a profound impact. I mean I can still now visualise the house, and the woman, and the many calls I made to that household. So that must have been '55 or something like that and it made quite an impression on me, care of people. Not just care of the dying, because one was looking after many elderly people who were dying very peacefully, I mean that was a normal part of general practice, but dying in pain, and again . . . a relatively young woman, I think she must have been in her, probably, mid-forties or something like that, made quite a profound impression on me at the time. And stimulated me to read, to see what there was that one could do to help. And there was very, very little in the literature in those days to give any indication. So that was the sort of background; you went against sort of traditional teaching and therapeutics to try and help a patient. But reading around in those days, reading the literature; there was nothing else to guide you.[12]

It was to be more than a decade before the first twentieth-century studies on these matters began to appear and, during the 1950s, even anecdotal publications on the care of the dying were rare indeed. At the British Medical Association's annual meeting held in Newcastle-upon-Tyne in July 1957, a plenary session took place on the subject and was reported in the British Medical Journal.[13] Dr Ian Grant's comments at the conference were later published in full. Drawing on over 30 years' experience in general practice but no published work, he concludes with this about his dying patients: 'They require kindness most of all, and they first and foremost wish and hope to find a comprehending and sympathetic friend in the physician.'[14] Again, the duty of the general practitioner was seen as that of bringing contentment and comfort to dying patients and not to simply strive to prolong life. A plea was made for more hospital accommodation for the moribund, and Grant argues that the welfare state should make it a priority 'to provide adequate hospital and nursing care for those who have served their country well and whose life is now drawing to a close'. Morphine continued to be the preferred drug in cases of terminal malignant disease, but in his view, which perhaps reflected wider sentiment, it should be withheld as long as possible to counteract problems of tolerance. In cases of desperation, however, the 'first duty is to relieve pain and to induce merciful oblivion'.

There was considerable tension in this debate about the benefits and hazards associated with the liberal use of morphine. A widely read article by Clifford Hoyle, published in 1944 and based on a lecture given at Horton Hospital in 1941, had characterized the physician as the sole arbiter of pain relief for the dying. If this meant hastening the death of the patient, with no prior discussion with patient or family, then this was a matter about which the doctor should keep his own counsel. While it remained illegal to end the life of the patient in a deliberate fashion, albeit for kind and medical reasons, it was rarely questioned, or acted upon in law. However, it could be brought about by rapidly escalating the dose of morphine.[15] In similar fashion to *The Practitioner* articles of 1948, Dr W. N. Leak had argued that morphine is the drug of choice when death draws near. It is unclear whether the 'overdose' referred to here is deliberate or not:

> There is no drug to touch it for dying folk and . . . contrary to common belief morphine does not hasten the end unless the patient is abnormally sensitive or an overdose is given'.[11]

However, other influential authors, particularly those from the United States and those with surgical backgrounds, advised that *all* other means of controlling pain (both pharmacological and non-pharmacological) should be pursued before resorting to the use of morphine. A surgeon from Illinois reported in 1956 that 'we are often loath to give liberal amounts of opiates because the drug addiction itself may become a hideous spectacle and actually result in great misery for the patient'.[16] This position, encouraged by sustained investment in work directed at finding a non-addictive analgesic by the US National Research Council,[17] clearly had a transatlantic influence, and the advice about withholding morphine in favour of new alternatives was promoted in UK textbooks and other publications.[18] Much of the fear came from a lack of knowledge about how to use morphine properly. Professor Duncan Vere reflects on his experience in London and is scathing in his comments.

> I will say that until about 1965 in hospitals—general hospitals and general practice— there was entrenched ignorance, a tremendous amount of severe pain. Patients who were in severe pain, or dying with pain, were often given the Brompton Cocktail (or Mist Obliterans as it was politely known), and it was a matter of patients being rendered so that they did not know what they were doing by doctors who certainly did not know what they were doing.[19]

The dominance of the specificity theory of pain was another major contributor to the ambivalence about the medical use of morphine for cancer pain in the mid-twentieth century. The theory argues for a specific pain system that carries messages from receptors in the skin to a pain centre in the brain. Accordingly, a logical treatment was to attempt to interrupt the pain system by means of nerve blocks or surgical sectioning of the spinal cord or brain. The development of these procedures flourished as surgery and anaesthesia reached their ascendant position in the hierarchy of medical specialities, which took hold after World War II.

For a prolonged period after World War II, serious efforts were made in the United States to find an alternative analgesic that was as effective as morphine, but with less addictive potential. These studies were led by Dr Ray Houde, Ada Rogers, and later Dr Kathleen Foley at the Sloan Kettering Institute for Cancer Research in New York. Houde's team conducted multiple long-term crossover trials, comparing new analgesics with morphine in cancer patients. The study patients, who acted as their own controls,[20] received medication for moderate pain with rescue medication if the initial dosage did not relieve the pain. They had hourly visits from Rogers, the research nurse, through the day. One unanticipated outcome of this innovative work was the development of a patient-centred technology for testing analgesics, on which modern analgesic trails are now based. This involved entering and trying to understand the patient's pain experience. Another outcome was the gradual realization that morphine, when the dose was properly titrated and used regularly, was the best drug available and that all of the many substitutes tested could not compare to it.

John Bonica, chief of anaesthesiology at the Madigan Army Hospital in Washington during World War II, developed his interest in 'abnormal pain' from his experience of trying to treat wounded servicemen. After the war, he embarked on a formidable programme of personal research, encompassing material written about pain in medical, phenomenological, and historical literature. He later argued that pain is what individuals feel, think, and do about the symptoms they perceive, and that patients in pain need their doctor's 'sympathy and kindness'. He published the first textbook of pain medicine in 1953, and later on in his influential career, he corresponded with Cicely Saunders and worked with other clinicians interested in pain and palliative care.

Saunders's philosophy for the care of the dying had many parallels with Bonica's work. Against accepted wisdom, she insisted on the absolute necessity of administering opiates regularly to patients with pain due to cancer. Her previous experience as a nurse meant that, when working as a volunteer at St Luke's home in Bayswater, she sought to understand why the nurses did not follow medical instructions to only give pain relief 'as required', instead giving it 'by the clock' every four hours.[21] She went on to argue that opiates used in this way were not addictive, and that patients receiving such medications could live out their lives in comfort and quality. Saunders also argued that opiates administered orally (as opposed to those given by injection) were effective and that they worked by relieving pain, not just by masking it.

Medicine and euthanasia

Parallel to this type of commentary and developing medical practice for pain and end-of-life issues was the discussion within medicine on the question of euthanasia. The Voluntary Euthanasia Legislation Society had been founded in 1935, the year it held its first public meeting at BMA House (home to the British Medical Association). The following year, a bill was introduced into the House of Lords seeking to legalize the voluntary euthanasia of willing adults suffering from fatal disease accompanied by severe pain. The 1936 bill was unsuccessful and, in 1950, a further attempt was made to bring it to the statute book, again without success. On the latter occasion, four medical peers (Lord Horder, Lord Webb-Johnson, Lord Haden-Guest, and Lord Amulree) all spoke against it. A leading article in *The Lancet*, echoing the words of Lord Horder in the debate, commented that 'the good doctor will distinguish between prolongation of life and the unnecessary prolongation of the act of dying'.[22] By such means, it supported the contrivance to obscure the role of the doctor at the dying patient's bedside. At the same time, it acknowledged that public interest in the issue of euthanasia remained considerable. In a letter in response to *The Lancet* article, Dr C. K. Millard, the founding honorary secretary of the Voluntary Euthanasia Legalisation Society, acknowledged that the opposition of medical peers 'was very unfortunate from our point of view and scarcely gave the motion a chance'.[23] However, he went on to remind readers that an eminent surgeon, the late Lord Moynihan, had founded the society and that currently it had the support of 170 distinguished members of the medical profession, 30 of which had knighthoods.

Paradoxically, as evidence began to accrue on the current state of care for the dying, medical opinion against euthanasia hardened, as seen in this excerpt from a 1961 lead article in *The Lancet*:

> If the known means to make death, when it comes, easy and happy were applied by individual and collective effort with intelligence and energy, could not all but a few deaths be made at least easy and, in our ageing population, even happy? And should we not avoid this pressure to assume the right—even the duty—to take life, with all the implications and consequences that assumption carries?[24]

The writer was referring here, not just to the recently published report by Glyn Hughes, but also to a new study by Arthur Norman Exton-Smith and to the writings of Cicely Saunders, which were now beginning to appear in the medical literature. Exton-Smith was among the first since the joint committee to gather systematic evidence on the conditions of dying patients, while Saunders, from her earliest publications, was a vehement opponent of euthanasia, and a tenacious advocate of new thinking and a more positive approach to the care of the dying.

New evidence

Exton-Smith,[25] a physician at London's Whittington Hospital, reported his observations on a series of 220 patients, aged 60–101 years, in which he found that 25 per cent died within the first week of admission to hospital and 82 per cent within three months. Exton-Smith's purpose was to assess the pain and distress experienced by this group of patients, who had a range of malignant and non-malignant diseases, including conditions of the cardiovascular, locomotor, and central nervous systems. He argued, following Worcester,[26] that a 'natural death' in old age is experienced by but a few. Interestingly, given the hospice movement's subsequent emphasis on cancer, he suggested that this was less likely to be a cause of pain and suffering in the elderly than in younger patients, and that 'processes which lead indirectly to death are associated with most pain and suffering'—in other words, the chronic conditions. Nevertheless, effective analgesia in the form of narcotics was usually denied to these patients because of fear of habit formation. Exton-Smith noted that 'the suffering of this group of patients was aggravated by the fact that they were all mentally alert and recognised their helplessness'.[26] Echoing Glyn Hughes, Exton-Smith called for more comprehensive inpatient facilities, allied to hospitals, for terminally ill patients who could not be cared for at home.

Exton-Smith and Saunders had been in contact with each other since 1959, when he had visited her at St Joseph's Hospice in Hackney, in the East End of London. Subsequently she had commented on the draft of his paper in *The Lancet*, as had Dr Leonard Colebrook of the Voluntary Euthanasia Legalisation Society. At this time, and following initial training as a nurse and almoner, Cicely Saunders was working at the hospice as a medical research fellow, undertaking clinical work, and compiling detailed information on a series of patients admitted there.

Her first publication on the care of the dying appeared in 1958 in *St Thomas's Hospital Gazette*,[27] and the following year the *Nursing Times* published a series of six of her articles on the subject.[28] Like the earlier medical commentary of the 1950s, these articles relied heavily on individual case descriptions and were anecdotal in style. At the same time, they contained a level of detail that quickly indicated something more substantial. There was a narrative quality about the descriptions which reflected Saunders's interest in carefully listening to the patients' stories, and the studies she began led on to papers that reported a growing series of patients, from 340 in 1960[29] to 1 100 by 1967.[30] A striking feature of these papers was their articulation of the relationship between physical and mental suffering, seen in almost dialectical terms, each capable of influencing the other.[31] Through such writings, Cicely Saunders was also able to characterize a particular strategy for the care of the dying.

> The provision of an institution primarily devoted to what is often called terminal care should not be thought of as a separate and essentially negative part of the attack

on cancer. This is not merely the phase of defeat, hard to contemplate and unrewarding to carry out. In many ways its principles are fundamentally the same as those which underlay all the other stages of care and treatment although its rewards are different.[32]

To this extent she differed from Glyn Hughes in advocating that more special homes for the dying should be created as independent facilities, rather than within the ambit of hospitals. She also departed increasingly from Exton-Smith's focus on the dying aged, fastening her attention on those in the final stages of cancer, especially those with the most complex problems. She put it as follows, in a letter to Exton-Smith in 1960:

> Carcinoma of cervix I think is the most difficult both from the point of view of pain and of general distress; and I think that carcinoma of breast with bone secondaries probably comes second to that. In both these groups it is the patients between 40 and 60 yrs. who tax our skill.[33]

It may be no exaggeration to suggest that this brief remark captured a much wider division that was now beginning to take place between those who would concentrate their efforts on the care of elderly people in general, which included their dying, and those who would focus in particular on people, of any age, dying from a particular disease, namely cancer. The separation between these areas of specialization was to prove remarkably consequential in later years.[34] It was no doubt strengthened by the very different social constructions and meanings surrounding *old age* and *cancer*, which were appearing within the wider social consciousness. That said, there was considerable interplay at the time between the chief protagonists, as Cicely Saunders recalls:

> Dr Exton-Smith, who was looking after geriatric patients at the Whittington Hospital in Highgate, was asked by the Chairman of the Voluntary Euthanasia Society to look at the pain at the end of life among his patients, and he got in touch with me and said [let's] meet up with Dr Colebrook who was Chairman, and we had lunch together at the Royal Society of Medicine, and I said: 'Well you must come and do a round at St Joseph's', which we did and at the end of it he said: 'Well, you know, if everybody could have this sort of care I could disband the Society,' [chuckles] and he wrote to me, not saying quite that, but saying that this was solving a lot of the problems, but alas it's going to be a long time before it's going to be really widely spread. But he remained as a friend to the end of his life.[35]

Saunders was to become instrumental in defining a new knowledge base of care for those dying from malignancies. In 1960, her chapter on the management of patients in the terminal stage, published in Ronald Raven's six-volume set *Cancer*,[36] contained reference to 40 published works; by 1967, her pamphlet on *The Management of Terminal Illness*[37] included 184 references. By such means, a new field of healthcare practice—*terminal care*—began to be defined. Moreover, based on her experience as nurse, almoner (medical social worker), and doctor, the field was to be multidisciplinary in orientation. The early papers by Saunders draw on other contributions, less well known, but important in shaping this new discourse of terminal care. These include Margaret Bailey's survey of patients with incurable lung cancer, conducted at the Brompton and Royal Marsden Hospitals;[38] as well as a survey of public opinion on cancer;[39] and a study of delayed help-seeking among cancer patients, which noted that 'the fact of palliative treatment is not understood, and hospitals appear to be trying to cure all their patients and failing in a high proportion of cases'.[40]

Evidence from the United States was also harnessed, including a study of terminal cancer care among 200 patients in Boston,[41] and a paper on social casework with cancer patients.[42] It was from the United States in particular that concerns emerged on more psychosocial issues, such as truth-telling,[43] anxiety and depression,[44] and anticipatory grief.[45] These were further supported by the early psychiatric work of Colin Murray Parkes on bereavement and mental illness.[46] Cicely Saunders describes her introduction to his work:

> I read an article of his in 1965 and I wrote to him saying that I was working with the sisters who worked with families very intuitively. I knew the staff needed to look very carefully at our families, and the needs of bereaved people, although I felt that really good terminal care would make quite a difference to the course of bereavement. And he was really excited and rang me up and I went and had lunch with him and John Bowlby. From '65 he went out and spent a year in Harvard. And I met him out there and we shared some of the ideas then.[47]

By the mid-1960s, research papers on the care at home of people with terminal cancer were being produced by Eric Wilkes, the Derbyshire general practitioner who later founded St Luke's Hospice in Sheffield.[48,49] In one, he observed the following:

> There seems to be no valid reason why hospital provision for terminal care is so inadequate, or for the National Health Service to lean so heavily on the few Curie Foundation Homes and the devoted but over-worked religious institutions specialising in this work.[50]

The entry of Wilkes into the debate was not insignificant. He was a formidable character. Born into a Jewish family in Newcastle-upon-Tyne in 1920, he went to King's College, Cambridge, in 1937 to read English. He left Cambridge in 1939–1940 with a war degree and joined the army as a Signaller. After the war, he followed through earlier thoughts of a medical career by returning to Cambridge to study medicine. His early medical training was conducted at St Thomas's Hospital, London (1947–1952). After general medical, obstetric, and paediatric training, he made the decision to leave hospital medicine for a career as a country GP in Baslow, Derbyshire. Eric Wilkes had heard of Cicely Saunders at St Thomas's Hospital, and attended one of her talks on care of the dying in Sheffield in the 1960s.

> I'd not known her because she was senior to me, she qualified before me . . . but I had heard of her and of her interests, and I heard her lecture once so I thought, 'Well', you know, 'will it work outside of London?' Because in London the primary care was worse than anywhere else in the country. It was the world of the lock up surgery, the doctor who didn't speak very good English, the man who referred everything to hospital if it wasn't obviously just wanting a certificate off work. This was the stereotype from someone educated at a London teaching hospital, but there was too much truth in it for comfort. And so . . . I contacted her and did a round with her at St Joseph's and I was impressed by her, 'cause she's a very impressive and charismatic lady . . . But it was very 'hospital'. It was very 'hospital' indeed and I thought that we could probably involve a slightly broader community base, with all the quality control of nursing standards, the common policies of care that a hospital would have, in darkest Sheffield. And this festered in my mind for a year or so . . . [50]

Also closely associated with the transition from anecdote to evidence was Dr John Hinton, who had qualified in psychiatry from London's Maudsley Hospital in 1958. As a trainee doctor, he had developed an interest in the psychiatric problems of terminally ill patients. His paper on the physical and mental distress of the dying, written in 1962 and published the following year,[51] was based on research conducted in the period of 1959–1961 at a teaching hospital. Hinton pointed out that before Exton-Smith, only William Osler,[52] over 50 years earlier, had described the incidence, severity, and relief of distress among the hospitalized dying. Like Cicely Saunders, Hinton was inclined to a conversational approach to data collection; his 1963 research paper is based on interviews with 102 patients thought unlikely to live for more than 6 months, along with controls. Those in the dying group were more commonly depressed and anxious, and half were aware that their illness might be fatal. Physical distress was more prevalent in those with heart or renal failure (57 per cent) than in those with malignancies (37 per cent), and in general was more severe and unrelieved for longer within the dying group. He describes how the study came about and was conducted.

> Dr Clifford Hoyle put in helpful words with the board to get permission for me to see the patients if the consultants were willing. I was made an honorary . . . senior registrar at King's so I could pop round, and I joined in with some of the general medical rounds. And then I started interviewing the patients in the ward, with control, in the same order of an individual who hadn't got a fatal disorder but some sort of quite serious parallel disorder, and noted things were likely to affect their mood and state, which included how much pain they had, something about their family background, something about their religious beliefs, social class and so on, and then pop back

and see them from week to week to see how they fared. And I just sort of carried on pursuing that for a couple of years, certainly until I'd interviewed over a hundred patients in each group. I think what I saw as important, I think quite a lot of people saw as important at that time, is that if one was going to learn about terminal care and be able to teach it, there should be a factual basis of knowledge. And people at hospitals and teaching hospitals were still looking a bit askance at what they saw as a religiously inspired element, as if therefore people who had gone in with a sense of religious vocation, their evidence, such as it was, was biased and you really couldn't take that as the sort of facts you would teach students, or the sort of thing that ought to carry much weight against what one's own personal experience, or what otherwise people had said. And so it was important to bring this evidence together which had some air of respectability, scientific respectability to it. And so that, I think, is why the initial paper had been fairly well received, because it did seem to be factual, it was set out in a scientifically respectable way and it could carry weight. When I started out on the study I could find very little, by the time I'd come to writing up the study there were about six factual things, papers or little pamphlets published, and by the time I'd finished writing the book I'd discovered more and more were being done, which was good.[53]

Just as the Exton-Smith paper had stimulated comment in *The Lancet*, now the *British Medical Journal* took notice in a lead article, 'Distress in dying', acknowledging the absence of 'objective inquiries into this matter', and praising Hinton for building on the contribution of Exton-Smith. The article focused in particular on mental distress and the need for doctors, described as 'at a disadvantage in this respect compared with nurses and patients' relatives', to pay attention to the problem of such distress in their dying patients. By so doing, 'we should re-examine the comfortable supposition that the majority of our dying patients are not suffering overmuch, or they are not pondering the outcome just because they do not ask the most dreadful question of all'.[54]

In response, a letter from Cicely Saunders to the *British Medical Journal* underscored the importance of giving patients the opportunity to talk (so much a feature of her methodology and of Hinton's approach), seeing this as the pathway to the relief of both mental and physical suffering. More generally, however, this was an opportunity, building on a lead article in one of the world's most eminent medical journals, to press the wider case for terminal care homes.

> In spite of what is already being done in this field there remains a need for more units planned for those patients who do not need the resources of a large hospital and who cannot be at home. There is also a need for more research and still more teaching in this unusually neglected subject. It is hoped that a hospice being planned by a recently founded charity will be able to stimulate further interest and skill in this important part of medical care.[55]

The countervailing argument, however, was also in evidence. A letter published on the same page from Maurice Millard likewise welcomed the work of

Exton-Smith and Hinton, but proposed that those 'not inhibited by dogmatic religious views' should use these papers as an opportunity to 'think again about our "Hippocratic" ethical opposition to permissive euthanasia—that is at the request of the sufferer—when all the resources of physical, mental, and spiritual help have been exhausted'.[56]

In fact, Hinton did not offer objections to euthanasia on religious grounds (though Saunders certainly did). In his important paperback *Dying*, published in 1967, Hinton included a lengthy and balanced discussion of the subject. Acknowledging powerful arguments in favour of euthanasia, he also pointed to the need for a bulwark against the erosion of human values that prohibit the deliberate taking of life. At the individual level, judgements would become too complex, particularly in relation to the question of whose interests were being served by euthanasia—patient, friends, relatives, or professional carers? Acknowledging these difficulties, Hinton concluded his discussion on the subject by introducing the question of improving care for the dying.

> As long as we can truly say that for the patient merciful death has been too long in coming, there is some justification for euthanasia. It seems a terrible indictment that the main argument for euthanasia is that many suffer unduly because there is a lack of preparation and provision for the total care of the dying.[57]

This, of course, begged many questions. Although some development in ideas about terminal care was taking place in the late 1950s and early 1960s, this was not being matched by any significant innovation in service delivery. While *The Lancet* and *British Medical Journal* could endorse the importance of research and even hint that a new approach might undermine the case for voluntary euthanasia, no powerful medical lobby had sought to raise the profile of terminal care within the NHS, or call for the implementation of the kind of ideas set out in the Glyn Hughes report. Indeed, the overall provision of any form of specific care aimed at the dying was still sparsely distributed and remained in the hands of groups that were largely religious and charitable in organization.

Change and continuity

Within the period in Britain between 1948 and 1967, it is possible to identify two sets of characteristics in thinking and practice relating to terminal care. One emphasizes significant departures from previous discourses and gives prominence to innovation and change. The other draws attention to continuities with the foregoing period and indicates the persistence of elements from an earlier set of thinking about the care of the dying.

Four particular innovations can be identified, characterizing a new and distinctive disposition towards the care of the dying and constituting an emerging specialized focus within medicine and healthcare.

(1) A shift took place within the professional literature of care of the dying, from idiosyncratic anecdote to at least the beginnings of systematic observation. A series of studies made some claim to the collection of evidence (through surveys, the collation of official statistics, case note reviews, and patient interviews) about the social and clinical aspects of dying in the context of the British National Health Service. In 1948, the Physician in Ordinary to His Majesty the King could introduce a medical symposium on death and dying with no more than a series of anecdotes about the deathbed remarks of former prime ministers and bishops. Yet, within 15 years, leading articles in *The Lancet* and *British Medical Journal* were drawing on the evidence of recent research to suggest ways in which terminal care might be promoted and arguments for euthanasia might be countered.

(2) A new valorization of dying began to emerge that sought to foster concepts of dignity and meaning. This transition is illustrated, for example, in the shift from a discourse that sees the emotional relatives of a dying person as awkward troublemakers to one where individual subjectivities are acknowledged in 'a philosophy concerning death which has helped all of us to see death as an essential part of life and as life's fulfilment'.[58] Enormous scope was opened up for refining ideas about the dying process and exploring the extent to which patients should and did know about their terminal condition.

(3) An active rather than a passive approach to the care of the dying was promoted with increasing vigour. Within this, the fatalistic resignation of the doctor that 'there is no more we can do' was supplanted by the determination to find new ways of doing everything. We see here not an anti-medical stance on death and dying; rather a response to perceptions of the medical neglect of the dying, and potentially an expansion of medical dominion.

(4) A growing recognition of the interdependency of mental and physical distress created the potential for a more embodied notion of suffering, later expressed most successfully in the concept of 'total pain'. This constituted a profound challenge to the body–mind dualism, upon which so much medical practice of the period was predicated.[59]

At the same time, two powerful continuities are in evidence that serve as a bridge between earlier traditions and the emerging modern discourse of terminal care. The first of these can be seen in the way both periods reveal a sense of paternalism associated with the personality and influence of the doctor. Thus, Hugh Barber, a contributor to the 1948 symposium, could observe, 'It is a poor doctor who cannot find a thought suitable for the occasion',[60] while Saunders could quote the patient who thanked her 'not just for your pills, but for your heart'.[61] In each case, though expressed with different degrees of subtlety, the personality of the doctor is construed as a therapeutic instrument.

Secondly, the new thinking on terminal care drew directly on foregoing ideas of religious care and solicitude, coupled with charitable endeavour. In this sense, it reached back directly to some of the principles that had preceded the British National Health Service and that the welfare state had sought to usurp. This association with charity and voluntarism had a profound influence in turn in shaping the subsequent development of the modern hospice movement.

We have been considering here a particular stage in the history of British public policy. These were the golden years of postwar social democracy, the principles of which are summarized by Anthony Giddens.[62] Here we see the pervasive involvement of the state in social and economic life, with an emphasis upon collectivism, demand management, the confined role of markets, egalitarianism, modernization, and comprehensive welfare 'from the cradle to the grave'. Each of these elements, as it worked its way through the NHS, helped to produce a particular model of healthcare organization. This was one based on confidence in improvement, high levels of central planning, and a suspicion of voluntarism. Moreover, it gave particular succour to a form of medicine that emphasized cure and rehabilitation, which was becoming increasingly heroic and hubristic in character. One aspect of this was medical specialization where, as Geoffrey Rivett notes, the main growth was not in the traditionally glamorous fields, but in 'anaesthetics, radiology, pathology, psychiatry, and later, geriatrics'.[63] All of this had implications for terminal care.

Certainly, the goal of policy was to provide comprehensive welfare, free at the point of delivery, to all who needed help. In practice, the early years of the NHS were preoccupied with organizational matters, as the architect of the plan, William Beveridge, 'did not disclose how his airy assumption of a national health service could be implemented'.[64] This problem fell to Bevan, who displayed considerable skill in bringing the complex array of hospital provision under state control, and in remunerating general practitioners through state capitation fees. But as costs exceeded predictions by as much as 40 per cent in the first two years, severe strain was placed upon the budget of a nation still in the throes of economic constraint. Accordingly, there was little new hospital construction before 1995, while at the same time in 'the first phase of the NHS, despite formulaic expressions of good intention by ministers, it is difficult to avoid the conclusion that general medical practice was treated by the health departments as a receding backwater'.[65] The inclusivist ambitions of policy and the desire to provide care right to the grave were severely limited. In such circumstances, the priorities were acute care and rehabilitation. Care at the very end of life occupied a much lower place in the pecking order.

Nor, as we have seen, was terminal care of much interest to those doctors who were already in mid-career when the NHS was founded. Rather, it was the doctors who trained entirely in the postwar era that began to show a substantial interest in the issue: Cicely Saunders, John Hinton, Eric Wilkes, and Colin Murray Parkes, in particular. From backgrounds in hospital and general practice, in general medicine and psychiatry, these were the first individuals in Britain to establish studies about an aspect of care that had previously belonged in the realm of medical folklore. Loudon and Drury put it as follows in writing about the history of general practice.

> Unfortunately, we know little about the care of the dying in general practice before the 1960s, except that it was shrouded in silence. Few talked about it, wrote about it, or were taught anything about it as students.[66]

As they also note, terminal care as a branch of medicine requiring its own training and skills was virtually unheard of before 1960.

This leads onto a fascinating legal case, which came to court in 1957, amid a flurry of public interest and curiosity. It has been beautifully described and contextualized in an article by Caitlin Mahar.[67] On 18 March 1957, around the time Cicely Saunders was preparing her first article for publication in the *St Thomas's Gazette*, the middle-aged general practitioner John Bodkin Adams, of Eastbourne in the south of England, was charged, and subsequently acquitted of the murder of an elderly patient, Edith Alice Morell. The case is a landmark in the ethico-legal literature, for in his summing up, Justice (later Lord) Devlin took the view that it was lawful for a doctor to administer pain-relieving drugs, even though it was known that such a practice in this instance would hasten death. For Mahar, however, the case has wider ramifications of a historical nature. It reveals to us how at this time a branch of medicine was emerging that had a legitimate role in the care of the dying, where specific, what we might call proto-specialist skills, were emerging. The case was not simply an exercise in medico-legal ethics, but served to frame medicine's role in relation to the dying person and, thereby, began to set in train the medicalization of dying as well as to 'draw back the veil' on the practice of terminal care in this period.

David Armstrong has considered the notion of a silence being lifted from dying and death and a new emergent discourse.[68] He echoes the sense of growing medical jurisdiction over the deathbed at this time and is not convinced by sociological commentators such as Geoffrey Gorer,[69] Barney Glaser, and Anselm Strauss,[70] who wrote in the first half of the 1960s that death in modern culture was emerging from the status of taboo into a new era of openness. Rather he sees the new subjectivity of the dying person as an instrument of power, rooted in medical interrogation and the compulsion to speak. Certainly, the discourse of terminal care that began to consolidate in the early 1960s was partly based upon the narratives of dying people who had participated in the studies described in this chapter. That cohort of terminal care founders (patients and clinical researchers) did indeed open up a new discourse and began to carve out a territory capable of specialist recognition. Yet, they did so despite, rather than because of, the prevailing policy context. Attention to the development of terminal care in the period 1948–67, therefore, encourages us to be cautious about viewing the postwar NHS as a modernist bureaucracy dominated by technical reasoning. In the fissures between the new organizational structures of the health service and against a legacy of medical anecdote and paternalism on the care of the dying, a new field began to emerge. It sought to rekindle charitable endeavour as a supplement to state provision; it revived concerns with spiritual matters; and it commenced to carve out a field of technical expertise based on research evidence. But it also strengthened a transition to a new era in which the norms of medical practice came to be a source of power and one in which the ability to administer powerful pain-relieving drugs, even in the knowledge that this would hasten death, became legitimized. In the period from 1948 to 1967, *terminal care* under the NHS had experienced a challenging beginning, which would make the expansionist years that were to follow all the more remarkable. Yet, within the cracks of disinterest, seeds were germinating, and new practices were being explored that would soon have a profound effect.

Notes

1. **Klein R** (1983). *The Politics of the National Health Service*. London, UK: Longman.
2. **Harris J** (1996). 'Contract' and 'Citizenship'. In: Marquand D, Seldon A (eds.). *The Ideas That Shaped Post-War Britain*. London, UK: Fontana.
3. **Webster C** (1996). *The Health Services since the War, Vol II; Government and Health Care, the National Health Service 1958–1979*. London, UK: The Stationery Office.

4. **Quoted in Abel-Smith B** (1964). *The Hospitals 1800–1948: A Study in Social Administration in England and Wales*, p. 481. London, UK: Heinemann; and Murphy C (1989). From Friedenheim to hospice: A century of cancer hospitals. In: Granshaw L, Porter R (eds.). *The Hospital in History*, p. 234. London, UK: Routledge.

5. **Clark D** (1998a). Originating a movement: Cicely Saunders and the development of St Christopher's Hospice, 1957–67. *Mortality*, 3(1):43–63; Clark D (1998b). An annotated bibliography of the publications of Cicely Saunders–1. 1958–67. *Palliative Medicine*, 12(3):181–93.

6. Joint National Cancer Survey Committee of the Marie Curie Memorial and the Queen's Institute of District Nursing (1952). Report on a National Survey Concerning Patients with Cancer Nursed at Home. Chairman, Ronald Raven. London, UK.

7. **Glyn Hughes HL** (1960). Peace at the Last. A Survey of Terminal Care in the United Kingdom. London, UK: The Calouste Gulbenkian Foundation.

8. **Gough-Thomas J** (1962). Day and night nursing for cancer patients. *District Nursing* (November):174–5.

9. Review of Glyn Hughes HL, *Peace at the Last* (1960). *Lancet* 275:195.

10. **Horder L** (1948). Signs and symptoms of impending death. *Practitioner* 161(962):73–5.

11. **Leak, WN** (1948). The care of the dying. *Practitioner* 161(962):80–7.

12. Hospice History Project: interview with John Berkeley by David Clark, 18 June 1997.

13. Summary of proceedings, British Medical Association Annual Meeting (1957). Newcastle upon Tyne. *British Medical Journal* (3 August):286.

14. **Grant I** (1957). Care of the dying. *British Medical Journal* (28 December):1539–40.

15. **Hoyle C** (1944). The care of the dying. *Post-Graduate Medical Journal*, 20:119–123.

16. **Cole W** (1956). Foreword. In: Schiffin MJ (ed.). *The Management of Pain in Cancer*. Chicago, IL: Year Book.

17. **Acker CJ** (2002). *Creating the American Junkie: Addiction Research in the Era of Narcotic Control*. Baltimore, MD: John Hopkins University Press.

18. **Baszanger I** (1998). *Inventing Pain Medicine: From the Laboratory to the Clinic*. New Brunswick, NJ: Rutgers University Press.

19. **Vere D** (2004). In: Reynolds LA, Tansey EM (eds.). *Wellcome Witnesses to Twentieth Century Medicine, Vol. 21: Innovation in Pain Management*, p. 15. London, UK: Wellcome Trust Centre for the History of Medicine at UCL.

20. **Meldrum ML** (2003). The property of euphoria. In: Meldrum ML (ed.). *Opioids and Pain Relief: A Historical Perspective*, pp. 193–211. Seattle, WA: IASP Press.

21. **Reynolds LA, Tansey EM** (eds.) (2004). *Wellcome Witnesses to Twentieth Century Medicine, Vol. 21: Innovation in Pain Management*, pp. 10–11. London, UK: Wellcome Trust Centre for the History of Medicine at UCL.

22. **Euthanasia** (1950). *British Medical Journal* (9 December):1318–9.

23. **Millard CK** (1950). Euthanasia. Letter. *British Medical Journal* (23 December):1447.

24. **Euthanasia** (1961). *Lancet* (12 August):351–2.

25. **Exton-Smith AN** (1961). Terminal illness in the aged. *Lancet* (5 August):305–8.

26. **Worcester A** (1935). *The Care of the Aged, the Dying, and the Dead*. Springfield, IL: Thomas.

27. **Saunders C** (1958). Dying of cancer. *St Thomas's Hospital Gazette*, 56(2):37–47.

28. **Saunders C** (1959a). Care of the dying 1. The problem of euthanasia. *Nursing Times* (9 October):960–1. Saunders C (1959b). Care of the dying 2. Should a patient know . . .?

Nursing Times (16 October):994–5. Saunders C (1959c). Care of the dying 3. Control of pain in terminal cancer. *Nursing Times* (23 October):1031–2. Saunders C (1959d). Care of the dying 4. Mental distress in the dying. *Nursing Times* (30 October):1067–9. Saunders C (1959e). Care of the dying 5. The nursing of patients dying of cancer. *Nursing Times* (6 November):1091–2. Saunders C (1959f). Care of the dying 6. When a patient is dying. *Nursing Times* (19 November):1129–30.

29. **Saunders C** (1960a). Drug treatment of patients in the terminal stages of cancer. *Current Medicine and Drugs*, 1, no. 1 (July):16–28.

30. **Saunders C** (1967a). The care of the terminal stages of cancer. *Annals of the Royal College of Surgeons*, 41 (Supplementary issue; Summer):162–9.

31. **Saunders C** (1964a). The symptomatic treatment of incurable malignant disease. *Prescriber's Journal*, 4, no. 4 (October):68–73.

32. **Saunders C** (1964b). The need for institutional care for the patient with advanced cancer, Anniversary Volume. Cancer Institute, Madras:1–8.

33. **Cicely Saunders**, letter to AN Exton-Smith, 2 September 1960.

34. **Seymour J, Clark D, Philp I** (2001). Palliative care and geriatric medicine: Shared concerns, shared challenges. [Editorial.] *Palliative Medicine*, 15:269–70.

35. Hospice History Project: Cicely Saunders interview with David Clark, 2 May 2003.

36. **Saunders C** (1960b). The management of patients in the terminal stage. In: Raven R (ed.). *Cancer*, vol. 6, pp. 403–417. London, UK: Butterworth & Company.

37. **Saunders C** (1967b). The management of terminal illness. Part three: Mental distress in the dying patient. *British Journal of Hospital Medicine* (February):433–6.

38. **Bailey M** (1959). A survey of the social needs of patients with incurable lung cancer. *The Almoner*, 11(10):379–97.

39. **Paterson R, Aitken-Swan J** (1954). Public opinion on cancer. *Lancet*, 267 (23 October):857–61.

40. **Aitken-Swan J, Paterson R** (1955). The cancer patient: Delay in seeking advice. *British Medical Journal*, 1 (12 March):623–7.

41. **Abrams R, Jameson G, Poehlman M, Snyder S** (1945). Terminal care in cancer. *New England Journal of Medicine*, 232(25):719–24.

42. **Abrams RD** (1951). Social casework with cancer patients. *Social Casework* (December):425–32.

43. **Brauer PH** (1960). Should the patient be told the truth? *Nursing Outlook*, 8 (December):328–33.

44. **Bard M** (1960). The psychologic impact of cancer. *Illinois Medical Journal*, 118(3):9–14.

45. **Lindemann E** (1944). Symptomatology and the management of acute grief. *American Journal of Psychiatry*, 101:141–8; **Aldrich CK** (1963). The dying patient's grief. *Journal of the American Medical Association*, 184 (4 May):329–31.

46. **Parkes CM** (1964). Recent bereavement as a cause of mental illness. *British Journal of Psychiatry*, 110:198–204.

47. Hospice History Project: Cicely Saunders interview with Neil Small, 7 November 1995.

48. **Wilkes E** (1964). Cancer outside hospital. *Lancet*, 1 (20 June):1379–81.

49. **Wilkes E** (1965). Terminal cancer at home. *Lancet*, 1 (10 April):799–801.

50. Hospice History Project: Eric Wilkes interview with David Clark, 13 October 1995.

51. **Hinton J** (1963). The physical and mental distress of the dying. *Quarterly Journal of Medicine*, 32 (January):1–20.

52. **Osler W** (1906). *Science and Immortality*. London, UK: Constable.

53. Hospice History Project: John Hinton interview with David Clark, 25 April 1996.
54. **Distress in dying** (1963). *British Medical Journal* (17 August):400.
55. **Saunders C** (1963). Letter re: Distress in dying. *British Medical Journal*, 2 (21 September):746.
56. **Millard M** (1963). Letter re: Distress in dying. *British Medical Journal*, 2 (21 September):746.
57. **Hinton J** (1967). *Dying*, p. 148. Harmondsworth, UK: Penguin.
58. **Saunders C** (1965a). The last stages of life. *American Journal of Nursing*, 65(3):75.
59. **Clark D** (1999). 'Total pain', disciplinary power, and the body in the work of Cicely Saunders, 1958–1967. *Social Science and Medicine*, 49(6):727–36.
60. **Barber H** (1948). The act of dying. *Practitioner*, 161 (August):76–9.
61. **Saunders C** (1965b). Watch with me. *Nursing Times*, 61, no. 48 (26 November):1615–7.
62. **Giddens A** (1998). *The Third Way*. Cambridge, UK: Polity Press.
63. **Rivett G** (1997). *From Cradle to Grave: Fifty Years of the NHS*, p. 10. London, UK: King's Fund.
64. **Clarke P** (1996). *Hope and Glory: Britain 1900–1990*, p. 22. London, UK: Penguin.
65. **Webster C** (1998). The politics of general practice. In: Loudon I, Horder J, Webster C (eds.). *General Practice Under the National Health Service 1948–1997*, p. 22. Oxford, UK: Clarendon Press.
66. **Loudon I, Drury M** (1998). Clinical care in general practice. In: Loudon I, Horder J, Webster C (eds.). *General Practice Under the National Health Service 1948–1997*, p. 121. Oxford, UK: Clarendon Press.
67. **Mahar C** (2015). 'Roy Porter student prize essay, 2012'—Easing the passing: *R vs Adams* and terminal care in postwar Britain. *Social History of Medicine*, 28:155–71.
68. **Armstrong D** (1987). Silence and truth in death and dying. *Social Science and Medicine*, 24(8):651–7.
69. **Gorer G** (1965). *Death, Grief, and Mourning in Contemporary Britain*. London, UK: Cresset Press.
70. **Glaser B, Strauss A** (1965). *Awareness of Dying*. Chicago, IL: Aldine.

Chapter 4

Cicely Saunders and her early associates: A kaleidoscope of effects

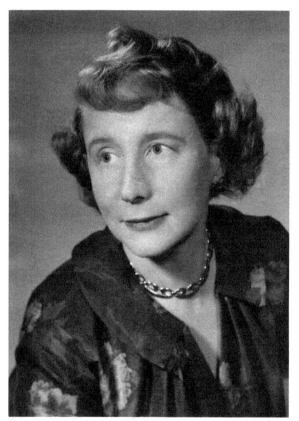

Figure 4.1 Florence Wald (1917–2008)
Florence Wald was Dean of Nursing at Yale University in 1963 when Cicely Saunders visited for the first time and delivered a lecture on the care of the terminally ill. The two struck up a friendship, which was to become deep and lasting. Wald and her associates went on to found the first modern hospice in North America, in Conneticut, where its work also helped pioneer the cause of Medicare funding for hospice care in the United States, which came into force in the early 1980s. Reproduced by kind permission of the Connecticut Women's Hall of Fame.

Changes in the wider context

The first decade of the National Health Service (NHS) in Britain had seen almost no traction in the development of state-provided care for the terminally ill and those with life-limiting conditions. Most doctors who offered a public opinion on the matter appeared rooted in a paternalist orientation to dying patients and their families and were generally fatalistic about what could be done, other than to make judicious use of morphine injections whenever possible. Where broader thinking and action had occurred—on matters of assessing need, formulating a policy response, and developing new services—these had all taken place *outside* the NHS and were spearheaded by charitable intervention and individually motivated endeavours. There was some limited contact between a small number of clinicians interested in these issues and, in a few cases, this extended to international exchanges of ideas and publications, study visits, and symposia. By the early 1960s some of this was consolidating. This chapter focuses on the specific contribution of Dr Cicely Saunders and her colleagues. It reveals how she drew, in a syncretistic fashion and internationally, on a wide range of clinical, religious, and cultural influences to formulate her particular approach to the care of the dying. Its elements could then, in turn, be rotated, like the pieces in a kaleidoscope, to produce differing results in different contexts. The end product was always recognizable, whether called hospice or palliative care, but its precise formulation could be a matter for local determination.

Working outwards from the homes for the dying

We have seen that in post-World War II Britain there was an increasing likelihood for dying people to spend their final hours in hospital rather than at home. At the same time, opinions varied on the form of institutional terminal care that should be provided to an ageing population, and concern about the experience of late-stage cancer patients was growing. During these years, small numbers of institutional homes were providing care for the dying, in the main outside the NHS, and in each case drawing on older traditions of religious care or philanthropy. After 1948, most of these continued to function in the shadow of the NHS. A few new developments had occurred in the immediate pre- and postwar period. In Scotland, the Irish Sisters of Charity had opened another hospice in 1950—St Margaret's at Clydebank. In addition, there were eight newly established Marie Curie residential cancer care homes, which were partly, but not entirely, concerned with terminal care. Elsewhere, in Birmingham the Taylor Memorial Home of Rest, first established in 1910 as a home for women with incurable internal malignancy, had been assimilated into the NHS as part of the Dudley Road Group of Hospitals. The Tarner

Home had opened in Brighton in 1936 and concentrated mainly on those close to the end of life.

These homes and hospices made up at best an incomplete patchwork. They were not a comprehensive system of service provision, nor did they see themselves as centres for excellence in teaching or research. Their influence was limited. Nevertheless, in some instances they had developed a cumulative wisdom that could provide the context for innovation. At St Luke's, for example, ideas about giving analgesia on a regular basis to prevent the recurrence of pain had become well established, and were described by the visiting physician Dr J Cameron Morris in an article[1] that appeared in the St Mary's Hospital Gazette in 1959. St Luke's also played host to a special symposium on the care of the dying held at St Mary's Hospital Medical School in May 1961, at which the responsibilities of the doctor (Dr P. Graeme), the almoner (H. Muras), and the chaplain (Revd R. Yale) were considered[2]; this must count as one of the earliest multidisciplinary symposia of its kind. Similarly, under the leadership of Sister Paula, the newly built (1957) Our Lady's Wing at St Joseph's, Hackney, had begun to attract interest from medical students and other visitors who, like Cicely Saunders, were impressed by the attention to individual care given there.

> Every new patient is greeted by one of the Sisters: 'You're welcome, Mr X.' He is welcomed into a place that will be home rather than just another hospital . . . He is welcomed by someone who is really interested in him as a person, in his soul and in his mind as well as his body. His physical burden will be lifted and his individual ways . . . will also be respected as far as possible.[3]

Despite the heavy emphasis upon charity and, in some instances, the idiosyncratic use of country mansions in inaccessible places, the homes for the dying made their contribution to the modern hospice movement that was soon to follow. Although they appeared at odds with most of the principles of a modern health service run on bureaucratic lines, these early homes nevertheless provided an enduring quality of self-help and voluntarism, which came to be reworked in a new context. Certainly, their influence on the development of Cicely Saunders's thinking was extremely important. While training in medicine, she visited and studied them. However, it was in a crucial seven-year period (1958–1965) while working at St Joseph's that she developed both her central clinical ideas and her plans for the creation of a new form of institutional provision for patients at the end of life—plans that would prove massively consequential.[4, 5]

Cicely Saunders—the person, the motivations, and St Christopher's Hospice

It is time to say more about the life of Cicely Saunders,[6] a woman who by the early 1960s was making a significant impact on discussions about care of the dying in British medicine and healthcare. Cicely Saunders was born in Barnet, Hertfordshire, on 22 June 1918, and at the age of 20 went to read Politics, Philosophy, and Economics at Oxford University. Two years later, she interrupted her academic studies to become a student nurse at the Nightingale Training School at London's St Thomas Hospital. When a back injury forced her to leave nursing, she returned to Oxford, and qualified in 1944 with a diploma in Public and Social Administration. She then commenced training as a hospital almoner, or medical social worker.

In 1948 while at the London Hospital, she cared for a dying Jewish émigré, David Tasma.[7] In a matter of weeks, following regular visits by her to the hospital, a profound bond developed between them. He had told her 'I only want what is in your mind and in your heart', and they discussed the possibility that one day she might found a special place more suited to those in his condition. Their exchanges served as a fount of inspiration, and they later became emblematic of Saunders's wider philosophy of care, but beyond them lay a great deal of further searching, both intellectual and spiritual. When he died on 25 February 1948, Tasma left Saunders with a gift of £500 and the encouragement: '*Let me be a window in your home.*'

Afterwards, she became determined to learn more about the care of those with a terminal illness. From the late 1940s, she worked at St Luke's as a volunteer, beginning to acquire knowledge of terminal care practice and drawing on the writings of Dr Howard Barrett, who had been a dominant figure in the work there until his death in 1921. In St Luke's she saw demonstrated some of the principles of pain relief, which she would later do much to promulgate. She then made the important decision to study medicine, starting in 1952, and qualifying in 1957 at the age of 38. In her final months as a medical student she drew together a comprehensive paper on the care of the dying,[8] describing four case studies of cancer patients with advanced disease, covering their medical histories in the years 1950–1956, and drawing on the experience of working at St Luke's, as well as visits to other London terminal care homes. The paper included sections on general management, nursing, the terminal stage, and pain. She also explored the value of special homes for terminally ill patients, refuting the notion that these are 'dismal and depressing places' and arguing for the importance of specialist experience in such areas as pain, fungating and eroding growths, mental distress, fear, and resentment. She wrote about the importance of telling the patient and relatives about the diagnosis and prognosis, and about the spiritual care of the patient and family.

In 1958, with funding from the Sir Halley Stewart Trust, Saunders was able to focus exclusively in this area and took up a position as research fellow at St Mary's School of Medicine, conducting work at St Joseph's Hospice in

Hackney, in the new hospital wing. It was here between 1958 and 1965 that Cicely Saunders taught herself as much as she could about the little-explored field of terminal care, and over time built up a nascent network of international contacts. She also formed her key ideas and specific clinical practice, laying down what were to become the fundamentals of *modern* hospice care. In particular, she became interested in the regular giving of analgesics and was attracted to the pain-relieving mixtures that were in use in London at that time. She also became fascinated by the relative merits of morphine and diamorphine for pain control, and her knowledge of new approaches emanating from the growing field of pain medicine steadily increased.[9]

At St Joseph's, she had an opportunity to put these ideas into practice and to develop a wider view of pain in the context of the whole person's suffering. Here she experienced a culture of religious solicitude that fostered her belief in the dignity of dying and the care of both body and soul. She also began teaching and, crucially, formulated her ideas about how all of this could be translated into a modern context with the potential for wider influence. She resolved to establish her own hospice, built for the purpose and founded on what she had learned from the London homes for the dying, and others she had studied at a distance.

Formulating the idea

By the end of the 1950s, Saunders was well established in the intention of dedicating the rest of her life to developing a modern approach to the care of the dying. She viewed this work as a matter of personal calling. She had studied medicine as a third profession, specifically to do something about the problem of pain in patients dying of cancer. In 1959, she was 40 years old, unmarried, and a committed Christian whose evangelical orientation was beginning to broaden. She had gained experience in the care of the dying as a nurse, social worker, volunteer, and researcher. However, at this time she was still seeking to clarify her initial ideas, striving to create a programme for action, and working hard to realize her vision.[4]

Crucial to this process was the question of the religious and spiritual foundation of the institution she was to establish. The issue had come early onto the agenda, after she had first raised it in 1959 while on a personal retreat at the Mother House of the Church of England, order of St Mary the Virgin, at Wantage, Berkshire. Subsequently, as she assembled around her a group of friends and associates who might help in her quest to found a new home for dying people, she quizzed them in turn on the question of religious priorities. Throughout the early part of 1960, there were numerous meetings, and extended correspondence with a clutch of evangelically inclined Anglican friends. By the end of the year, enough clarity had emerged that was sufficient to take the project forward. Though the protagonists were likely unaware of it, their deliberations were also to have a profound influence upon the later development of what became known as the hospice movement.

The first clear evidence of Cicely Saunders's strategic intentions about the formation of a new type of hospice came in the second half of 1959, when over the space of a few months she circulated a 10-page document to several associates, seeking their reaction. Entitled *The Scheme*, it set out *de novo* the structure and organization of a modern terminal care home containing 60 beds, together with staffing levels, capital and revenue costs, and contractual arrangements. By the end of the year, the 'home' in question had a name: St Christopher's Hospice. In this place, the patron saint of travellers would thus accompany those making their final earthly journey. Soon, a small but enthusiastic group of supporters had formed, including Dr Glyn Hughes, author of the recent report on the state of terminal care in Britain; Betty Read, head almoner at St Thomas's Hospital; and Jack Wallace, an evangelical friend and lawyer. The group was soon joined by Evered Lunt, Anglican bishop of Stepney; Sir Kenneth Grubb of the Church Missionary Society; and, very significantly, Dame Albertine Winner, deputy chief medical officer. Led by their enthusiasm, and the inspiration and energy of Cicely Saunders herself, they set about raising funds to bring the enterprise to realization.

Shirley du Boulay,[10] in her biography of Cicely Saunders, correctly argues that it was the connection with Dr Olive Wyon, then a retired theologian living in Cambridge, which did much to clarify a major issue that Cicely Saunders was grappling with at this time—the precise character of the proposed venture as a *community* and, in particular, the relationship between its religious orientation and medical practice. Among Olive Wyon's interests were the new religious movements and communities that had developed after World War II across Western Europe,[11] and it was her knowledge of these new waves of religious development that was to prove so helpful. Cicely Saunders first wrote to Olive Wyon on 4 March 1960 at the suggestion of Sister Penelope at Wantage. Her letter set out some of the background.

> The problem about which I wrote to Sister Penelope, is the question of the 'Community' which some people seem to see envisaged in my plan. I am tremendously impressed by the love and care with which the Irish Sisters give to our patients—something more than an ordinary group of professional women could ever give, I think. But I was not really thinking of anything nearly so definite as a real new Community, I think I was using the term in a much less technical way. I asked Sister Penelope if I was attempting the impossible to hope that a secular group of people without any kind of rule would be able to hold together and give the feeling of security, which I want so much to help our patients ... So I am really

faced with two problems. On the spiritual side, I know that the spiritual work is of paramount importance and while it goes hand in hand all the time with our medical work, it is the only lasting help that we can give to our people ... I feel that the work should be a definitely Church of England one rather than interdenominational and that it must be widely based in the Church, and not just in one wing. Then the other problem is this question of a Community of those who work there. I think myself that this matter should be held in abeyance; I may have adumbrated it in my scheme, but I had not been thinking of going any further than pray for the right people to come, and wait for the leading of the Spirit should He want us to draw together more definitely.[12]

In just over a week, Cicely Saunders had visited Olive Wyon, and came away feeling supported. She had been encouraged to make contact with the Sisters of Commaunaté at Grandchamp in Switzerland, and she wrote soon afterwards to the foundress, Sister Geneviève, who replied with information about the community and an invitation to attend a retreat in the summer. Her relationship with Grandchamp is an interesting one, but it does not seem to have strengthened Saunders's convictions about establishing her hospice as a form of new religious community. Initial attempts to make a connection with Grandchamp were surrounded with difficulties. In July 1960, a visit was postponed as she felt unable to leave Antoni Michniewicz, a patient for whom she had been caring over the past seven months at St Joseph's Hospice and who was now nearing death. In June of the following year, despite hesitation due to her father being unwell, it was possible to make a retreat there, but during this visit, she received the news that her father had died. Nevertheless, her links with the sisters at Grandchamp, who undertook to offer prayers for St Christopher's, continued for many years thereafter.

However, in 1960, two issues required resolution. The first was dealt with straightforwardly. The second remained unclear, and continued to be so, even as St Christopher's moved towards its opening day. First was the question of the precise religious character of the hospice. The debate was initially about in which theological wing of the Church of England the hospice should be located, but quickly ecumenical ideas and the influence of wider discussions about Christian unity became apparent. This was the extent of interfaith considerations; Britain in these years was still some way from addressing multicultural issues, and the question of non-Christian religions was not given any acknowledgement. That would come later. To a considerable extent, the issue was resolved pragmatically; a major source of charitable funds, the City Parochial Foundation, was showing an interest in the project, but the Foundation was unable under its terms of trust to give to a purely Anglican venture. As Saunders noted in a letter to her brother on 30 August 1960, 'I very much prefer something that is "inter" rather than "un-"',[13] referring here to the question of the denominational character of St Christopher's. Betty West, the mother of a friend from medical school, had captured this sentiment months earlier in a letter encouraging her not to be too dismayed by the apparent diversity of Christian influences that were helping to form St Christopher's: 'Could it be do you think, that in heaven our ways don't seem quite so different as they appear to us—and who knows that the edges might well melt away or not matter so much.'[14] By the end of 1960, the issue was settled and Cicely Saunders wrote the following to Olive Wyon on 6 December 1960:

> We have decided that it shall be an interdenominational foundation, although we will have something in the documents stating as firmly as possible that it must be carried out as a Christian work as well as a medical one . . . I found that I just couldn't think it was right to be exclusive. First of all, I could not be exclusively evangelical and thought that perhaps it would therefore have to be Anglican to keep it safe from heresy or secularisation. But then it didn't seem right to be that either, and in our legal Memorandum stands the statement: 'there shall be a chapel available for Christian worship', and I do not think that really we could be much broader than that![15]

For the second question however, which was that of St Christopher's as some form of community, no such categorical statement appeared. Indeed, there was a sense that this issue remained something to be explored and later encountered, even as the work of the hospice got under way. Whereas on the question of denominational identity, Saunders had felt that her supporters and collaborators were taking a broader view than her own, on this second issue it was as if they constrained her from the possibility of a more strongly communal orientation. The almoner Rosetta Burch expressed this clearly in a letter of 16 June 1960:

> To the outside world you must be first and foremost a medical concern . . . You are a Christian doctor not a spiritual leader with a medical vision. You have lots of experience of working with others on a professional basis but God has never given you the experience of being a member of a Community. Don't you think he would if that were to loom large in his plan?[16]

So it was that Cicely Saunders was able to write to Olive Wyon at the end of 1960 that 'it does not seem to have been right to think much more along the lines of a Community for this Home at the moment. I think that if we are to be drawn together in this work, that it will happen when we get there'.[15]

It is now clear that 1960 was an intensely formative year for Cicely Saunders. It was a year of deep reflection and consultation with others on the precise nature of her vision for St Christopher's Hospice. It was also the year in which the death of one particular patient, Antoni Michniewicz, created in her a

powerful and abiding sense of loss for a relationship that never came to frui-
tion, yet at the same time made her feel that she was capable of giving a true
authenticity and imperative to her subsequent work.[10] The issues that she had
explored at such length with her friends and associates during that year would
continue to tax her imagination and energy, but a clear and pragmatic turn
had occurred, which enabled the purposes of St Christopher's to be explained
succinctly to the wider public, including potential donors.

A few years later the supporters of St Christopher's, who had been meeting
since 1962 under the guidance of the bishop of Stepney (in what they called 'a
community of the unalike'), sought to clarify and set down in a statement the
basic principles of their work. It was at one of these meetings in June 1964 that
Olive Wyon 'made an excellent digest of my woolly thoughts', Cicely Saunders
later wrote in a letter to Wyon.[17] The result was a document entitled *Aim and
Basis* that was to have currency at the hospice for many years in the future.[18]
Within it, St Christopher's Hospice is defined as a religious foundation based
on the full Christian faith in God, with five listed underlying convictions.

1. All persons who serve in the hospice will give their own contribution in
   their own way
2. Dying people must find peace and be found by God, without being subjected to special pressures
3. 'Love is the way through', given in care, thoughtfulness, prayer, and silence
4. Such service must be group work, led by the Holy Spirit, perhaps in
   unexpected ways
5. The foundation must give patients a sense of security and support, which
   will come through a faith radiating out from the chapel into every aspect
   of the corporate life

The *Aim and Basis* provided St Christopher's with a statement of its underpinning motivation, which was reviewed from time to time in later years. The
discussions that preceded it, however, were to shape the work of the hospice
for many years to come. They reveal a profound sense of purpose coupled with
a rigorous approach to debate and discussion, which were essential in establishing the dominant themes in the world's first modern hospice.

Nevertheless, other energies were also required at this time. Saunders was
starting to receive visitors at St Joseph's and some of these developed into
wider connections and networks. One chilly day in November 1960, she received a visit from Dr K. J. Rustomjee, of Colombo, Ceylon. He had arrived
at St Joseph's Hospice in Hackney, eager to meet the enthusiastic doctor who
had been working there for the past three years improving her understanding
of terminal care, and also attracting attention for her publications in *Nursing*

Times[19] and a substantial chapter in Ronald Raven's recent six-volume edition on *Cancer*.[20] The two bonded immediately and soon 'Rusty' and she were in regular contact by airmail. A prodigious worker, he had done much to champion the need for cancer care in Ceylon. His interests spanned the entire spectrum, from disease prevention, to treatment and terminal care. In particular, Dr Rustomjee harboured his own ambition to establish a terminal care home in Colombo. Some years before, the Ceylon Cancer Society, of which he was president, had pledged to the then Prime Minister S. W. R. D. Banderanaike that the Society would establish such a home for the shelter, comfort, and peace of terminal cancer patients. By the time he and Cicely met in 1960, plans were well advanced, and by early 1961, an elephant was deployed to clear the site in preparation for building.

In their correspondence, Saunders and Rustomjee exchanged news and updates on their parallel projects. While her letters were carefully typed by her secretary of the time, Jenny Powley, his were handwritten. Hers were quite formal, his less so. Nevertheless, they did exchange pleasantries about the weather, bouts of illness, and events of the day. Over the years, she updated him on the fundraising work for St Christopher's and the successes and disappointments along the way. She also supplied him with a steady stream of reprints of her publications from the period.

At the same time, he shared with her the details of the home being built in Ceylon, its facilities, and how it was to be staffed. He then sent a full album of photographs depicting the opening ceremony, of 19 November 1962, with its ritual lamp-lighting and Buddhist ceremonial paraphernalia. Dr Rustomjee had many connections. When he visited St Joseph's in 1960, he was *en route* to Ceylon from the United States where he had undertaken a wide-ranging tour of organizations and facilities engaged in cancer care. On this same visit, he had also attended the Fourth National Cancer Conference, which had taken place over three days in September at the University of Minnesota, Minneapolis. He wrote up the whole experience in a report sent to Cicely Saunders in February of the following year. When in summer 1962, she contemplated making a similar visit, he was quick to step in and make the necessary introductions. These included a connection to Mildred Allen at the American Cancer Society, as well as to the Home of our Lady of Good Counsel in Minnesota. The following year Cicely Saunders headed to the States herself, followed in his footsteps for part of the way and, on concluding her trip, she did as her friend by preparing a detailed report that she could pass on to others. Her connection with the American Cancer Society was to be long lasting and beneficial.

By the time Cicely Saunders met with Dr Rustomjee, she was already actively engaged in communicating her ideas to those who had the material wherewithal to turn them into reality.[4] By early 1961, there were architectural drawings of the hospice and an estimated cost of £376 000, although in the inflationary environment of the times the architect warned that prices were rising daily. By 1966, with building well underway at the chosen location in Sydenham and the project budget now estimated in excess of £400 000, there was still a considerable shortfall in funds and the national financial climate was not favourable. By early 1967, the overall budget stood at £480 000; but by June a team of staff had been appointed, the building commissioned, and the first patients were beginning to arrive. By opening day, 24 July 1967, all debts had been cleared.

There was also a growing critical mass of friends, acquaintances, supporters, and colleagues gravitating around the hospice founder and her ideals. Dr Mary Baines is a good example. She had been at medical school with Cicely Saunders, as had Tom West and Gillian Ford, who also became closely involved with St Christopher's. Baines and Saunders were active in the Christian Union, but after graduation they lost touch with each other. Mary Baines recalls how they were reconnected.

> I'll never forget this . . . it was in 1964 and I was just at home, I think it was a Sunday evening, Ted [her husband] was out and by chance, I turned on the radio, and there was my old friend Cicely Saunders, whom I'd lost touch with since medical student days. And she was giving *This Week's Good Cause* appeal on behalf of the hospice she was going to found. And I sent her three pounds, which was a lot of money then, and especially for an impecunious clergy wife and became a 'Friend of St Christopher's'. And then a really extraordinary thing happened really, in that Ted was invited to become a vicar in Beckenham, which is three miles from here. This was in April '67. So we moved up to this area before St Christopher's was opened. And before coming up, I had arranged, and gained, another part-time GP job in Norwood, which is not very far from here. I then came to the opening of St Christopher's in July '67 and at that time met up with Cicely again. And she sent me a letter which I've got a copy of, saying, and it was a very clever letter, and I've laughed about it with her many times, saying that as I was a local general practitioner, and would be sending patients to St Christopher's, would I like to come round one afternoon and have a private look round with her? And of course it was a great big hook. And I fell for this. So I guess it would have been somewhere, August/September, that sort of time, that I came, and she then asked me whether I would like to join her at St Christopher's . . . And I didn't think I wanted to work with the dying, and all sorts of very good reasons, because it was a very unusual thing. And I sent this letter to her, and even suggested the name of a friend of mine who might be interested in the job, as I patently wasn't! But then we thought it over, and prayed it over, and talked it over, and it did seem the right thing to do . . . And joined here in April '68. So that's how it happened.[21]

An article published in *The British Hospital Journal and Social Service Review* soon after the opening amounts to a prospectus for St Christopher's. The hospice 'will try to fill the gap that exists in both research and teaching concerning the care of patients dying of cancer and those needing skilled relief in other long-term illnesses and their relatives'.[22] On opening, the hospice contained 54 inpatient beds, an outpatient clinic, and also 16 beds available for the long-term needs of staff and their families. There would be an emphasis on providing continuity of care for those able to return home and there were plans for a domiciliary service. Relatives' involvement in care would be encouraged. Research on pain, developed at St Joseph's, would be extended. The hospice was to be 'a religious foundation of very open character', and there was a sense that the whole endeavour amounted to an elaborate pilot scheme, which could have extremely far-reaching implications.

Indeed, Cicely Saunders and others around her, even before the opening of St Christopher's, had an intuition that this was a project far greater than building a single new hospice, taxing though that may have proved. Colleagues wrote from America urging her to realize that she had two obligations: one, to develop the work of her own organization, and the other to spread her learning further afield. Therefore, the practical accomplishment was about more than St Christopher's Hospice alone. Links had already been established with a wide range of hospitals and nursing and theological colleges, and there were plans for exchange visits with colleagues in Yale, Harvard, and other centres in the United States. Within a few years, voluntary, independent terminal care services would proliferate, and the modern hospice 'project' would have a growing influence on policy and practice. A nascent movement[4] was under way, the starting point of which, most marked in the British context, was outside rather than within the formal healthcare system. For this movement to flourish and grow, it would need Cicely Saunders to apply enormous levels of personal energy, commitment, and resilience.

Three visits to the United States: 1963, 1965, and 1966

A striking feature of Cicely Saunders's practice during the formative years of St Christopher's was the way in which she forged links with and drew strength from colleagues in America. She made three key visits in the 1960s that yielded a huge amount in terms of knowledge, insight, and collaboration. The first, in the spring of 1963, was a *tour de force*, covering the East and West Coasts and making connections with individuals from a variety of disciplines who would become influential in forging modern ideas about 'hospice care' across the United States. Afterwards she compiled a detailed report of her experiences and went to considerable trouble to send copies to many people she had met. Indeed, she soon ran out of copies, as demand outstripped supply, and she underestimated the level of interest her report would attract. Three of those who she encountered on the trip were asked to become vice presidents of St Christopher's Hospice. The first was Professor Gordon Allport, a contact made through her brother, Christopher, who was chair of psychology at Harvard University and executive secretary of the Ella Lyman Cabot Trust, which supported the visit to the United States. Second was Theodate Soule, who was a consultant to the Hospital Social Service Fund in New York; and third was the Revd Almon Pepper, director of the department of Christian Social Relations at the Protestant Episcopal Church in New York, who subsequently attended the laying of the foundation stone for St Christopher's in 1965.

For a lone Englishwoman who had never before travelled to the United States—a country at that time in considerable foment over civil rights and international relations issues—it was a remarkable tour, lasting eight weeks. Taking in New York, Yale, Boston, Washington DC, Los Angeles, San Francisco, and Vancouver, she visited 18 different hospitals of varying types, as well as the National Institutes of Health in Maryland. Along the way, she met with doctors, psychiatrists, nurses, social workers, social scientists, and hospital chaplains. As she noted in the introduction to her report, 'I found it a great asset that I was able to go in my threefold capacity of nurse, social worker, and doctor. It made my own approach a broad one and also made me "one of them" when I discussed problems with each of the different professions'.[23] There are sections in the report dealing with pain in terminal cancer; the mental pain and distress of dying patients; relatives and their problems; homecare programmes; nursing homes; and the work of chaplains.

Several of those she met on this visit became long-standing colleagues and friends, and over time, an elaborate network of individuals concerned with the care of the dying began to develop. In the early 1960s, letter writing was their main means of communication, coupled frequently with an enthusiastic exchange of reprints from recent publications. In these years, Cicely Saunders was a prolific letter writer and her correspondence gives remarkable insight into the energy with which she pursued her links with the United States and the benefits that flowed from them. Her personal papers contain no less than 15 archive boxes of correspondence with US colleagues, much of it covering the period up to 1967.[24]

Regular correspondents on the US West Coast were Dr Herman Feifel, chief psychologist at the Veterans Administration in Los Angeles and author of key early work on aspects of death and dying,[25] as well as Esther Lucille Brown, a social anthropologist working with the Russell Sage Foundation. Brown was a frequent source of letters and ideas, with specific interests in improving the quality of nursing care. On the East Coast, Florence Wald (Figure 4.1), then dean of nursing at Yale; Professor Gordon Allport; and Carleton Sweetser, chaplain at Memorial Hospital, New York, all became close colleagues.

The link with Yale was to be particularly significant. Cicely Saunders's first visit had been at the invitation of Dr Bernard Lytton, a former surgeon at the London Hospital, from where he had visited St Joseph's Hospice once a week. On moving to Yale and learning of her planned visit to the United States, he invited his friend to lecture at the university. At Yale, she spoke first to the student council in the school of medicine and then, by special request, repeated the talk the following day to the faculty of postgraduate nursing. It was at the second lecture that she met Florence Wald, who remarked afterwards, 'this is what we have lost, and this is what we need'.[23] Florence Wald explains:

> Virginia Henderson was doing an annotated index of all the nursing literature from the 1900s. Everything that was written in English, and so when she saw the name Cicely Saunders she knew what she was doing. I knew nothing about her at all and she said, 'Well you must go and hear her.' And I said, 'Well, I'm stuck because I'm supposed to be introducing the speaker at another forum and I don't feel as if I can get out of that.' So she said, 'Well, I'll go and I'll report back to you,' which she did and just said, you know: 'We've got to get this woman to speak.' She was talking about how she's taken care of the dying patients, and our faculty and our students were struggling very much with the intensive treatment that was going on and on for patients and how they were debilitated by this and the . . . inability to stop using those kinds of therapeutics. And so I immediately got in touch with Bernie Lytton and Cicely agreed to meet our students in faculty the next day, and I gathered as many people from the hospital as I could in the departments of social work and so forth, and she did the same presentation. And of course it just 'wowed' us. And then you have to realise that in that same month in May 1963 that's when the marches of Martin Luther King began in Selma . . . and Alabama. And it was in that summer that doctors and nurses also began to join in the fight against segregation. So that, you know, it found us at a time when the kinds of things that we were suffering, there suddenly seemed to be a way to move.[26]

As Joy Buck, the historian of American nursing, has noted, Wald was at a critical point in her own life in 1963. She was an advocate for major reforms in nursing education and the clinical role of the nurse and, like Cicely Saunders, believed that professional nurses should eschew non-nursing tasks to give more focus to care at the bedside. She was also deeply sceptical of the drive within medicine to prioritize technology and cure over an emphasis on care of the person. Wald believed the hospice concept offered the perfect vehicle by which she and other reformers could achieve a 'brave new world' in health-care with nursing and medicine working together as equals at the helm.[27]

Saunders's second visit to the United States began in May 1965 in New York with a lecture at the Postgraduate Center for Mental Health, followed by speaking engagements at Yale, and meetings at the Massachusetts General Hospital with Professor Lindemann, a psychiatrist and an early bereavement researcher who developed the concept of *anticipatory grief*. On this occasion, as before, financial assistance from the Ella Lyman Cabot Trust was made available, mediated through the good offices of Gordon Allport. Saunders observed to Esther Lucille Brown: 'I cannot be too grateful to them, for not only did they help me very substantially on my last trip but they also sent me a most generous gift as "seed money" for St Christopher's. I am most un-deservedly fortunate in the people who support us.'[28] In the case of Gordon Allport, there was also an emotional and intellectual debt, for it was he who in 1963 had first introduced her to the writings of the Austrian psychiatrist and concentration camp survivor Viktor Frankl, in particular *Man's Search for Meaning*,[29] which was to prove very influential upon her thinking in the coming years.

American colleagues also proved to be useful sounding boards about events and developments taking place back in London. After writing to Esther Lucille Brown about leaving St Joseph's in the autumn of 1965, her friend wrote back: 'It must have been a wrench to leave St Joseph's after seven years there. I believe, however, that this is a most auspicious moment for you to sever ties and prepare yourself psychologically for initiating your new pro-gram in your own new hospital.'[30] On another occasion when the finances of St Christopher's had taken an upturn, Brown wrote: 'Isn't it marvellous how financial sustenance at this very trying moment has been coming to your rescue. I do hope that it will continue . . .'[31]

Regular correspondents all received the newsletter, which contained details of the development of St Christopher's; this was clearly an important chan-nel of communication and often featured in the exchange of information and the words of encouragement that were such a feature of the letters to and from Saunders's American colleagues. Perhaps resulting from the cultural disposition of the Americans with whom she made contact, there was a ten-dency for her to receive greater recognition of the wider import of her work from across the Atlantic than she found at home. In due course, the UK–US traffic became two-way, with American visitors arriving in London to visit St Joseph's and the still-to-be-opened St Christopher's with increasing regu-larity. Anselm Strauss, for example, a San Francisco-based sociologist and pioneering researcher on awareness contexts in dying,[32] visited her in the autumn of 1965 and many others followed.

Saunders's third sojourn to North America began in April 1966 with six weeks at Yale, before moving on to Cleveland and then Vancouver. She began her lecture at the Yale School of Nursing as follows.

> This is the third time I've been at Yale, and like St Thomas's Hospital, I think you must begin to feel that every time you get rid of me, I come back in another capacity. This time I've chosen the title, 'The Moment of Truth', not because I just want to discuss the perennial question, 'Should you tell the dying patient the truth?' (which is not really the right question anyway), but because meeting dying patients and facing the fact of death does concern all of us, whether we're nurses, doctors, social workers, psychologists, or of any other discipline; I think perhaps almost most of all, when we're just members of the family. This moment is, or should be, a moment of truth, not just a matter of words, who says what and when, but something much more deep and far-reaching than that in its implications, implications which, I think, are relevant to the whole of life.[33]

While at Yale, Saunders also met with two major figures in the emerging psychiatry of dying and bereavement: Elisabeth Kübler-Ross, who was visiting from Chicago; and Dr Colin Murray Parkes (with whom she had already become acquainted in London), who was spending a year in Harvard. Their first encounter brought together a remarkable triad of names that were to become synonymous with the modern care of the dying and bereaved. Kübler-Ross was at that time working as a psychiatrist at the Billings Hospital and University of Chicago, where she had begun to embark on a series of important and widely acclaimed works on death and dying.[34] Parkes was later to work closely with Saunders at St Christopher's, where he brought his psychiatric perspective not only to the care of patients and families, and to research, but also to the support of the staff. Speaking in 1996, he recalls some of the early contacts in the field.

> It must have been about 1964 I made my first visit to America. I was lecturing on bereavement at Billings Hospital in Chicago where I'd been invited by Knight Aldrich who was the Professor of Psychiatry there. And he said, 'Well, I've got an interesting trainee, a junior psychiatrist working here on the subject of psychological reactions to terminal illness.' And he introduced me to this lady, Elizabeth Kübler-Ross, and I actually sat behind a one-way vision screen and watched her interviewing patients. She was collecting information for what was subsequently her book, *On Death and Dying* it was called, in which she described the stages of dying.[35]

Cicely Saunders continued her frequent visits to Yale, and in June 1969, she was awarded the degree of Doctor of Science from the university. Her friendship with Florence Wald was also to grow and thrive over many years, particularly as developments for America's first hospice, in New Haven, got underway. Likewise, Colin Murray Parkes got involved with St Christopher's from the outset and became a lifelong colleague.

Publications in the United States

In February 1964, Cicely Saunders received an invitation from the Episcopal Church Center in New York to write for *The Living Church,* an American journal, on the topic of 'Facing death'. The theme of the article[36] was the denial of death, and in it Saunders suggested that acceptance of one's mortality was a route to finding meaning in life itself. She described the case of a young woman, about to die, who wanted to assist her children and husband through the process, and the reactions of the staff. The paper rejected the apparently 'swift and easy' solution of euthanasia in these cases and suggested that religious peace may come to dying people in such circumstances, even those who seem most indifferent and recalcitrant before the end.

Inspired by this, Dorothy Nayer, associate editor of the *American Journal of Nursing,* then wrote to Cicely Saunders requesting an article that would help readers come to terms with their attitudes about death and assist them in their service to dying patients and their families. Characteristically, a detailed correspondence ensued. Saunders checked on various themes that might be explored in the article, discussed the use of illustrations, and asked for advance copies of two papers by Anselm Strauss that were to appear in the journal at a later date. The editor was delighted with the result. Illustrated by impressive line drawings, the article[37] took as its theme the idea that the last stages of life should not be seen as defeat, but rather as life's fulfilment. Using case illustrations from St Joseph's Hospice (although the name appeared incorrectly in the text), it focused on the nursing aspects of care, especially the responsibility of telling or not telling the patient about the prognosis. Readers were as enthusiastic as the editor, and nurses from around the country wrote in with their endorsement. Typically, each received an individual and detailed reply from Saunders. Her association with this publication continued, and in December 1971 the journal ran a special feature on 'Christmas at St Christopher's'; indeed, some of those who had read the original article in 1965 were still writing in with requests to visit the hospice many years later.

The third American publication for which Cicely Saunders wrote in the decade before St Christopher's Hospice opened was the journal *Geriatrics.* This took the form of an extended letter, produced by invitation.[38] In it she gave details of the developing plans for St Christopher's and the goal of making an impact on the lack of interest in research, teaching, and care relating to the dying. It emphasized the concept of a 'hospice' as a resting place for travellers and pilgrims, something between a home and a hospital, and also noted that the project had already established international links, particularly with the United States.

By late 1965, Saunders's reputation in the United States was growing rapidly. Media attention followed, along with requests for her help and guidance, as well as for her to speak at meetings and write for other publications. In May 1966, she took part in a series of lectures at Western Reserve University in Cleveland, Ohio (later published[39]), titling her talk 'The Moment of Truth: Care of the Dying Person'. The other lecturers included Lawrence Leshan ('Psychotherapy with the Dying Patient'); Anselm Strauss ('Awareness of Dying'); Robert Kastenbaum ('Psychological Death'); and Richard Kalish ('The Dying Person: Impact on Family Dynamics').

By autumn 1966, there was a sense of an emerging critical mass of interest not only in her work, but also in the wider field to which she was contributing. By now, what Robert Kastenbaum referred to as 'our little death newsletter'[40] had evolved into the journal *Omega*, and was reproducing her article 'A medical director's view', which had appeared first in the journal *Psychiatric Opinion*.[41] These early publications in the United States spanned several key disciplines and audiences: the church, nursing, medicine, and psychiatry. America was learning about the work of Cicely Saunders and she was learning from America.

Perhaps more than anything, it was the opportunity America afforded for access to a range of disciplines and perspectives that was so important to Saunders as she, in her own words, picked up ideas like a sponge. Here she could meet chaplains, such as Carleton Sweetser, struggling with the care of the dying in a modern hospital setting, and social workers, like Theodate Soule at the United Hospital Fund of New York. In addition, there were psychologists, sociologists, and anthropologists who, unlike most of their contemporaries in Britain, were also contributing to developments in the field of care for the dying.

There was also the new cadre of pain specialists, such as Stanley Wallenstein and Ray Houde, at Memorial Hospital, New York, and Henry Beecher at Massachusetts General Hospital, from whom she received encouragement and inspiration for her own studies. It resulted in a rich mixture of influences and skills, and one that was later to become such an important aspect of the modern multidisciplinary specialty of hospice and palliative care. There was a sense of forces coming together, of new possibilities. A special relationship was forged between Cicely Saunders and her American friends and colleagues during the mid-1960s. The relationship was part of an extraordinary groundswell of interest in the care of the dying and the bereaved, out of which new social movements and professional specialities were quick to emerge, not only in Britain and the United States, but worldwide. Moreover, in this process the activities at St Christopher's were to prove a key demonstrator.

Making St Christopher's work

The opening of St Christopher's Hospice marked the culmination of one aspect of Cicely Saunders's vocation, but also the mere beginning of its true purpose. For now, the work of the hospice had to be developed in earnest, and its ideas and principles would require testing in practice. Above all, it would begin to serve as a source of inspiration to so many others in Britain and around the world. From the opening of the hospice in the summer of 1967 to the autumn of 1985, a period of 17 years, Cicely Saunders was its medical director. The job involved a huge quantum of daily clinical work and numerous organizational responsibilities, as well as financial concerns, which were never far away. There was also the need to attract appropriate staff, and in this, her methods were often direct. She had attended medical school with Tom West, who later joined the Church Missionary Society; when she heard he was resigning from the mission field, she quickly wrote to him.

> And when Cicely Saunders heard that I had given in my notice, she wrote and offered me the job of her deputy at St Christopher's. I wrote back and said that I was delighted and flattered to take this very honourable job on. I had been home on such occasions as the laying of the foundation stone for St Christopher's. I had followed the progress, through my mother and through Cicely, of the building, and thought and prayer behind St Christopher's, and I was deeply honoured. But I did say I can't join you for two years, therefore, there's not much future in this offer. And she wrote back and said, 'In that case we'll wait for you,' which I often think is the greatest compliment that Cicely ever paid me. The other thing that she did, which was wonderful, was in the six months or year before I left Northern Nigeria, she sold a rug which she'd inherited from her father and came out to see me in my context, saying, 'You're going to spend the rest of your working life in my place, I think I better come out and see your place before you leave it!' And that was good. So in 1972 I left Nigeria and came back, and started a job as deputy to Cicely in 1973, by which time, of course, St Christopher's was up and going. And I reckon that I came in as, not perhaps the second wave, but as the one and a half wave of new appointments.[42]

For Saunders these years were filled with regular travelling, lecturing, and writing. They were times of growing recognition for the movement that she and her colleagues had initiated and of the global contribution she was making to improvement in the care of the dying. With this came a measure of fame that Cicely Saunders might hardly have contemplated in 1959. Quite quickly, there were awards and honours, plaudits, and frequent publicity. At the same time, her personal life became more rewarding and eventually led to marriage. These were expansive years, professionally and personally rich, and lived to the full.

At St Christopher's, new staff continued to be appointed, procedures and policies were developed and refined, and the credibility of the service in the local area was confirmed. The hospice became a training ground for many doctors who would subsequently shape the direction of hospice care elsewhere in the United Kingdom and further afield. At a symposium in October 1970, an overview of the work of St Christopher's emphasized several points.[43] Despite a continuing reliance on charitable grants and gifts, the NHS now contributed two-thirds of the running costs; indeed, the research programme, together with the experimental outpatient and domiciliary service were at that time wholly supported by NHS funding. The hospice included 54 inpatient beds and the Drapers' Wing had 16 'bed sitting rooms' for elderly people. A teaching unit was now under construction. By 1970, some 400 patients died at the hospice each year, and between 40 to 60 patients were discharged home, at least for a short time. Soon, the majority of patients had their first encounter with the hospice's services in their own homes.

At the same time, plans for other hospices modelled substantially upon St Christopher's were beginning to emerge—in Sheffield, Manchester, Worthing, and elsewhere in the United Kingdom. There was a constant flow of communication between the staff of St Christopher's and others across the United Kingdom with similar aspirations. As this collectivity of enthusiasm developed, policymakers began to take a closer interest in the subject, and the first national symposium on the care of the dying was held in London in November 1972, with the proceedings published in the *British Medical Journal*.[44]

A paper by Cicely Saunders that appeared in 1968 in a Catholic quarterly elegantly captured St Christopher's orientation to care for those in the last stages of life.[45] It called for a positive approach that sees this as a time not of defeat, but of life's fulfilment, recognizing that there will be many different paths to life's ending. Here comfort and care become the prominent aims in a 'middle way' between too much and too little treatment, where understanding and compassion are vital. In subsequent years and first articulated in the American paper of 1966, we see in Saunders's thinking a growing attention to notions of *personhood,* particularly in the family context. This greater focus on families was regarded as an important distinction between care at St Christopher's and earlier work at St Joseph's. The emphasis on *person* speaks in turn of a growing influence from psychology and theology. Saunders was increasingly interested in how the *person* is seen always as someone in inter-relationship with others, and how the person, thus seen, is *being* in the face of physical deterioration. At such moments, 'full time concern for the patient' becomes essential. Elsewhere, this is neatly captured in the statement that professional work in this area has two key dimensions: 'We are concerned *with persons* and we are concerned *as persons*.'[46]

Nevertheless, such caring, it was acknowledged, could be costly to those who gave it. At St Christopher's, emphasis was placed upon the development of a multidisciplinary team that could work together to explore the needs of individual patients at the deepest level, but which could also support and enrich itself—not only through the inclusion of a range of professional per-spectives, but also of volunteers, as well as the children of staff, and the elderly residents living in the Drapers' Wing. A sense of community was fostered that might serve to ameliorate the emotional consequences of work involving constant exposure to loss, sorrow, and bereavement. In this context, atten-tion was needed to support the staff and this was fostered at St Christopher's through small-group discussion, and the regular involvement and psychiatric perspective of Colin Murray Parkes.

Between 1970 and 1974, a working party of the Church of England Board for Social Responsibility sought to develop an Anglican contribution to the debate on euthanasia. Saunders drafted two chapters in the group's report.[47] All members endorsed the recommendations, including: (1) the undesirabil-ity of extending the term 'euthanasia' to incorporate the withdrawal of artifi-cial means of preserving life, or to include the use of pain-relieving drugs that may marginally shorten life; (2) the assertion that if all care of the dying was at the highest standard, then there would be no *prima facie* case for euthanasia; and (3) the belief that such standards are more hindered by ignorance than by money and staff shortages. A few years later, Cicely Saunders was active in commenting on and expressing opposition to Baroness Wootton's *Incurable Patients Bill*, which came to the House of Lords in 1976, and about which Saunders feared the *right* to die might be interpreted by some as a *duty* to do so. Likewise, in 1977 and 1978, she took part in debates at the Royal Society of Health and the Union Society, Cambridge, where in each case, motions in support of the legalization of euthanasia were defeated. Her position was clear: euthanasia is not a matter of desisting from active treatment; it is a kill-ing act and the person who requests it has been failed in some way by others. She did acknowledge, however, that both sides in the euthanasia debate have a vendetta against pointless pain and impersonal indignity, although their solutions were radically different in character.

From the outset, there was an emphasis on the science and the art of caring at St Christopher's. The early research programme had three predominant themes:

1. Psychosocial studies of grief and bereavement
2. Evaluation of St Christopher's approach in relation to other care organizations
3. Pharmacological work on the relative merits of different narcotics and their management[48]

These endeavours marked a consolidation of the work by the early founders of modern terminal care in the late 1950s and early 1960s.[49] Nevertheless, in a 1973 volume on health services research, the state of this emerging field could be stated quite starkly: 'The position of terminal care in this country is at present unsatisfactory.'[50] Although interest in research into terminal care was growing, much of it remained descriptive and anecdotal, and high quality work was desperately needed to promote a rational approach to the care of the dying. Small achievements could be significant, as when Cicely Saunders was asked to write a chapter on terminal care for a volume on the scientific foundations of oncology,[51] the editors thought it necessary to justify their reasons for including a contribution from such an underdeveloped medical field, where scientific foundations were only just being laid.

By 1978, some important evidence was emerging from research studies conducted at St Christopher's. Work by Colin Murray Parkes showed that unrelieved pain, as reported later by families, was found among 8 per cent of patients at St Christopher's Hospice, compared to 20 per cent of those in local hospitals and 29 per cent of those being cared for at home.[52] Building on the work of the St Christopher's research fellow, Dr Robert Twycross, it was also possible to state beyond reasonable doubt that morphine had become the preferred analgesic over diamorphine, and that the previously much heralded mixtures containing alcohol and cocaine should be discontinued.[53] We shall learn more of this work in Chapter 5.

Cicely Saunders could also observe that whereas 'science tries to look at things in their generality in order to *use* them; art tries to observe things—and people—in their individuality in order to *know* them'.[43] The photographs that she used in her lectures and publications illustrated the importance of welcoming patients and the involvement of the staff's own children in the life of the hospice. Patients were encouraged to write about their experiences in prose and poetry; others made drawings and paintings that served as a window on suffering. Such an approach was also fostered through the sense of St Christopher's as a community in which many who served felt supported by some form of religious commitment.

By 1976, *Nursing Times* was publishing a revised and updated set of Cicely Saunders's articles that had originally appeared in 1959 and had caused so much interest at that time.[54] There was a sense that the field of terminal care was beginning to consolidate. There were opportunities to review changes that had occurred over the previous 17 years and to address new debates and issues, such as 'living wills', 'furore therapeutics', and 'meddlesome medicine'. By now, the increasing use of the term *palliative care*, coined by Balfour Mount in 1974, was coming to denote the transferability of ideas developed in the hospice into other settings, including hospital and home, as well as a broadening reach beyond those imminently dying.

The introduction of the term has been well documented.[55] Inspired by reading the works of Elizabeth Kübler-Ross and Cicely Saunders, the Montreal-based surgeon Balfour Mount had visited St Christopher's in 1974 and been impressed by what he saw there. On his return to the Victoria Hospital, however, he found himself unconvinced by the term 'hospice', which in French Canada had overtones of an impoverished and undignified home for the moribund. He pondered on an alternative term that might find wider applicability. His ruminations on the issue soon bore fruit.

> And I remember thinking that, as I considered various options, I was actually shaving one morning and thought that if there are intensive care units and coronary care units and surgical intensive care units, there could be a *palliative* care unit. That seemed to have a nice ring to it; and a palliative care service. I wasn't at that point too sure about the etymology of the word 'palliative' but I liked the concept. Of course to palliate at that point was in common usage, meaning to treat for goals other than cure, and particularly locally we talked about palliative radiation therapy, and it was simply meant that it was acknowledged to be non-curative. And so that took me to the *Oxford English Dictionary* and to a little search into the origins of the term and to the Latin word *pallium*, to cloak and to hide and so forth and so on. And it seemed to me that it passed from 'to cloak or to hide' to 'to improve the quality of', and that seemed to be *exactly* what it was that we were trying to do. So it seemed to me a perfect term. . . One of the advantages of getting in on the ground floor of something is you can shape it anyway you want and tell people: 'This is the way it needs to be done' and you have some advantage. I wrote Robert Twycross and perhaps Cicely, but certainly Robert's response I remember very clearly: he wrote back immediately to say, 'I do not like your term *palliative*, it won't do at all,' and proceeded to give me a critique as to why it wouldn't do. And as I recall Cicely's reaction to the term initially was not very positive as well, but later she wrote a letter to say, you know, 'I have to say I was wrong, the term is excellent.'[56]

It seems that Saunders adopted the term rather quickly. Within a few years of Mount's original visit to St Christopher's, she was using it freely in her own writing and referring to the Montreal palliative care unit as its source. It was a significant step. The terminology had now changed and the focus of care had moved beyond its original locus, that of the hospice, to encompass other settings.

In 1978, Cicely Saunders's first book—which many had awaited for so long—finally appeared. It was an edited volume, with contributors who had been involved directly with the work of St Christopher's. Her first chapter was important in opening up a debate about the relationship of terminal care to the 'cure' and 'care' systems, arguing that no patient should be inappropriately locked into one or other system.[53] By the early 1980s, she was at even greater pains to suggest that the 'terminal' condition of a patient may not be an irreversible state,[57] and 'active', 'palliative', and 'terminal' care could each be seen as overlapping categories.

The professional and clinical achievements of these years, however, cannot be allowed to mask the organizational issues and difficulties that also had to be overcome. There were losses and stresses that from time to time affected the whole of St Christopher's. In 1970, Dr Ron Welldon, the hospice's first research fellow, suddenly died, the news reaching Saunders just as she was about to give a lecture in the United States. The following year, the death of Lord Thurlow after a period of illness marked the loss of a chairman in whom she had great confidence and who had been such a support to her in the hospice's formative years. There was also unwelcome publicity following the screening on German television of a film about the hospice. There were periodic financial crises, including a major one in 1974. In addition, some visitors to the hospice, on writing about their experiences, were critical about staff morale and the management culture, some describing it as authoritarian and inflexible, and concerned only for the patients and not for the staff. Yet, in 1979 a foundation group at St Christopher's that was formed to review the early statement of *Aim and Basis* drafted by Olive Wyon could find little reason for any significant reorientation.

In 1980, St Christopher's held its first international conference. It was characterized as the hospice's *Bar Mitzvah* and involved participants from 17 different countries.[58] The contributions contained a growing conviction that the work of hospice should be integrated with general medical practice, forming a complementary resource and service. There was now an expanding confidence that the ideas and influences developed in the world of charitable hospices were beginning to affect the mainstream healthcare system.

Life, faith, and work at St Christopher's

Following a rather dramatic religious experience in the 1940s, Cicely Saunders had moved in Christian evangelical circles for several years, yet she was also at ease in the Roman Catholic ambience of St Joseph's Hospice. She was inclined to worship intently and to read widely. Her personal beliefs and ideas about religion were central to her plans for St Christopher's. It is through the evolving sense of a personal *calling* that we see this most visibly. Strongly evidenced in her early correspondence about the idea of St Christopher's, where many passages refer to a sense of being drawn by God to this work, within a few years it was as if the *whole project* had taken on a sense of something predetermined and part of a greater purpose. The nurturing of the oft-repeated phrase of David Tasma—'*Let me be a window in your home*'—contributed to this. It was akin to a 'foundation myth' that served constantly to reinforce the origins and purpose of the hospice. There is a sense in which if David Tasma had not existed, it might have been necessary for her to invent him. Yasmin Gunaratnum has written eloquently about David Tasma and Cicely Saunders. She shows how 'the dark coordinates' of his life have been left unexamined in the build-up of oft-repeated anecdotes about him. Why did Cicely Saunders have recourse to an outsider, a migrant, for the formation of her thinking? Did he serve as a foreign founder whose timely departure from the narrative prevented him becoming disruptive and unruly? As Gunaratnum explains: 'In bringing David Tasma's fractured story with her into the public domain, it has been put into a relation with injustices suffered by other dying people, allowing pain to be many things, weighty in its historical content, but not without company.'[59]

In this context, there could be no straightforward and simplistic blueprint for the hospice and the 'window' it contained. The precise character of St Christopher's religious status had required careful consideration. Undoubtedly, St Christopher's became an organization of Christian motivation; but in opting for a strategy of practical action in the world, rather than an ethic of caring located outside it, Saunders and her colleagues gave birth to an idea capable of wide adaptation and development across many cultures and settings.

It is now clear that during the years leading up to 1967, the hospice movement was already in formation. The opening of St Christopher's in July of that year should be seen not as the start of the modern hospice initiative, but as the culmination of a project that made that initiative possible. Although the term *hospice movement* had not yet appeared in the lexicon of terminal care in 1967, its foundations were firmly established. From 1958 to 1968, between the ages of 40 and 50, Cicely Saunders had undertaken a remarkable personal project. Harnessing her own faith, her private sorrows, her professional skills, and her indomitable energies, she had gathered around her the support of friends and colleagues who, with her, made St Christopher's Hospice possible.

These years inevitably made huge demands on her personal resources. A life devoted to giving also needs to receive support and nourishment, both through the realm of faith or meaning, and in relationships with others. Cicely Saunders was capable of prodigious quantities of work at this time, but she could also be vulnerable to illness. A life lived in the public domain needs to foster some private areas for reflection, recuperation, and intimacy. In 1968, Cicely Saunders's mother died in St Christopher's; she had remained active up to the end, and it was a loss that could be accepted by her daughter. However, just over two years after the hospice opened, there was a long period of sick leave for its founder, from the autumn of 1969 to March 1970.

From 1963 onward, her relationship with the artist Marian Bohusz-Szyszko had been developing, slowly and intermittently. He was born in Poland in 1901 and had studied fine art and painting at the universities of Wilno and Cracow, and at the Warsaw Academy of Fine Arts. He spent most of World War II as a prisoner of war before making his way to Italy in 1945. Subsequently he settled in London, where in the autumn of 1963 he held a major retrospective at the Drian Galleries in Porchester Place. Here his work had come to the attention of Cicely Saunders. She fell in love with the paintings and then with him. She became his patron, and his work was prominently displayed in the hospice from the outset. He had professed his love for her, but was not free to marry. His long-estranged wife in Poland was still alive, he continued to support her financially, and his Catholic faith precluded any divorce. It seemed an arrangement that suited him, but over time, a suitable solution evolved. In 1969, Cicely Saunders moved from Lambeth to Sydenham to live closer to the hospice. There, with Polish friends of Marian, she purchased a house where the two couples could share accommodation. They thought of it as their 'kibbutz', and it was to prove a lasting domestic arrangement. In 1975, Marian's wife died, but it was not until 1980, 17 years after they had first met, that Cicely Saunders and Marian Bohusz-Szysko married. She was 61 and he 79. At first, their news was kept secret to all but a tiny group of close friends, but gradually it became public and delighted many. Her last five years as the hospice medical director were spent as a married woman. Secure in her status, she had never been so content with her personal life.

Wider influence

Between 1967 and 1985, Cicely Saunders produced, individually and with others, around 85 publications; they appeared in several languages and in numerous countries.[5, 60] She wrote for clinical journals and prestigious textbooks, for religious publications, and for the wider public. Three clinical and organizationally oriented books on hospice and palliative care appeared, and one of them was soon produced in a second edition. There was also a collection of poems and prose pieces produced for patients, families, and professionals encountering suffering and disease—an early example of a contribution to the *medical humanities* as an aid to teaching.[61] Her work appeared in the proceedings of symposia and conferences, it was described in magazines and newspapers, and it became the subject of documentary films. Links with overseas colleagues produced a growing cross-fertilization of ideas.

Over this period, there was also growing reflection on the state of the 'movement', which was developing around hospices and similar centres. As her work matured, Saunders reflected more on the early origins of homes and hospices for the dying. She also had increasing evidence that palliative care was something that could be developed in many modes and settings—extended beyond its initial successes with cancer patients to include those with non-malignant conditions, such as motor neurone disease, and in due course, the challenge of caring for people with AIDS. Above all, its major purpose came to be seen as the improvement of care within the mainstream setting, not through the continuing proliferation of hospice units, many of them independent charitable organizations, but rather through education and training, and the broader diffusion of appropriate knowledge, skills, and attitudes. Accordingly, we see at this time the first discussions taking place about the creation of national representative bodies to promote the interests of hospices and those who work with them, such as Help the Hospices and the Association of Palliative Medicine.

Of course, St Christopher's Hospice had a vital role to play. Initially it was the only centre for specialized education and training in the new field of terminal care. There was a tidal wave of requests from around the world to visit, to work, and to spend time at the hospice. Initially these were encouraged, even fostered. By 1975, there were 2 000 visitors per annum; special hours were set aside for visitors each week, and in due course, some tours were conducted in French. However, some enthusiasts could be a cause of irritation, and Saunders was not well disposed to those who made extravagant journeys to St Christopher's at the expense of overlooking growing expertise nearer to home.[62]

There were also many people who wished Cicely Saunders would come to them. In her years as medical director, she visited North America around a dozen times, developing close professional links as well as an enduring friendship with Balfour Mount and the palliative care service at the Victoria Hospital, Montreal, and at the international conference that he hosted every two years starting in 1976. She also made visits to many other countries, including Yugoslavia, Belgium, Australia, Israel, and South Africa. Her network of collaborators expanded, and her influence and reputation grew, as she was increasingly acknowledged as the 'founder' of the modern hospice movement.

It is apparent that Cicely Saunders did not see her vision as something that could only be bounded by the discipline of medicine. The concept of 'total pain', for example, which she formulated in her writings of the late 1950s and early 1960s, adopted a wide-ranging definition of suffering, taking into account physical, emotional, psychological, social, and spiritual elements (see Chapter 5). These were to be addressed through the combined skills of a multidisciplinary team of carers, including volunteers, with active attention to family involvement. In seeking to establish a foundation outside the parameters of the British National Health Service in the form of an independent, charitable hospice, Saunders also displayed scepticism about the ability of the mainstream healthcare system to foster her ambitions. In the early 1980s, looking back on the period described here, she again recalled David Tasma's reference to the window: 'We moved out of the National Health Service with a great deal of its interest and support, in order to build round that window. We moved out so that attitudes and knowledge could move back in . . .'[58]

Moving out meant establishing an inpatient hospice followed by a home-care service that would become a centre for the development of three activities: clinical care, teaching, and research. In Britain, others quickly followed along similar lines, although few combined these three elements at the same level. In the United States and elsewhere, the ideas were developed and adapted according to local context and quite quickly a separate trajectory emerged for 'hospice' based on homecare and a federal system of funding. The notion of 'community' developed in the St Christopher's model was elaborated in various ways. The multidisciplinary team became emblematic of hospice care; there was a great deal of emphasis on the active relationship between hospices and their local communities. As the work developed, it took on the character of a reformist social movement, challenging prevailing attitudes, practices, and modes of organization. At St Christopher's, which served as the locus of an international movement for many years, the idea of community remained important and continued to be worked through in various ways.

The real importance of the early thinking that led to St Christopher's, how-ever, is evident in what was decided *against*. The ideas not pursued and those allowed to recede are themselves significant. In particular, it was confirmed that this would not be an endeavour located in a narrow evangelical wing of the Church of England, where the primary purpose would be to proselytize. Nor was it to be a new religious community where a dedicated few, operating outside of the secular world, would care for the dying in their own special way. Instead, it became a foundation underpinned by the Christian religion, where the contributions of various disciplines were also fostered; where critical reflec-tion through research and teaching could take place; and where others came to develop their own ideas and skills. Without such omissions and commissions, it is difficult to envision the subsequent development of the international hospice-palliative care movement. The success of the vision, as defined, notwithstand-ing its Christian focus, was that it could be emulated or elaborated, and this made possible its global spread in the following years. It was also the engine for the initial articulation of a new field of medicine—one with the potential to de-velop its own separate interests and skills, which would gain wider recognition from the medical establishment, as we shall see in Chapters 5 and 6.

Notes

1. **Cameron Morris J** (1959). The management of cases in the terminal stages of malig-nant disease. *St Mary's Hospital Gazette*, 65(4):4–6.
2. **Graeme P, Muras H, Yale R** (1961). The terminal care of the cancer patient. *St Mary's Hospital Gazette*, 67(4):118–125.
3. **Saunders C** (1962). Working at St Joseph's Hospice, Hackney. Annual Report of St Vincent's, Dublin, pp. 37–9.
4. **Clark D** (1998). Originating a movement: Cicely Saunders and the development of St Christopher's Hospice, 1957–67. *Mortality*, 3(1):43–63.
5. **Clark D** (1998). An annotated bibliography of the publications of Cicely Saunders–1. 1958–67. *Palliative Medicine*, 12(3):181–93.
6. **Clark D** (2002). *Cicely Saunders. Founder of the Hospice Movement: Selected Letters 1959–1999*. Oxford: Oxford University Press; Clark D (2006). Introduction. In: Saunders C (ed.). *Selected Writings 1958–2004*, pp. xiii–xxvii. Oxford, UK: Oxford University Press.
7. **Saunders C** (1981). The founding philosophy. In: Saunders C, Summers D, Teller N (eds.). *Hospice: The Living Idea*, p. 4. London, UK: Edward Arnold.
8. **Saunders C** (1958). Dying of Cancer. *St Thomas's Hospital Gazette*, 56(2):37–47.
9. **Clark D** (1999). 'Total pain', disciplinary power, and the body in the work of Cicely Saunders, 1958–1967. *Social Science & Medicine*, 49:727–36.
10. **Du Boulay S** (1994). *Cicely Saunders: The Founder of the Modern Hospice Movement*, rev. ed. London, UK: Hodder and Stoughton.
11. **Wyon O** (1963). *Living Springs: New Religious Movements in Western Europe*. London, UK: SCM Press.
12. **Cicely Saunders**, letter to Olive Wyon, 4 March 1960.

13. Cicely **Saunders**, letter to Christopher Saunders, 30 August 1960.
14. **Betty West**, letter to Cicely Saunders, 11 February 1960.
15. Cicely **Saunders**, letter to Olive Wyon, 6 December 1960.
16. **Rosetta Burch**, letter to Cicely Saunders, 16 June 1960.
17. Cicely **Saunders**, letter to Olive Wyon, 11 June 1964.
18. *St Christopher's Hospice Aim and Basis* (1964). Mimeograph, revised.
19. **Saunders C** (1959a). Care of the dying 1. The problem of euthanasia. *Nursing Times* (9 October):960–1; Saunders C (1959b). Care of the dying 2. Should a patient know . . .? *Nursing Times* (16 October):994–5; Saunders C (1959c). Care of the dying 3. Control of pain in terminal cancer. *Nursing Times* (23 October):1031–2; Saunders C (1959d). Care of the dying 4. Mental distress in the dying. *Nursing Times* (30 October):1067–9; Saunders C (1959e). Care of the dying 5. The nursing of patients dying of cancer. *Nursing Times* (6 November):1091–2; Saunders C (1959f). Care of the dying 6. When a patient is dying. *Nursing Times* (19 November):1129–30.
20. **Saunders C** (1960). The management of patients in the terminal stage. In: Raven R (ed.). *Cancer*, vol 6, pp. 403–417. London, UK: Butterworth and Company.
21. Hospice History Project: Mary Baines interview with Neil Small, 10 July 1996.
22. **Saunders C** (1967f). St Christopher's Hospice. *British Hospital Journal and Social Service Review*, 77:2127–30.
23. **Saunders C** (1963). Report of Tour in the United States of America (Spring), unpublished.
24. **King's College**. Archive Catalogues: Saunders, Dame Cicely. Available at http://www.kingscollections.org/catalogues/kclca/collection/s/10sa88-1, accessed 7 July 2014.
25. **Feifel H** (1959). *The Meaning of Death*. New York, NY: McGraw-Hill.
26. Hospice History Project: Florence Wald interview with Neil Small, 29 February 1996.
27. **Buck J** (2009). 'I am willing to take the risk': Politics, policy, and translation of the hospice ideal. *Journal of Clinical Nursing*, 18(19):2700–9.
28. Cicely **Saunders**, letter to Esther Lucille Brown, 16 February 1965.
29. **Frankl V** (1962). *Man's Search for Meaning*. Boston, MA: Beacon.
30. **Esther Lucille Brown**, letter to Cicely Saunders, 30 November 1965.
31. **Esther Lucille Brown**, letter to Cicely Saunders, 17 November 1966.
32. **Glaser B, Strauss A** (1965). *Awareness of Dying*. Chicago, IL: Aldine.
33. **Saunders C** (1966). Unpublished text of lecture at Yale School of Nursing (28 April).
34. **Kübler-Ross E** (1969). *On Death and Dying*. London, UK: Routledge.
35. Hospice History Project: Colin Murray Parkes interview with David Clark, 10 January 1996.
36. **Saunders C** (1964). Death. *The Living Church*, 26 (July):8–9.
37. **Saunders C** (1965). The last stages of life. *American Journal of Nursing*, 65(3):70–5.
38. **Saunders C** (1966). Terminal patient care. *Geriatrics*, 21(12):70–4.
39. **Saunders C** (1969). The moment of truth: Care of the dying person. In: Pearson L (ed.). *Death and Dying: Current issues in the treatment of the dying person*, pp. 49–78. Cleveland, OH: Case Western Reserve University Press.
40. **Robert Kastenbaum**, letter to Cicely Saunders, 13 October 1966.
41. **Saunders C** (1966). A medical director's view. *Psychiatric Opinion*, 3(4):28–34.
42. Hospice History Project: Tom West interview with Neil Small, 28 January 1997.
43. **Saunders C** (1971). The patient's response to treatment. A photographic presentation showing patients and their families. In: *Catastrophic Illness in the Seventies: Critical Issues and Complex Decisions*, pp. 33–46. Proceedings of the Fourth National Symposium, 15–16 October 1970. New York, NY: Cancer Care.

44. **Saunders C** (1973). A death in the family: A professional view. *British Medical Journal*, 1(844):30–1.
45. **Saunders C** (1968). The last stages of life. *Recover* (Summer):26–9.
46. **Saunders C** (1972). A therapeutic community: St Christopher's Hospice. In: Schoenberg B, Carr AC, Peretz D, Kutscher AH (eds.). *Psychosocial Aspects of Terminal Care*, pp. 275–89. New York, NY and London, UK: Columbia University Press.
47. **Saunders C** (1975). Member of Church of England Board of Social Responsibility Working Party. *On Dying Well: An Anglican Contribution to the Debate on Euthanasia*. London, UK: Church Information Office.
48. **Saunders C** (1967). *The Management of Terminal Illness*. London, UK: Hospital Medicine Publications Limited.
49. **Clark D** (1999). Cradled to the grave? Terminal care in the United Kingdom, 1948–67. *Mortality*, 4(3):225–47.
50. **Saunders C, Winner A** (1973). Research into terminal care of cancer patients. In: **McLachlan G** (ed.). *Portfolio for Health 2. The Developing Programme of the DHSS in Health Services Research*, pp. 19–25. Nuffield Provincial Hospitals Trust. London, UK: Oxford University Press.
51. **Saunders C** (1976). The challenge of terminal care. In: Symington T, Carter R (eds.). *The Scientific Foundations of Oncology*, pp. 673–9. London, UK: Heinemann.
52. **Murray Parkes C** (1979). Terminal care: Evaluation of in-patient service at St Christopher's Hospice Part 1. Views of surviving spouse in effects of the service on the patient. *Postgraduate Medical Journal*, 55:517–22.
53. **Saunders C** (1978). Appropriate treatment, appropriate death. In: Saunders C (ed.). *The Management of Terminal Malignant Disease*. London, UK: Edward Arnold.
54. **Saunders C** (1976). Care of the dying—1. The problem of euthanasia. *Nursing Times*, 72:1003–5.
55. **Mount B** (1997). The Royal Victoria Hospital Palliative Care Service: A Canadian experience. In: Saunders C, Kastenbaum R (eds.). *Hospice Care on the International Scene*. New York, NY: Springer.
56. Hospice History Project: David Clark with Balfour Mount, 14 March 2001.
57. **Saunders C** (1981). Current views on pain relief and terminal care. In: Swerdlow M (ed.). *The Therapy of Pain*, pp. 215–41. Lancaster, PA: MTP Press.
58. **Saunders S, Summers D, Teller N** (1981). *Hospice: The Living Idea*. London, UK: Edward Arnold.
59. **Gunaratunum Y** (2013). *Death and the Migrant: Bodies, Borders and Care*. London, UK: Bloomsbury.
60. **Clark D** (1999). An annotated bibliography of the publications of Cicely Saunders— 2. 1968–77. *Palliative Medicine*, 13:485–501.
61. **Saunders C** (1983). *Beyond All Pain: A Companion for the Suffering and Bereaved*. London, UK: SPCK.
62. **Clark D** (2001). A special relationship: Cicely Saunders, the United States, and the early foundations of the hospice movement. *Illness, Crisis, and Loss*, 9(1):15–30.

Chapter 5

Defining the clinical realm

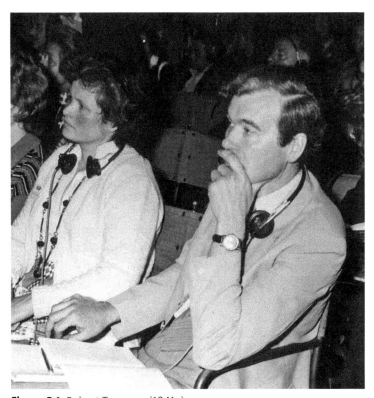

Figure 5.1 Robert Twycross (1941–)
On completion of his further medical training, Twycross took up a position as clinical research fellow at St Christopher's Hospice, in London in 1971. Here he embarked on a groundbreaking series of studies on the actions of morphine, in combination with other agents, on pain caused by advanced malignant disease. His studies revolutionized the practice of cancer pain relief and led to the abandonment of complex mixtures, such as the Brompton Cocktail. After establishing his own palliative care unit in Oxford, he went on to teach extensively and in particular to influence the work of the World Health Organization as it began to engage with pain and palliative care as global, public health issues. He is pictured here with his wife Deidre Twycross at the First World Congress on Cancer Pain, held in Venice in 1978.

A loose web of activity

The pioneers of hospice and palliative care in the 1960s and 1970s carried a heavy burden. Anyone associated with this work was likely to be involved in lobbying, advocacy, and innovation in service delivery, as well as being drawn into fundraising and capital development. Clinicians had to forge a loose web of activity, values, and aspirations into a recognizable and definable clinical domain. This meant characterizing the patients who could most benefit from the new and developing approaches—the paradigm case being the person dying of cancer. It also meant understanding and codifying patients' main clinical signs and symptoms, taking into account that these might be social, psychological and spiritual, as well as physical. In particular, it called for a detailed understanding of pain. This led to some rich areas of pharmacological as well as phenomenological insight, to efforts to describe and measure pain, and to innovative approaches in pain relief. Such work found these pioneers engaging in radical new methods for the use of strong opiates and, in time, building new research-based knowledge and understanding of these drugs. By the early 1980s, these efforts were taking on significant international dimensions and the World Health Organization (WHO) began to support innovation in global cancer pain relief. Gaining recognition for this newly acquired knowledge through publication in established journals and the creation of specialist outlets, as well as in the building of affinities between colleagues, ideas, and practices, were all crucial elements in defining palliative medicine as a distinctive area of clinical intervention.

The terrain of palliative medicine

By the mid-twentieth century, innovative treatments were proliferating in medicine and there was an increasing emphasis upon the cure and rehabilitation of those with serious illness. From oncology to cardiology and geriatrics, from psychiatry to paediatrics, new fields were opening up with their own defined boundaries, internal status hierarchies, codified claims to knowledge, and specific skills and technologies. It was important, therefore, that the growing interest in hospice and palliative care should articulate with these developments. To survive and thrive, hospice doctors would also need to speak the language of the modern medical establishment. That was not always to their liking.

As we have seen, there was sometimes a sense of scepticism towards research. For some, letters of thanks from grateful relatives were the only reassurances needed that the provided care was along the right lines. Moreover, some saw the hospice as a place to connect with patients in a way that modern medicine increasingly prevented. For them, hospice care came to signify a reaching out to those in the terminal phase of illness, often in a manner influenced by religious or personal and social commitments, with the goal of engaging the fundamentals of human mortality—making the departure from life dignified, meaningful, and free from suffering. This version of hospice care also had wider goals. Yes, it was about medicine, services, and systems of care. But it also spoke to a specific social agenda: the recognition of death as a part of the fabric of life, and the need for medicine and healthcare to re-engage with the care of dying and bereaved persons. It was therefore less pre-occupied with research and evidence in the sense understood by biomedicine. The notion that the hospice could provide a new approach to care at the end of life, one that might make roots and take hold elsewhere in the healthcare system, if perhaps slightly altered in the process, was a goal for some of these twentieth-century hospice doctors, but not all. As palliative medicine developed, however, and began to uncouple itself from some of the wider attributes of hospice care, the intent to engage with the healthcare system and find a place within it became much more central and explicit.

These differing priorities within hospice and palliative care had wide reverberations and often shaped the pathways of development in specific countries and contexts. In turn, there were also detractors and doubters outside the field, for whom hospice care could appear prescriptive and even proselytizing. It was perhaps too caught up in an idealism that would be difficult to apply beyond a limited number of services and initiatives run by committed activists. Some considered that it muscled in on the territory of the generalist—surely these services were what all good doctors were already offering? Viewed from the perspective of the public health system, it could also be seen as a limited approach, focused mainly on malignant and end-stage disease and, therefore, unlikely to be capable of meeting needs at the general population's level. As one British detractor later declaimed, hospices appeared 'too good to be true and too small to be useful'.[1] In America there was also concern about the 'death groupies' attracted to hospices, who were 'full of good intentions and slightly crazy ideas'.[2]

Not all physicians were sceptical, however, and the history of the modern hospice includes many examples of medical doctors who stepped off their professional tramlines to engage in a field where alternative approaches might be possible and where working alliances could go beyond the obvious networks of the medical system. Over time, some of these (though perhaps a minority) would gain fluency and a degree of acumen in assessing outcomes, modelling interventions against best evidence, and evaluating the costs and benefits of particular approaches. There was a need for a strategy and a way of thinking that would translate better into health system contexts and that would engage more effectively with professional agendas and public health orientations. This was to be the cornerstone of palliative care and, within it, of the emerging specialty of palliative *medicine*. However, there was much to be done before that point could be reached.

There were also generational and cohort aspects to the early pioneers. Members of the first cohort of British hospice doctors, who were already embarked on a medical career and became attracted to hospice care, were usually qualified in and committed to a particular strand of hospital medicine, or to general practice. Some had heard of Cicely Saunders as medical students. Many came to hospice care through locally organized groups, and the efforts of charitable bodies to develop hospice services. They took on the role of champions for hospice care in their local communities. They were the trusted local physicians who would get involved in lobbying the health authorities, giving public talks, and helping with fundraising. When the hospices became operational, they would often become the part-time medical directors. They were not trained in this line of medicine. Self-taught to a degree, some availed themselves of *ad hoc* opportunities to spend time at St Christopher's Hospice, as well as the other hospices that began to appear in the United Kingdom from the early 1970s onwards. Dr Tony Crowther, a GP and later medical director of St Luke's Hospice, Sheffield, is such an example. He describes here his first encounter with the Cicely Saunders approach, while working as a trainee doctor in a London teaching hospital in 1961. It was more than a decade later that he became actively involved with his local hospice.

> One of my jobs [as a houseman] was to ring St Joseph's Hospice in Hackney and ask for patients to be transferred there. And that was the time when Cicely Saunders was working there . . . And she actually rang us one day and said 'I'd like to show you round, do a ward round with you.' And we did this ward round, and I'll always remember, she introduced us to a patient with cancer of the stomach who was reading a book, sitting up in bed, with totally inoperable carcinoma. And we came away from the bed, and I was the bright-eyed, bushy-tailed houseman who said, 'Excuse me, Dr Saunders, but I haven't seen any fridges for blood or drip sacks to give blood, and yet that man with a cancer of the stomach might have a haematemesis, a massive haematemesis,' which is what we'd been taught in pathology. And, of course that just isn't true, massive haemorrhages are actually amazingly rare in terminally ill patients. And she said, 'Well, it's unlikely, but if he did, he'd have an injection of morphine and he would either die of his haemorrhage comfortably and unaware of what was happening, or if he didn't die from it then we would think about and consider transfusion the next day.' And I thought, 'Wow! What commonsense. That's humanity, that's normality', because I'd only ever been taught resuscitation and putting drips up and saving lives, and I thought, 'Wow! That is brilliant'. And then— I suppose—I forgot about it.[3]

There was however a growing public interest in this kind of approach, a rising interest in how suffering at the end of life could be avoided, how the stigmatizing elements of a death from cancer could be overcome, and what local people of all stripes could do about it in their communities. By the close of the 1970s, hospice philosophy had captured the imagination of people in many parts of the United Kingdom. Fifty-eight hospices were founded between 1981 and 1984, compared with 36 during the whole of the previous decade. Part of the appeal for many of these individuals was a determination to draw attention to the problem of pain at the end of life, and particularly for those dying from cancer. Moreover, this became a rather special focus and rallying call.

The problem of cancer pain

The liberal use of pain medication could alarm doctors who had been socialized into using morphine with extreme caution. Since the early twentieth century, greater regulation of the use of opiates in several countries meant that patients could find it difficult to get adequate pain relief. Both doctors and patients were concerned about the possibility of addiction to strong drugs. Reinforcing this perspective, the endurance of pain without resort to powerful narcotics was portrayed as a test of moral fortitude and, in the case of cancer, an inevitable aspect of advanced malignancy.[4] Treatments that interrupted the pain system by means of nerve blocks or surgical sectioning of the spinal cord or brain had therefore gained favour, meaning that the use of morphine for pain was seen as a last resort.[5] The new hospice and palliative medicine doctors sought to promote a different orthodoxy, and this involved forging a connection with the parallel (and also emerging) field of non-surgical pain medicine.

In 1953 in the United States, John Bonica published the first textbook of pain medicine, in which the role of morphine was reappraised. He wrote: 'In spite of what has been and will be said, it is my opinion that narcotic drugs, particularly morphine, when *properly used* have no pharmacological rivals in the management of intractable pain associated with inoperable disease.'[6] His groundbreaking work was followed by other studies—for example, one in Boston on terminal cancer care among 200 patients[7] and a paper on social casework with cancer patients.[8, 9] There were also studies from Britain on public opinion about cancer and the late presentation of cancer patients.[10, 11] All of these offered insight into the problems, pain, and suffering of patients and families affected by advanced disease, particularly cancer, which would influence future activists in palliative care.

Before the 1970s, however, cancer pain had generally received little international attention as either a clinical or a public health problem, and it was often regarded as an intractable, not fully controllable, consequence of the disease.[4, 12] From the early 1970s, John Bonica had been driving the development of the International Association for the Study of Pain (IASP). He had gathered together an international group in 1973, in Issaquah, Washington, near his base in Seattle. Buoyed with enthusiasm, IASP held its first World Congress in Florence in 1975 and the first issue of the journal *Pain* was published in the same year. Pain specialists Dr Kathleen Foley from the United States and Dr Vittorio Ventafridda from Italy organized a follow-up meeting on cancer pain immediately after the congress in Florence, and this was attended by 150 people.[13] Research presented at this and subsequent conferences suggested that physicians had the means to relieve even severe cancer pain, and that the principal factors contributing to poor pain management were legal barriers against opioid use, and a lack of knowledge in pain management on the part of clinicians. Soon the National Cancer Institute in the United States was supporting work on the epidemiology of cancer pain in a collaborative study involving five centres there, as well as St Christopher's Hospice in London and the National Cancer Institute in Milan. Some of those involved went on to contribute to the first International Symposium on Cancer Pain held in Venice in 1978.[14]

The problem of cancer pain was being tackled from two directions. On the one side were figures from the hospice movement, notably Dr Robert Twycross (Figure 5.1), who was undertaking research at St Christopher's. On the other was the growing cadre of pain specialists who were grouping under the banner of IASP. Although operating out of different clinical settings and frameworks, there was at least some overlap between them. It was this coming together of pain specialists with hospice medicine specialists and relevant oncologists that led to the development of improved methods for managing pain.[15] The Venice meeting was supported by the private foundation of the industrialist Floriani family of Milan who, encouraged by Ventafridda, was taking a special interest in pain and hospice care. Held on 24–27 May 1978 on one of the Venetian islands, it became a landmark event in the history of the field and resulted in a hefty volume, edited by Ventafridda and Bonica.[16] As Marcia Meldrum has observed, it was the site of a stand-off between Robert Twycross of St Christopher's and Ray Houde of Memorial Sloan Kettering. They had clashed on three key issues: the question of 'tolerance' to opiates, the rule of giving analgesia 'by the clock', and the benefits of parenteral versus oral administration of morphine. Perhaps urged on by the presence at the meeting of Cicely Saunders, Twycross saw little evidence of tolerance and advocated for careful titration of the drug, arguing forcibly for a rigid approach to regular giving.[17] This approach soon began to shape the emerging discussion at WHO.

In 1982, WHO enlisted the aid of these hospice care leaders and cancer pain specialists, plus pharmaceutical manufacturers to develop a global Programme for Cancer Pain Relief. It would be based on a three-step analgesic 'ladder' with the use of adjuvant therapies, and incorporating the use of strong opioids as the third step. The idea was reputedly sketched on a paper serviette by Ventafridda in the cafeteria of WHO in Geneva.[15] This was an early sign of cancer pain coming to be characterized or 'framed' as a public health issue. One of the key participants in these discussions, Kathleen Foley, the neurologist and pain specialist from Memorial Sloan Kettering Hospital, New York, and subsequently a major leader in the global development of palliative care, describes the context, and how the work was undertaken.

> In 1981, I was at Memorial Sloan Kettering and had been there for about six years, and had been working on developing a clinical pain research programme, and that worked on identifying the nature of pain and the epidemiology of pain in cancer patients, and John Bonica and Jan Stjernswärd, who was then the Director for the Cancer Programme of the WHO, had decided that we needed to address cancer pain at an international level. And so really I would say that the concept, or the idea of pain as a public health issue and one that the WHO should consider really originated with Jan Stjernswärd, with John Bonica—and in fact Mark Swerdlow, who was an early, an important contributor to those early discussions and those initiatives—and Vittoria Ventafridda . . . And we basically sat days on end talking about developing a simple monograph on cancer pain relief. I had *enormous* difficulties with that because I didn't think anything was simple and everyone kept wanting to make it simple, so I must say that I was taught about public health in that meeting from the perspective of understanding that, if you wanted to move an agenda forward at a public health level, then you had to make it simple. And really to their credit, I would say that it was Jan Stjernswärd who kept pushing hard about making it simple and not being a content expert; and then Robert Twycross, who was clearly a content expert, and who had a wonderful ability to make things simple, and who was willing to make it simple even if he wasn't so sure they were right; and myself who was somewhere in between. But what came out of that meeting was, what we called the *Methods* for Pain Relief—and we called them methods because we were working under a WHO umbrella with the Floriani Foundation, but not in a very official capacity. And so that, if you really wanted a document, you would need an expert panel, and you couldn't call them *guidelines* before you had tested them as guidelines. It was the first of the meetings that led to an expert panel, meeting in Geneva, in which Robert wrote the first draft of the document and then everyone critiqued it, re-wrote it, advised about it. But really again, to Robert's credit, he wrote a very extensive and detailed document that was heavily edited and changed and simplified even more but I think it carries a very strong imprint of his teachings and workings and writings. And typically the way those panels worked was that you came and stayed in Geneva for five days and you worked in the days at the meeting and then you worked at night to revise the documents. So it was quite intense, and quite extensive, and it was like, typically, whenever we met. We got through that process and then we had a document that required lots of editing and I—and this is a total aside—but hilariously funny, I was on a trip with my family and I remembered Jan meeting me at the train station as my family and I were driving by, and we sat in this

train station to finish off the editing of it while my husband and kids, you know, went God knows where to do what while we sat there for four hours attempting to get this document finished, and it finally was finished.[18]

The crucial meeting at the Villa d'Este on Lake Como outside Milan took place in October 1982. Marcia Meldrum has listed the five key people present. They were becoming familiar to one another following the conferences in Florence and Venice.

> Anesthesiologist Mark Swerdlow, Stjernswärd's chief consultant, who had founded the first formal pain organization, the Intractable Pain Society, in Manchester in 1967; oncologist Vittorio Ventafridda, the energetic pain specialist at Italy's National Cancer Institute, whose efforts had brought the WHO group to Milan, his home city; palliative care physician Robert Twycross, who had conducted innovative drug research studies for Cicely Saunders at St. Christopher's Hospice in London in the 1970s; neurologist Kathleen Foley, who had published the first taxonomy of cancer pain syndromes and who had been trained in pain research at Memorial Sloan Kettering Cancer Center in New York; and pharmacologist Anders Rane of Stockholm.[17]

The group was becoming very focused on the global scale of the problem associated with cancer pain relief. There was a lack of medical education on the subject; a wariness of clinicians in engaging with the use of strong opiates; and major barriers that existed in laws and established procedures that combined to restrict access to appropriate medication in many parts of the world.

On the back of these efforts, WHO representatives launched an international initiative to remove legal sanctions against opioid importation and its use, relying on national coordinating centres to organize professional education and to disseminate the core principles of the 'pain ladder'. The WHO programme met with only partial success, however. Opioid consumption between 1984 and 1993 rose dramatically in 10 industrialized countries, but showed much smaller increases in the rest of the world,[19] and significant differences in the pattern and the extent of opioid use were seen to continue within and between global regions.[4]

Nevertheless, the interest of WHO raised further debate about the relationship between palliative care and oncology. It was increasingly recognized that curative care and palliative care were not mutually exclusive and that as long as few options for curative oncological treatment existed for many patients in the developing world, the allocation of resources should shift towards a greater emphasis on palliative care.[20] Cancer pain was coming to be defined as a *public health* issue and, as that occurred, the scope to widen involvement—beyond the immediate world of hospice—was in turn opening up.

Researching the new model of care

The rise of hospice and palliative care in a distinctly modern guise took place against a backdrop of a modest but growing clinical, educational, and research interest.[21] For Cicely Saunders, this effort was about establishing the modern science and art of caring for patients with advanced malignant disease. She focused her attention on patients in the final stages of cancer, especially those with the most complex problems, and she played a key role in defining a new knowledge base of care for those dying from malignancies. Her writings relied heavily on individual patient experiences, which she was assiduous in collecting.[22,23]

She also inspired those around her to attend to the business of research in the newly opened St Christopher's Hospice. Here she stuck to the maxim of a 'middle way' between too much and too little treatment. St Christopher's Hospice sought to establish itself as a centre of excellence in a new field, giving equal weight to clinical care, education, and research. In the early days, it was associated with some major clinical and organizational studies that did a great deal to advance the field.

Research took place on the science of pain control and the underlying pharmaco-kinetic mechanisms at work in the administration of strong opiates. This began with the close scrutiny of the methods of pain relief favoured within the early hospices and terminal care homes, in particular the use of the so-called Brompton Cocktail.[24] This had been gaining popularity throughout the twentieth century and had appeared in print for the first time in the 1950s—a mixture of morphine hydrochloride, cocaine hydrochloride, alcohol, syrup, and chloroform water, but with many local variants and names.

Such mixtures had become widely adopted and were made available for the patient to drink on demand, or at regular intervals. In 1952, the Brompton Hospital had produced its own supplement to the National Formulary and the mixture appeared in print for the first time under the name Haustus E. (Haustus meaning a draught or potion, and E. perhaps elixir).

- Morphine hydrochloride 1/4 grain
- Cocaine hydrochloride 1/6 grain
- Alcohol 90 per cent 30 minims
- Syrup 60 minims
- Chloroform water to 1/2 fl. oz

This version was then listed in Martindale's Extra Pharmacopoeia in 1958. In 1976, it had appeared in the British National Formulary and gradually it had come to be known by several different names: Brompton Cocktail; Brompton

Mixture; Mistura euphoriens; Mistura pro moribunda; Mistura pro euthanasia; Saunders's Mixture; Hoyle's Mixture. Indeed, when the first modern hospices opened in the United Kingdom, they too adopted their own nomenclatures, as at Sheffield where there was St Luke's mild, then St Luke's moderate, followed by St Luke's 'individual'. As the use of the mixture proliferated, its contents became more variable. The alcohol could take the form of gin, whisky, or brandy, and might be included in various quantities according to preference. A phenothiazine began to be added, either prochlorperazine or chlorpromazine, for both antiemetic and sedative purposes. Further afield in France, there is evidence that an antihistamine, such as promethazine, was also being included in what were then called 'lytic cocktails'.[25] Above all, some practitioners in the United Kingdom favoured diamorphine over morphine; some even dropped the cocaine, and used morphine and diamorphine together in the mixture.[26]

Robert Twycross and the Brompton Cocktail

In her early writings, Cicely Saunders had been eager to promote this rather exotic mixture, but it was the St Christopher's research fellow Robert Twycross who set out to scrutinize the potion in detail in what became a series of classic studies, the first of their kind undertaken in the hospice setting. Twycross first met Cicely Saunders in 1963. The following year, while still an undergraduate at Oxford University, he had created the Radcliffe Christian Medical Society simply to give a pretext to invite her to speak in Oxford. Then five years later in 1968, he received an invitation to join her team at the newly opened St Christopher's. He declined the offer, however, in favour of completing his Membership of the Royal College of Physicians, and it was not until 1971 that he finally went as a clinical research fellow to the hospice. He describes the events as follows.

> There was an international conference organised by the SCM, the Student Christian Movement, which was in Bristol in the first few days of 1963, which was the big freeze-up. It froze on Christmas Eve and it continued freezing for a couple of months. And we somehow managed to get to Bristol despite the amount of snow between here and there. And in this international student conference, in addition to the keynote addresses and that sort of thing, there were workshops. And one series of workshops was on 'Health and Healing' and it was groups—group discussion— and there were sufficient senior members to have a senior member sitting in, I think, with each discussion group. And the senior member in the group I was in happened to be Cicely Saunders. And obviously she said a few things which happened to resonate with me—that was why I arranged this meeting at the medical school, in Osler House. So, less than eighteen months later, Cicely Saunders came to speak on 'The Management of Pain in Terminal Cancer'. That meant that I went into her black book as a doctor, or a future doctor, who might well be interested in hospice care.

And that meant that a couple of years after I qualified, which must have been some time in 1968, she wrote and said would I be interested in applying for a Clinical Research Fellowship, and I wrote back saying, 'Well, it's very nice of you, but I've decided to take my MRCP [Member of the Royal College of Physicians], so I've got to finish that.' And I sort of forgot about it. And then a couple of years later, when the Research Fellow they appointed died tragically, I think within two years of taking up his post, I got another letter in December 1970 saying would I like to consider applying for the Research Fellowship now, which I did. So that was one strand; the link from '63 to the letter in December 1970. I was following a typical medical career . . . But after House jobs, when I was going for Registrar posts, a little voice inside would say, 'That's a step further away from St Christopher's, that's a step further away from St Christopher's.' And it would just flash out of the sub-conscious and recede again. So there must have been something going on down there, so that when this letter came, the famous letter in December 1970: 'Would you like to consider applying for the Clinical Research Fellowship?' I read the letter twice and gave a laugh to myself and said, 'Yes.' And obviously there was an interview and that sort of thing and I came into the post in March . . . March 1st, 1971.[27]

There, continuing the early research initiated by the late Dr Ron Welldon, Twycross subjected the Brompton Cocktail to unparalleled clinical and scientific scrutiny. Over the next few years, his work focused on a number of areas: standardization of the mixture; the relationship between the active constituents and the vehicle; the storage properties of the mixture; the role of cocaine within it; and also the relative efficacy of the morphine and diamorphine. Indeed, between 1972 and 1979, Twycross produced 39 publications on these and related themes.

In his 1973 paper 'Stumbling blocks in the study of diamorphine', which appeared in the May issue of the *Postgraduate Medical Journal*, he reported on the limited shelf life of the drug in solution; its potency ratio *vis-à-vis* morphine; the lack of research into its oral administration; the insensitivity of current assays; the determinants of undesirable side effects; and between-sex comparisons of metabolic handling.[28] The following year, in a paper written with colleagues from the Epsom Hospital Laboratories, he began to advance the case for the oral administration of strong narcotics, demonstrating from a study of urinary excretion that 'an orally administered solution of diamorphine hydrochloride is completely absorbed by the gastrointestinal tract, but a solution of morphine sulphate is only two-thirds absorbed'.[29] This difference, he suggested, could be allowed for in the dosage.

In addition, in 1974, Twycross reported on a survey of 90 teaching and district general hospitals in the United Kingdom that showed marked variation in the composition of what he was now calling 'elixirs' for the relief of pain and suffering in terminal cancer. He welcomed, therefore, the introduction of a standard diamorphine and cocaine mixture to the British Pharmaceutical

Codex, but raised questions about its 'keeping' properties. Another issue concerned the acceptability to patients of a mixture that might be experienced as either extremely sickly or unacceptably alcoholic. Above all, the paper pointed to the need to 'evaluate objectively the contribution of cocaine in the pharmacological effect of the mixture'.[30]

Across the Atlantic, others were being influenced by the British hospice movement's adoption of the Brompton mixture, as well as the developing ideas of Cicely Saunders on the nature of pain. In Canada, Balfour Mount, Ronald Melzack, and colleagues began a series of studies at the newly opened palliative care unit in Montreal. Early descriptions suggested that 'the Brompton mixture provides convenient and uniform pain control without important adverse effects'.[31] It was found that the mixture relieved the pain of 90 per cent of patients in the palliative care unit and 75–80 per cent of those in the general wards and private rooms, an interesting sidelight on the added benefits of the palliative care setting. It was concluded that the results were consistent with the gate-control theory of pain, and that the Brompton mixture 'does not act on only a single dimension of pain but has a strong effect on the sensory, affective, and evaluative dimensions together'.[32] So far, it seemed, the traditional elixir, albeit with greater specificity as to its makeup, had survived the transition from old-style care of the dying to the new world of palliative care.

Then an important breakthrough came in two papers published by Robert Twycross in 1977. The first appeared in the journal *Pain*.[33] Here, a controlled trial of diamorphine and morphine was reported, in which the two drugs were administered regularly in a version of the Brompton mixture containing cocaine hydrochloride in a 10 mg dose. A total of 699 patients entered the trial and, of these, 146 crossed over after about two weeks from diamorphine to morphine, or vice-versa. The previously determined potency ratio of 1.5:1 was used. In the female crossover patients, no difference was noted in relation to pain or other symptoms evaluated, but male crossover patients experienced more pain and were more depressed while receiving diamorphine, suggesting that the potency ratio was lower than expected. Twycross concluded that if this difference in potency is allowed for, then morphine is a satisfactory substitute for orally administered diamorphine, but that the more soluble diamorphine retained certain advantages when injections were required and doses were high.

In the second trial,[34] which was reported in a letter to the *British Medical Journal*, the morphine and diamorphine elixirs were compared with cocaine added and without it. There were 45 satisfactory crossovers, and since the trends within the morphine and diamorphine groups were similar, they were combined for purposes of analysis. The study showed that introducing a 10 mg dose of cocaine after two weeks resulted in a small but statistically significant difference in alertness; but stopping cocaine after this period had no detectable effect. Twycross adjudged that at this dosage, cocaine is of borderline efficacy and that tolerance to it develops within a few days.

As a result of this work, the routine use of cocaine with patients at St Christopher's was abandoned and, in particular, morphine was prescribed alone in chloroform water, or together with an antiemetic where indicated. Supporting evidence came two years later from the Canadian researchers, who also reported a double-blind crossover in which a standard Brompton Cocktail containing morphine, cocaine, ethyl alcohol, syrup, and chloroform water was compared with morphine alone in a flavoured water solution. Pain was measured using the then recently developed McGill Pain Questionnaire, and ratings of confusion, nausea, and drowsiness were obtained from the patients and their relatives, and nurses. The study showed no significant difference between the cocktail and the oral morphine alone; both relieved pain in about 85 per cent of patients, with no differences in confusion, nausea, or drowsiness. The Canadians adopted the name 'elixir of morphine' for the morphine solution.[35]

In 1979, as one of three chapters he wrote for the important trilogy *Advances in Pain Research and Therapy*, edited by John Bonica and Vittorio Ventafridda, Twycross drew together his summative statement on the matter.[36] There had been, he suggested, a tendency 'to endow the Brompton Cocktail with almost mystical properties and to regard it as the panacea for terminal cancer pain'. Generously, he allowed that if the physician is aware of the potential side effects of the main ingredients, then its use might be maintained. However, set against this was the disadvantage to the pharmacist, the potential unpalatability to the patient, the higher financial costs incurred, and the restricted potential for the physician to manipulate the doses given. The Brompton Cocktail, it turned out, was no more than a dressed-up way of administering oral morphine to cancer patients in pain. It was about to depart from the received wisdom of the new palliative care community.

It is not difficult to see the fall of the Brompton Cocktail as part of a wider sea change in the science and art of the emerging palliative care field. We might capture this as a shift from a 'traditional' mode of thinking and practice, to one that is distinctly 'modern' in character. Potions, mixtures, and elixirs carry ancient associations, reaching back to earlier periods in the history of medical practice. They can be invested with mystical, or even alchemical properties. Yet, their actions can be as cloudy as their appearance. The conjoining of substances and liquids has an intuitive, even hubristic quality—a medicine of faith, rather than fact. At the same time, as the varying names of this particular mixture reveal, the purpose of its use was also somewhat ambiguous. Was it intended to induce euphoria? Did it respond to, or propentiate, moribundity? Most intriguing of all, was it intended to bring about 'easeful' death, or actually to hasten demise?

There seems to be no doubt that the Brompton Cocktail was spoken about euphemistically by doctors and nurses, and patients and families were aware of this. Such ways of communicating are hard to abandon—witness the McGill term 'morphine elixir' for a mixture that contained only the drug itself and water. However, in general, this did not continue. Instead, since the demise of the Brompton Cocktail, an allegedly more rational approach was adopted to the management of pain. Yes, drugs came to be used in combination (often in palliative care for purposes for which they were not licensed), but titration became the important watchword, something much harder to do with the varied ingredients of the cocktail.

Encouraged by Cicely Saunders at St Christopher's Hospice and mentored by Duncan Vere at the London Hospital, Robert Twycross saw the implications of all this. He 'deconstructed' the Brompton Cocktail. As his work was disseminated, it became clear that simpler, more predictable means of pain control could be adopted, that narcotics could be used safely, and in particular, that morphine was just as effective as diamorphine. Combining energies from Britain, North America, and Europe, a new field of pain medicine and research was opening up, a field with which the particular contribution of Dr Robert Twycross will always be associated.[24]

In 1976, Twycross moved to Oxford to lead his own NHS hospice. Here he continued his research into pain with new fellows working under his direction; first Dr Geoffrey Hanks and later Dr Claud Regnard.

> Well Geoff was brought in to continue the work on morphine and again there was a whole lot of descriptive work, much of which never got published in fact, a whole lot of descriptive work, because a lot of mine was descriptive. If you're doing controlled trials you've got time to fill in with descriptive work; the use of morphine, you know; what happens to the dose if you have someone on morphine for two years, you know; maximum dose, all that sort of thing; dose ranges; concurrent use of other drugs, and all that sort of thing. So he did that and he also dabbled in a number of controlled trials, some of which came to a successful conclusion and some of which didn't because of a lack of suitable patients. He was enticed away to the Marsden. He was undoubtedly the right person for the right job; someone who'd previously been in pharmaceutical medicine and had the right qualifications and no doubt could fight his corner at the Royal Marsden. I don't think anyone else at that time could have successfully established a palliative care unit in the Royal Marsden.
>
> Claud, again, came to do more work on morphine, but his other activities tended more and more towards lymphoedema, and in 1985, at his instigation, we set up the British Lymphology Interest Group and the first inaugural general meeting was in

the day centre dining room, which was before we had the Study Centre. We had an inaugural day conference of the British Lymphology Interest Group, which is another interesting aspect of the whole story; how lymphoedema has been grafted on at a number of hospices. He went to Newcastle, in '86.[28]

By the early 1980s, Twycross was making an increasing name for himself, not so much in research, but for his teaching and textbook publications. He took on the role of abstracter and synthesizer of published work, and his joint texts with Dr Sylvia Lack, who trained in palliative medicine at St Joseph's before moving to the Connecticut Hospice, became widely read as the field grew and the demand for training material expanded. He reduced his clinical commitments at Sobell House, Oxford, and became a clinical reader in palliative medicine at the University. As we have seen, by now he had a major international role, too, and was a key architect of the WHO pain ladder.

Total pain

If Twycross demolished the prevailing method of relieving pain, Saunders created a radically new approach to conceptualizing it.[37] A striking feature of Saunders's early work was its articulation of the relationship between physical and mental suffering. This reached full expression with the concept of *total pain*, which was taken to include physical symptoms, mental distress, social problems, and emotional difficulties. There can be little doubt that when Cicely Saunders first used this term she was in the process of bequeathing to medicine and healthcare a concept of enduring clinical and conceptual interest. The concept emerged from her unique experience as nurse, social worker, and physician—the remarkable multidisciplinary personal platform from which she launched the modern hospice and palliative care movement. It also reflected a willingness to acknowledge the spiritual suffering of the patient and to see this in relation to physical problems. Crucially, it was tied to a sense of narrative and biography, emphasizing the importance of listening to the patient's story and of understanding the experience of suffering in a multifaceted way. This was an approach that saw pain as the key to unlocking other problems, and as something requiring multiple interventions for its resolution.

The inseparability of physical pain from mental processes is alluded to by Cicely Saunders even in some of her earliest publications. In 1959, she could note: 'Much of our total pain experience is composed of our mental reaction . . .'[38] At this stage we have the idea of total pain in a weaker, more preliminary sense than was to emerge within a few years. Here it is a general descriptor, indicating that there may be several layers that have to be understood to have a full grasp of the problem of pain in the terminally ill. The specific context of this understanding is the stage of illness 'when all curative and palliative measures have been exhausted'.[22] This moment, at which modern medicine typically states that 'there is nothing more to be done',[39] thus becomes the starting point for an emergent medicine of terminal care, central to which is a multifaceted understanding of pain. This is a medicine concerned also with the meaning of pain. A cry simply to be rid of pain is not worthy of humans, who must question the pain that is endured and seek meaning in it. Seen this way, pain breaks the yoke of material values and allows the finest human sentiments to shine through.

In this sense, pain has become something indivisible from both the body and the wider personality. Therefore, it can be observed that 'the body has a wisdom of its own and will help the strong instinct to fight for life to change into an active kind of acceptance that may never be expressed in words'.[40] The following narrative, from a 1964 paper in *Nursing Mirror*, describes for the first time the key elements of what came to be viewed as 'total pain'. It is about Mrs Hinson, a patient cared for at St Joseph's Hospice, Hackney. It was later quoted extensively within the palliative care literature, becoming emblematic of the whole principle of care within the emerging specialty.

> One person gave me more or less the following answer when I asked her a question about her pain, and in her answer she brings out the four main needs that we are trying to care for in this situation. She said, 'Well doctor, the pain began in my back, but now it seems that all of me is wrong.' She gave a description of various symptoms and ills and then went on to say, 'My husband and son were marvellous but they were at work and they would have had to stay off and lose their money. I could have cried for the pills and injections although I knew I shouldn't. Everything seemed to be against me and nobody seemed to understand.' And then she paused before she said, 'But it's so wonderful to begin to feel safe again.' Without any further questioning she had talked of her mental as well as physical distress, of her social problems and of her spiritual need for security.[41]

That same year, 1964, in a paper for *The Prescribers' Journal,* the phrase 'all of me is wrong' was used more formally to introduce the concept of total pain in its stronger and definitive sense—to include physical symptoms, mental distress, social problems, and emotional problems.[42] Although often overlooked by writers of subsequent publications, this is the foundational piece in which total pain is *fully* described by Saunders for the first time. In a 1966 paper, a patient being admitted to St Joseph's used the phrase, 'it was *all* pain' and the author observed that this '"total pain" calls us to analyse, to assess and to anticipate'.[40] As early as 1959 she had acknowledged that pain in this multifaceted sense could not be relieved solely through analgesics.[39] Likewise, it posed greater challenges than could be overcome by the technologies of regular administration for pain relief. By 1967, a new conceptualization of pain had emerged: 'Pain demands the same analysis and consideration as an illness itself. It is the syndromes of pain rather than the syndromes of disease with which we are concerned.'[43]

In the early years at St Christopher's Hospice, the concept of total pain was further elaborated by researchers, clinicians, and by patients themselves. It entered into the fabric of daily life at the hospice and became a defining feature of its philosophy and approach. By 1985, when Cicely Saunders retired from the full-time role of medical director at St Christopher's to become its chairperson, palliative medicine was just two years away from specialty recognition in the United Kingdom. It is not unreasonable to view the concept of total pain as a major element within the conceptual armamentarium of the new discipline. Indeed, it may well be judged as one of the most innovative concepts yet to emerge from the field of palliative care.

When considering the writing of Cicely Saunders on total pain and related subjects, several publications in the period 1968–1985 merit our attention. The notion that chronic pain presents particular challenges to the clinician is regularly stated in her work from this time. In particular, it is seen as a problem on the level of meaning, for such pain can be timeless, endless, meaningless, bringing a sense of isolation and despair.[44] This is in stark contrast to the acute pain, familiar in teaching hospitals, which so often is seen as purposive—for example, in the diagnostic process as an indicator of problems, or postoperatively as a staging post on the road to recovery. An important chapter published in 1970 describes chronic pain as 'not just an event, or a series of events . . . but rather a situation in which the patient is, as it were, held captive'.[45] In terminally ill patients, a major challenge is to avoid the onset of such pain by active strategies of prevention, in particular the regular giving of strong analgesia in anticipation of, rather than in response to, the onset of pain. We see the maxim oft repeated, 'constant pain needs constant control'. At the same time, the value of listening is also emphasized, as in the patient who said 'the pain seemed to go by just talking'. If terminal pain can be regarded as an illness in itself, so the use of drugs is not simply a matter of technique but also the expression of understanding between one person and another.

Crucially, Saunders saw the relief of pain as the most vital component in confronting the issue of euthanasia—pain in the final stages of cancer had attracted the imagination of the public and was a regular theme in public debate.[46] It was therefore important to demonstrate to the public that pain could be avoided. The use of moderate doses of strong opiates was a core feature of this. For example, in the 1970s, only 10 per cent of patients cared for at St Christopher's Hospice needed a dose of more than 30 mg of diamorphine.

Moreover, it was found that by providing physical relief, opportunities then arose for communicating with the patient on a much deeper level, not least on the complex issue of what to disclose about the prognosis.

By 1973, it had become possible to refer in published writing to some of the research on pain being carried out at St Christopher's Hospice.[47] Pain was acknowledged to be a problem still inadequately tackled; whether in the patient's own home, or in a busy general hospital ward. One part of the problem was that the constant pain of terminal cancer was not alleviated by earlier teachings; to the effect that doses of narcotics should be spaced as widely as possible to avoid the onset of dependence. Fears about dependence also limited the availability of morphine and diamorphine in some countries, and double-blind trials at St Christopher's were designed to shed light on the relative merits of the two drugs. Another problem was that of titration, largely seen as a subjective process. However, by 1976 it was possible to refer to the use of radioimmunoassay as a method for measuring the level of drugs in the body, thus allowing Robert Twycross's research to show that the use of opiates with terminally ill patients does not need to continually escalate and might even decline.[48] By now, it was becoming clear from the work of Twycross that there was no observable clinical difference between morphine and diamorphine, although the latter was more favoured for injection because of its greater solubility.

Evidence of growing recognition for Cicely Saunders's approach can be seen in the invitation extended to her as well as to Twycross, to contribute to one of the volumes on research edited by international pain experts John Bonica and Vittorio Ventafridda, published in 1979, and based on presentations at the 1978 cancer pain symposium in Venice.[49] In the resulting chapter, she used patients' paintings and drawings, case histories, and research in combination to develop her argument. A series of patients' pictures was particularly telling. They show the feeling of being impaled by a red-hot iron, of total isolation from the world, of the implacable heaviness of pain or, in one case, the feeling that 'I am a scrap heap'. Another woman who had experienced a year of relentless pain from carcinoma of the pancreas drew it as a small rodent eating into the side of a tree trunk; the few traces of green at the top were described as 'my life trying to get through'. By attention to all aspects of such pain, the possibility of its relief came in sight. So, rather unusually, Cicely Saunders was able to state: 'Vital signs in a ward specializing in the control of terminal pain include the hand steady enough to draw, the mind alert enough to write poems and to play cards, and above all the spirit to enjoy family visits and spend the last weekends at home.' She went on to argue that good care of this kind could also be delivered in a variety of settings and was not dependent upon the availability of an inpatient hospice facility.

At the beginning of the 1980s, another substantial chapter appeared from the pen of Saunders, this time in Mark Swerdlow's collection *The Therapy of Pain*.[50] Here she cited examples from studies conducted between 1954 and 1978 that gave evidence of unrelieved terminal pain. By contrast, data on 3 362 patients cared for by St Christopher's between 1972 and 1977 showed that only 1 per cent had continuing pain problems, although more than three-quarters presented to the hospice with such problems. The achievement of these results, however, could occasion the phenomenon of 'staff pain', resulting from prolonged exposure to the suffering of patients and families facing death. Although the need for formal staff support was acknowledged and described, it was argued that 'the resilience of those who continue to work in this field is won by a full understanding of what is happening and not by a retreat behind a technique'. The same paper made the important point for those countries in which *diamorphine* was unavailable, that *morphine* was now the preferred analgesic of the two. It also noted that the use of mixtures containing alcohol and cocaine should be discontinued. Both pronouncements followed the work of Robert Twycross and Ronald Melzack. Three years later, having established the preference for morphine, it was possible to discuss new techniques for its administration through both slow-release formulation and the use of the syringe driver.[51]

The syringe driver

In the 1960s, electrically powered syringe pumps were used in medicine mainly to give intravenous cytotoxic drugs. In the United Kingdom, it was Dr Patrick Russell who in 1979 first described the use of the Graseby syringe driver to deliver continuous subcutaneous infusion (CSCI) in the hospice context—for pain and symptom relief. The idea was that by loading pain relieving and other drugs into an electric pump attached to a butterfly needle and inserted under the skin, it would be possible to deliver uninterrupted pain and symptom control over several hours to the patient without the need for regular injections. The syringe driver, used in this way, came to be viewed as almost indispensable to British palliative care practice, although it was not universally adopted elsewhere.[52]

Its inventor was the British bio-engineer Martin Wright, who had long been interested in innovative continuous infusion devices and had been approached by a paediatrician who wanted a portable infusion device suitable for use by her thalassaemic patients. Following the success of the syringe driver in thalassaemia, Wright (who also invented the peak flow meter) began to consider other applications for the pump. It was soon used to good effect in postoperative analgesia, insulin dependent diabetes, and the treatment of myasthenia gravis. But it was in the management of pain and other symptoms in palliative care that it was about to find its definitive and most enduring role; and this came about almost by chance.

Wright's own general practitioner, Patrick Russell, was a neighbour and family friend. Russell was also medical officer at Michael Sobell House, a hospice in the grounds of Mount Vernon Hospital, Northwood in the south of England. During one of their neighbourly discussions on medicine and patient care, Wright suggested that Russell might like to try using the syringe driver to administer CSCI to those hospice patients unable to take oral medication. Russell was keen to try it. In the first attempt, the syringe driver was used on a cachexic, nauseated man with lung cancer. As his pain resolved, the improvement in his quality of life was dramatic and he remained mobile until the day of his death. However, for Russell, it was another case that particularly convinced him of the syringe driver's worth.

> ... the one that was the most memorable for me was a young woman with advanced ovarian cancer who was clearly dying and she had a family holiday organised in Bognor with her two young children and her husband and she was desperate to go on this, but her pain control needs were very great. So we thought, well, we've got her on a syringe driver ... But how can we organise that? So in the end, of course this was in the very early days, we rang a health centre in Bognor and told them we'd got a patient coming down on holiday ... with a syringe driver who was having, I can't remember what dose of diamorphine in 24 hours now. They were a bit taken aback because they'd never heard of it, but we managed to persuade them that they would cooperate. The next problem was what to do about the fortnight's supply of diamorphine ... in fact, the police station cooperated and held it for us. So, off she went down to Bognor and the district nurses or practice nurse, changed the syringe driver every day and she came back really overjoyed with her holiday because she knew time was short and it had meant so much to her to have this holiday with those children ... and that's stayed in my mind ever since. For me that was the moment when I knew this had a big future.[53]

Pleased with the results they were having with the syringe driver at Michael Sobell House, Russell wrote a letter to the *British Medical Journal* (*BMJ*) describing their approach. Published on the 9 June 1979 and titled 'Analgesia in Terminal Malignant Disease',[54] it took the form of a response to a *BMJ* article by Drinkwater and Twycross[55] from earlier that year, advising that the oral route could achieve effective pain relief in almost all cases. Russell was in agreement with Drinkwater and Twycross and with the view that there was no longer a place for the Brompton mixture in modern palliative care, but he went on to describe the use of the syringe driver for the small number of people in whom the oral route proved impossible. He suggested the device could be used to administer drugs by the subcutaneous or intramuscular routes and that it was simple to use, effective, reliable, foolproof, and being small and lightweight, allowed complete mobility.

The UK hospice community soon expressed great interest in this new device. Russell and the medical director of Michael Sobell House, Robert Dickson, were asked to attend a national hospice conference to report their use of the syringe driver. Unfortunately, the chairman Eric Wilkes was unaware of the arrangements and no space was made available in the programme. Wilkes advised that those who wanted to know about the syringe driver would have to come back early from lunch and was perplexed when he returned to find a large crowd of people had gathered to find out more about what seemed to him merely a gimmick. The use of the syringe driver in palliative care proved to be more than a passing fashion however, and Russell's letter to the *BMJ* became the first of many publications on the use of this approach to symptom control. By 1989, a survey of UK palliative care providers found that most undertook CSCI in the management of symptoms and that Wright's syringe driver was used by the overwhelming majority (96 per cent).[56] Twelve years later, another study found this was still the case, with only a handful of units using any other devices.[57]

The syringe driver had become perhaps the central technology in the practice of British palliative care. It was soon to be matched by the emergence of new formulations of the key palliative care drug for pain relief—morphine.[58] In August 1979, a short letter was published in the *British Journal of Clinical Pharmacology*, in which researchers at Bard Pharmaceuticals, Aberdeen, reported 'formulation studies' performed by Napp Laboratories, which had resulted in the development of controlled release 10mg morphine sulphate.[57] A method had been found to bind the morphine to a wax-like substance that would slowly break down in the body, thereby affording continuous symptom relief over an extended period. Controlled release morphine formulations could be used when pain is constant. Their administration would reduce the number and frequency of doses needed by the patient. Controlled release could also complement more standard immediate release formulations, allowing immediate release morphine to be used for 'breakthrough' pain once a person was established on a sustained release product. The use of such tablets was a significant departure from the 'as required' mode of administering morphine, but an early analysis of the use of sustained release tablets in a hospice setting reported that such preparations brought an improved quality of life for patients and care givers.[59]

There was now a growing confidence within the world of hospice and palliative care that the complex and multilayered symptoms associated with terminal pain could be attended to effectively by a combination of the well-informed use of narcotics *and* a sophisticated understanding of the emotional, spiritual, and social problems that might also occur for those with terminal illness. By the mid-1980s, total pain had become firmly established as a central concept within the emerging palliative care specialty and was proving a useful concept in clinical work, in teaching, and (to a lesser extent) in research. Interesting then that, in 1983, Cicely Saunders published a small volume that contained poems, prayers, and other writings selected to help those facing life-threatening illness.[60] Her selections included work by concentration camp survivor and founder of logotherapy, Viktor Frankl; theologians Teilard de Chardin and Olive Wyon; English writers John Bunyan and D. H. Lawrence; as well as some patients from St Christopher's Hospice. It reflected important truths learned in a quarter century of close attention to the suffering of dying patients. It was entitled *Beyond all Pain*.

Burgeoning research and service development

This growing momentum for the study of pain was paralleled in the early 1960s with studies by Colin Murray Parkes on bereavement,[61] and by the mid-1960s, with research papers by Dr Eric Wilkes on terminal cancer at home.[62], [63] These works did much to raise interest in the problems of care for the dying, although it was still the case, as the psychiatrist John Hinton noted, that 'the large number of articles in which remembered experience is distilled into advice on the management of dying awesomely overshadows the few papers attempting to measure the degree of success or failure of treatment'.[64] Over time, however, there was a shift in publications about the care of the dying and a research-based approach to improving care at the end of life began to be more visible.[65] Within a few years, there was also sociological interest in these issues, found in ethnographic studies of the care of the dying in American hospitals,[66] and in surveys of bereaved relatives who were asked about the experiences of the deceased person in the last year of life.[67]

Evaluation research, focused on understanding the hospice service as a whole, began at St Christopher's even before the first patient was admitted. The psychiatrist Colin Murray Parkes built up over time a cohort of cases consisting of 276 patients who died of cancer in two London boroughs, 49 of whom were still under active treatment at the time of death. He found much unrelieved pain, whether the patient died in a hospital or at home, and as patients entered the study, he was able to show that people with serious pain problems were referred from the start to the hospice and their pain was largely relieved.[68] The study was repeated 10 years later as part of the ongoing evaluation of the hospice's work. Although pain and symptom control improved in the hospital setting over time, psychosocial needs and continuity of care continued to be better approached in the hospice.[69] Parkes describes the overall approach.

> We had to do research because that was the only way to sort of underpin the work. For the first five or six years at St Christopher's very little was published. I mean we were doing some drug trials, we were doing various things, but we were developing skills and techniques and ideas which we didn't dare to test out in any sort of empirical way because we hadn't yet got them right. We needed to develop a model that seemed to be working before we started testing it. And I think there's an important lesson here: I think if we'd been in too much of a hurry to do the evaluations, the evaluations would probably have been negative and it's quite possible that the entire hospice movement would have been discredited. It's always a danger if you're enthusiastic for something that you will, you know, well everybody says, 'Well, prove it', you know, 'You've got to evaluate.' And I agree with evaluation. I think we've got to evaluate, but we also have to acknowledge that, in this area, evaluation is actually very difficult. It's not a simple matter . . . there's a simple idea that you can get simple answers to complex questions, but where evaluation of anything as subtle as the care of the dying is concerned, with its multiform different aspects, it would be very surprising if there were a simple way of assessing the value of anything as complex as the quality of life of a person who's dying.
>
> I think that the fact that the first few trials were all sort of drug trials and trials of pain relief enabled the hospice to get off to a good start because in all of these, the results of those studies were very positive in showing how well the hospice was doing. I mean, my own studies, one of the studies I carried out was a comparison of relatives of patients who'd died in a hospice with relatives of patients who'd died from cancer in other hospitals in the vicinity. And in the early 1970s and late '60s, there were very big differences between them, largely due to the fact that in other hospitals in the vicinity people were still dying in agony. The pain was so bad that not only the patients but the families too were very depressed and so our measures of depression which correlated fairly highly with patients measures of pain were reflections of that issue. Once we got the pain relieved, the depression in the family improved. At that time we were not showing big differences between families on post bereavement outcome, and that sort of thing. It was only a few years later, when we got really sophisticated bereavement counselling going, that we were able to show differences between helped and unhelped groups of bereaved people.[70]

Planning and change

Hospital support teams for terminal care (as they were then called) were pioneered in the United Kingdom from 1976, when the first one opened at St Thomas's Hospital. A notable early casualty was reported in the *BMJ*,[71] but their subsequent development was given impetus by departmental guidelines published in 1987. Between 1982 and 1996, the number of hospitals with either a multidisciplinary palliative care team or a palliative care clinical nurse specialist grew from five to 275.[72] A review of the efficacy of hospital-based palliative care teams noted their continuing evolution and gave support to their work as well as encouragement for further evaluative studies.[73] Such teams varied widely in character, but they became the principal interface between oncologists and palliative care specialists in the hospital setting.

In Britain, this was an era of what has been called 'emotional planning' in hospice and palliative care services.[73] Ideas and proposals for new services often came forward at the local level, sometimes despite (rather than because of) the support of local health bureaucrats. Only gradually did formal guidance begin to appear, sometimes hastily cobbled together in the face of a rising tide of local hospice developments led by specially formed charities. A landmark of policy recognition came in 1980 with the report of the Working Group on Terminal Care produced by the Standing Sub-Committee on Cancer of the Standing Medical Advisory Committee.[74] It was known thereafter as the Wilkes Report, after its chairperson, who a decade earlier had founded St Luke's Hospice in Sheffield and gone on to become a professor of community medicine.

The Wilkes Report was a response to the significant developments that had taken place since the report two decades earlier by H. L. Glyn Hughes. Notwithstanding his role as a hospice founder within his own locale, Wilkes gave a cold shower to expansionist tendencies among hospices. The report argued that these were neither affordable (in cash) nor sustainable (in personnel), but rather the focus should be on encouraging the principles of terminal care throughout the health service, with good coordination between the sectors. If prescient in orientation, it did little however to stem the immediate tide of enthusiasm for the creation of new hospice organizations. The decade that followed was unprecedented for hospice growth.

Two major UK cancer charities were also important drivers of change at this point.

The variously named 'Macmillan' organization had begun in 1911 to support those affected by cancer. Until 1964, it was directly led by its founder Douglas Macmillan, and its main role was in distributing funds to patients and families affected by the disease. In the mid-1970s, it underwent a period of unprecedented expansion, becoming increasingly involved with palliative care and supporting training programmes, specialist professional posts, and academic positions, as well as capital and service developments. In 1975, the first Macmillan nurses were appointed to care for dying cancer patients at home and later in hospital. It also opened its first cancer care unit in Christchurch,

Dorset. Under the leadership of Major Henry Garnett, the charity went on to develop education programmes in cancer care and advanced pain control (1980), and then introduced the concept of Macmillan-funded doctors (1986). The engagement of what was fast becoming one of Britain's major charities (of any kind) was a major boost to palliative care and a key source of funding for medical positions in the emerging field.

Established in 1948, the Marie Curie Memorial Foundation had three objectives: a nursing and welfare service for patients in their own homes; the provision of residential nursing homes; and the encouragement and funding of scientific learning. As we have seen, it was also instrumental in 1952 in conducting a major survey of need among people with cancer. In the 1980s, the Marie Curie nursing homes underwent a transition to become specialist palliative care centres, and the charity supported a wide range of educational and research activities in palliative care. Under the leadership of another ex-military man, Michael Carleton-Smith, Marie Curie increased its income in 10 years from £9 million to £55 million; 5 000 Marie Curie nurses were seeing 19 000 patients a year and the 11 centres had 300 beds catering for some 4 000 patients annually.

In 1987, the British government published its first official circular on terminal care. District health authorities were called on to take the lead in planning and coordinating services for terminally ill people, and clear strategies with monitoring arrangements were required for this. From 1989 onwards, funding earmarked for hospice services was identified by central government. By 1993, the sums involved had doubled to £43 million. Letters of guidance were sent to health authorities explaining how they should manage their relationships with independent hospices and other providers of terminal care services. Palliative care, though still not the term of choice at this time, was beginning to enter the fabric of the National Health Service.[73] The work of defining its clinical realm and of how it could be organized was beginning to pay off.

A picture later emerges of hospice ideals and practices being disseminated into other settings. By the mid-1990s in the United Kingdom, there were over 1 000 specialist Macmillan nurses working in palliative care; approximately 400 homecare teams; and over 200 daycare and 200 hospital-based services, as well as some 5 000 Marie Curie nurses providing care in the home. This meant that these services came increasingly under the purview of planners and strategists. When the Expert Advisory Group on Cancer published its findings (the Calman–Hine Report) in 1995 and proposed major restructuring for cancer services, palliative care was not left out. The report defined the palliative care resources needed at the general population level (for 500 000 people, two consultants in palliative care were required; 25 specialist beds; 12 full-time clinical nurse specialists; and 200 specialist daycare places per week) and it recommended that palliative care should be embedded within the cancer teams and integrated with general practice.[75]

Other nondirect care organizations started to emerge as interest and activity grew, and the need for more coordinated approaches to development, planning, and service delivery were being recognized. Help the Hospices had come into being in 1984 as a national charity to support independent hospices by grant-giving and lobbying activities. However, within a few years, government perception was that the growing sector of hospice and palliative care, including the major national charities, needed a single voice to represent it. Amid heated debate among the various stakeholders, the National Council for Hospice and Specialist Palliative Care Services was founded in 1991. Its goal was to serve as a multidisciplinary body, representing the several professional groups of nurses, doctors, social workers, chaplains, volunteers, and others that were now organizing themselves. It also served to bring together the views of the major national charities, the independent hospice movement, and other key players. It was a daunting task for a sector still at the 'storming and norming' stage of its development. Scotland followed suit with the Scottish Partnership for Palliative Care, formed in 1991. These organizations were to endure over time and were key in bringing the field of palliative care practice into the world of health policy, planning, and politics.

Conditions of possibility

Over the decades described here, hospice and palliative care, and particularly the medical aspects of this work, became increasingly clarified and defined. There was high-level nursing leadership from within the British hospices, as well as from the associated national charities such as Macmillan and Marie Curie. Social work perspectives became more strongly articulated and religious care from chaplains of various faiths was seen as a core aspect of palliative care, rather than an optional element. The role of volunteers was emphasized in hospice organization, and beyond them sat a large workforce of fundraisers and supporters in the wider community. The field was evolving as a consciously multidisciplinary discipline. *Total pain* required more than a response from medicine; it called on carers skilled in each of its dimensions, who would have to work in consort to address the needs of the *whole person*. To this wider, more inclusive view of palliative care, the emerging discipline of palliative medicine could at times have an ambivalent orientation.

Up until now, the emerging knowledge base of hospice and palliative care had been demonstrated through mainstream medical, nursing, and other professional journals, but specialist outlets also began to appear. The *Pain Research News Forum* was first published in 1982, and by 1986 had evolved into the *Journal of Pain and Symptom Management*. The *Journal of Palliative Care* published its first issue, from Canada, in 1985. Then 1987 saw the launch of the first UK journal—*Palliative Medicine*—to be concerned solely with palliative care. Through these and other fora, a fertile ground for debate was opening that would characterize the specialty in the years ahead. Into this space also stepped other commentators, viewpoints, and sources of debate and scholarship. They were accompanied by some who took a wider view of thanatological matters, with contributions from the social and clinical sciences as well as the arts and humanities. The field was growing and its reach was expanding.

Within this wider culture of recognition, and as the 100th anniversary of Munk's key publication approached, important developments were taking place internationally. There was increasing acknowledgement that the benefits of good palliative care should not be confined to those in the affluent nations of the world while the cancer epidemic of the developing countries also required attention. Gradually, interest in these issues was spreading throughout many societies and cultures. The momentum for the new field was growing and formal recognition from the medical establishment now seemed within the grasp of its founders.

Notes

1. **Douglas C** (1992). 'For all the saints'. *British Medical Journal*, 304(6826):479.
2. **Butterfield-Picard H**, **Magno JB** (1982). Hospice the adjective, not the noun: The future of a national priority. *American Psychologist*, 37(11):1254–9.
3. Hospice History Project: David Clark interview with Tony Crowther, 3 December 1996.
4. **Seymour J, Clark D** (2005). The modern history of morphine use in cancer pain. *European Journal of Palliative Care*, 12(4):152–5.
5. **Baszanger I** (1998). *Inventing Pain Medicine. From the Laboratory to the Clinic*. New Brunswick, NJ: Rutgers University Press.
6. **Bonica JJ** (1953). *The Management of Pain: With Special Emphasis on the Use of Analgesic Block in Diagnosis, Prognosis, and Therapy*. London, UK: Henry Kimpton.
7. **Abrams R, Jameson G, Poehlman M, Snyder S** (1945). Terminal care in cancer. *New England Journal of Medicine*, 232:719–24.
8. **Abrams RD** (1951). Social casework with cancer patients. *Social Casework* (December):425–31.
9. **Bailey M** (1959). A survey of the social needs of patients with incurable lung cancer. *The Almoner*, 11(10):379–97.

10. **Paterson R, Aitken-Swan J** (1954). Public opinion on cancer. *Lancet* (23 October):857–61.

11. **Aitken-Swan J, Paterson R** (1955). The cancer patient: Delay in help seeking. *British Medical Journal* (12 March):623–7.

12. **Seymour J, Clark D, Winslow M** (2005). Pain and palliative care: The emergence of new specialities. *Journal of Pain and Symptom Management*, 29(1):2–13.

13. **Jones LE** (2010) *First Steps: The Early Years of IASP 1973–1984*. Seattle, WA: IASP Press. Available at http://www.iasp-pain.org/files/Content/ContentFolders/Publications2/FreeBooks/First_Steps_The_Early_Years_of_IASP.pdf, accessed 25 May 2015.

14. **Bonica JJ, Ventafridda V** (1979). *International Symposium on Pain of Advanced Cancer*. New York, NY: Raven Press.

15. **Reynolds LA, Tansey EM** (2004). *Innovations in Pain Management. Welcome Witnesses to Twentieth Century Medicine*, vol. 21. London, UK: Wellcome Trust.

16. **Ventafridda V, Bonica J** (1979). *International Symposium on Pain of Advanced Cancer*. New York, NY: Raven Press.

17. **Meldrum M** (2005). The ladder and the clock: Cancer pain and public policy at the end of the twentieth century. *Journal of Pain and Symptom Management*, 29(1):41–54.

18. Hospice History Project: Kathleen Foley interview with David Clark, 27 October 2003.

19. **Stjernswärd J, Joranson DE** (1995). Opioid availability and cancer pain—an unnecessary tragedy. *Supportive Care in Cancer* 3(3):157–8.

20. **Higginson I** (1993). Palliative care: A review of past changes and future trends. *Journal of Public Health*, 15(1):3–8.

21. **Clark D** (2002). Between hope and acceptance: The medicalisation of dying. *British Medical Journal*, 324:905–7.

22. **Saunders C** (1960). Drug treatment of patients in the terminal stages of cancer. *Current Medicine and Drugs*, 1(July):16–28.

23. **Saunders C** (1967). The care of the terminal stages of cancer. *Annals of the Royal College of Surgeons*, 41 (Supplementary issue) Summer:162–9.

24. **Clark D** (2003). The rise and demise of the "Brompton Cocktail". In: Meldrum ML (ed.). *Opioids and Pain Relief: A Historical Perspective. Progress in Pain Research and Management*, vol. 25, pp. 85–98. Seattle, WA: IASP Press.

25. **Meunier-Cartal RN, Souberbielle JC, Boureau F** (1995). Morphine and the "Lytic Cocktail" for terminally ill patients in a French general hospital: Evidence for an inverse relationship. *Journal of Pain and Symptom Management*, 10(4):267–73.

26. **'The Brompton Cocktail'** (1979). Editorial. *Lancet* (9 June):1220–1.

27. Hospice History Project: David Clark interview with Robert Twycross, 4 January 1996.

28. **Twycross RG** (1973). Stumbling blocks in the study of morphine. *Postgraduate Medical Journal*, 49 (May):309–13.

29. **Twycross RG, Fry DE, Wills PD** (1974). The alimentary absorption of diamorphine and morphine in man as indicated by urinary excretion studies. *British Journal of Clinical Pharmacology*, 1:491–4.

30. **Twycross RG** (1974). Diamorphine and cocaine elixir BPC 1973. *Pharmaceutical Journal* 212(5755):153, 159.

31. **Mount BM, Ajemian I, Scott JF** (1976). Use of the Brompton mixture in treating the chronic pain of malignant disease. *Canadian Medical Association Journal*, 115 (17 July): 122–4.
32. **Melzack R, Ofiesh JG, Mount BM** (1976). The Brompton mixture: Effects on pain in cancer patients. *Canadian Medical Association Journal*, 115 (17 July):125–9.
33. **Twycross RG** (1977a). Choice of strong analgesic in terminal cancer: Diamorphine or morphine? *Pain*, 3:93–104.
34. **Twycross RG** (1977b). Letter. Value of cocaine in opiate-containing elixirs. *British Medical Journal*, 2:1348.
35. **Melzack R, Mount BM, Gordon JM** (1979). The Brompton mixture versus morphine solution given orally: Effects on pain. *Canadian Medical Association Journal*, 20 (17 February):435–8.
36. **Twycross RG** (1979). The Brompton Cocktail. In: Bonica JJ, Ventafridda V (eds.). *Advances in Pain Research and Therapy*, vol. 2, pp. 291–300. New York, NY: Raven Press.
37. **Clark D** (1999). 'Total pain', disciplinary power, and the body in the work of Cicely Saunders, 1958–1967. *Social Science and Medicine*, 49:727–36.
38. **Saunders C** (1959). Care of the dying 3. Control of pain in terminal cancer. *Nursing Times* (23 October):1032.
39. **Saunders C** (1966). The care of the dying. *Guy's Hospital Gazette*, 80:136–42.
40. **Saunders C** (1965). Telling patients. *District Nursing* (September):149–54.
41. **Saunders C** (1964). Care of patients suffering from terminal illness at St Joseph's Hospice, Hackney, London. *Nursing Mirror* (14 February):vii–x.
42. **Saunders C** (1964). The symptomatic treatment of incurable malignant disease. *Prescribers' Journal,* 4, no. 4 (October):68–73.
43. **Saunders C** (1967). *The Management of Terminal Illness*. London, UK: Hospital Medicine Publications Ltd.
44. **Saunders C** (1969). The moment of truth: Care of the dying person. In: Pearson L (ed.). *Death and Dying: Current Issues in the Treatment of the Dying Person*, pp. 49–78. Cleveland, OH: The Press of Case Western Reserve University.
45. **Saunders C** (1970a). Nature and management of terminal pain. In: Shotter EF (ed.). *Matters of Life and Death*, p. 15. London, UK: Dartman, Longman, and Todd.
46. **Saunders C** (1970b). An individual approach to the relief of pain. *People and Cancer*, pp. 34–38. London, UK: The British Council.
47. **Saunders C, Winner A** (1973). Research into terminal care of cancer patients. *Portfolio for Health 2. The Developing Programme of the DHSS in Health Services Research*, pp. 19–25. Published for the Nuffield Provincial Hospitals Trust by Oxford University Press.
48. **Saunders C** (1976a). The challenge of terminal care. In: Symington T, Carter R (eds.). *The Scientific Foundations of Oncology*. London, UK: Heinemann.
49. **Saunders C** (1979). The nature and management of terminal pain and the hospice concept. In: **Bonica JJ, Ventafridda V** (eds.). *Advances in Pain Research*, vol. 2. New York, NY: Raven Press.
50. **Saunders C** (1981). Current views on pain relief and terminal care. In: Swerdlow M (ed.). *The Therapy of Pain*. Lancaster, PA: MTP Press.
51. **Saunders C, Baines M** (1983). *Living with Dying: The Management of Terminal Disease*. Oxford, UK: Oxford University Press.

52. Graham F, Clark D (2005). The syringe driver and the subcutaneous route in palliative care: the inventor, the history and the implications. *Journal of Pain and Symptom Management* 29(1):32–40.

53. Hospice History Project: Fiona Graham interview with Patrick Russell, 8 May 2003.

54. Russell PSB (1979). Analgesia in terminal malignant disease. *British Medical Journal*, 1:1561.

55. Drinkwater C, Twycross R (1979). Analgesia in terminal malignant disease. *British Medical Journal*, 1(6172):1201–2.

56. Milner PC, Harper R, Williams BT (1989). Ownership, availability and use of portable syringe drivers among hospices and home care services. *Public Health*, 103:345–52.

57. Leslie ST, Rhodes A, Black FM (1980). Controlled release morphine sulphate tablets: a study in normal volunteers. *British Journal of Clinical Pharmacology*, 9:531–4.

58. Seymour J, Clark D (2005) Evaluation in cancer pain relief: from private to public trouble? *International Conference for Health Technology Assessment*, Rome, Italy. Unpublished.

59. Slattery PJ, Boas RA (1985). Newer methods of delivery of opiates for relief of pain. *Drugs*, 30(6):539–51.

60. Saunders C (1983). *Beyond All Pain: A Companion for the Suffering and Bereaved.* London, UK: SPCK.

61. Murray Parkes C (1964). Recent bereavement as a cause of mental illness. *British Journal of Psychiatry*, 110:198–204.

62. Wilkes E (1964). Cancer outside hospital. *Lancet* (20 June):1379–81.

63. Wilkes E (1965). Terminal cancer at home. *Lancet* (10 April):799–801.

64. Hinton J (1965). Problems in the care of the dying. *Journal of Chronic Diseases*, 17:201–5.

65. Clark D (1999). Cradled to the grave? Pre-conditions for the hospice movement in the UK, 1948–67. *Mortality*, 4(3):225–47.

66. Glaser B, Strauss A (1965). *Awareness of Dying.* Chicago, IL: Aldine.

67. Cartwright A, Hockey J, Anderson JL (1973). *Life before Death.* London, UK: Routledge and Kegan Paul.

68. Murray Parkes CM (1978). Home or hospital? Terminal care as seen by surviving spouses. *Journal of the Royal College of General Practitioners*, 28:29–30.

69. Murray Parkes CM, Parkes J (1984). 'Hospice' versus 'hospital' care—re-evaluation after 10 years as seen by surviving spouses. *Postgraduate Medical Journal*, 60:38–42.

70. Hospice History Project: David Clark interview with Colin Murray Parkes, 10 January 1996.

71. Herxheimer A, Begent R, MacLean D, Philips L, Southcott B, Walton I (1985). The short life of a terminal care support team: Experience at Charing Cross Hospital. *British Medical Journal*, 290:1877–9.

72. Clark D, Seymour J (1999). *Reflections on Palliative Care.* Buckingham, UK: Open University Press.

73. Higginson IJ et al. (2002). Do hospital-based palliative teams improve care for patients or families at the end of life? *Journal of Pain and Symptom Management*, 23(2):96–106.

74. Working Group on Terminal Care [The Wilkes Report] (1980). *Report of the Working* Group on Terminal Care. London, UK: Department of Health and Social Services.
75. Expert Advisory Group on Cancer [The Calman-Hine Report] (1995). A Policy Framework for Commissioning Services: A Report by the Expert Advisory Group on Cancer for the Chief Medical Officers of England and Wales. London, UK: Department of Health and Welsh Office.

Chapter 6

Specialty recognition and global development

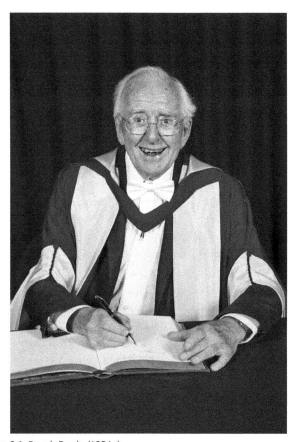

Figure 6.1 Derek Doyle (1931–)

Returning to Edinburgh in 1966 from work as a medical missionary in Africa, Doyle soon found himself caught up in plans to create the city's first modern hospice, St Columba's. He became the medical director from its opening in 1977 and quickly used this as a platform for wider teaching and promulgation of hospice ideas. He was instrumental in the formation of several key national and international advocacy organizations, and took a leading role in the creation of the specialty of palliative medicine, which was officially recognized in the United Kingdom in 1987.

Acceptance and spread

Any history of modern medical practice is, in part, a history of specialization. From the twentieth century onwards, it is also a history of globalization. Beginning in the nineteenth century and reflecting broader changes in what Emile Durkheim[1] described as 'the division of labour in society', medicine was undergoing forces of change often seen as both the inevitable and desirable outcomes of scientific progress and advancement. The generalist was giving way to the specialist, and new fields of clinical endeavour were being defined and circumscribed. For the historian George Weisz, these changes were driven by the unification of medicine and surgery, for only within an understanding of medicine as a single domain was it sensible to divide into sub-fields.[2] By such specialization, it was then possible to amass sufficient observations on a specific problem or aspect of medicine, which an increasing scientific rationality required. Moreover, this was in turn consistent with emerging views of the appropriate way to manage large populations, through the systematic accrual of information about a certain class of phenomena, problems, and their subcategories. We have already seen evidence of this in the writings of nineteenth-century physicians concerned with the care of the dying, interested in their symptoms, and how to describe and manage them. In the later decades of the twentieth century, this field of clinical interest underwent a transformational change; first in mapping out the scope of the activity, and then in raising questions about its potential for geographic spread. Increasingly, it did this from the standpoint of a recognized field of specialization that took on global dimensions.

In this chapter, we look in detail at the formation of palliative medicine as a medical specialty and at the global spread of the field. There were two elements to this process. First, palliative care had to be defined as an activity (and this came to be at differing levels of specialization or generality). With this would come the potential for recognition by the wider healthcare system, as well as from interested groups in society—for resource allocation; for education, training, and research; and for designated service development. Second, palliative medicine had to gain recognition from *within* the medical establishment itself to become accepted as a legitimate field of medical specialization, and to establish pathways for medical training, accreditation, and the regulation of standards.

Hospice growth—laying the foundations for specialization

St Christopher's Hospice, founded in 1967, quickly became a source of inspiration to others. As the first modern hospice, it was at the time unique in combining three key principles: specialist clinical care, education, and research. St

Christopher's differed significantly from the more modest goals of the other homes for the dying which had preceded it, and sought to establish itself as no less than a centre of excellence in a new field of care. The success of St Christopher's was phenomenal and it soon became the stimulus for an expansive phase of wider development.

In the United Kingdom, there was a golden period of hospice growth that peaked in the 1980s, with about 10 new hospices coming into existence each year. Established national charities then came alongside the emergent hospice movement, giving support and strength to the field of palliative care. This was an important phase in which a sense of critical mass was growing, when the activists of the day could move in from the margins and begin to identify a centre ground within the healthcare system that could be occupied successfully.[3]

From the outset, ideas developed at St Christopher's were being applied differently in other places. Cicely Saunders was also acting as part of an international network of like-minded people that covered North America, India and Ceylon, Australia, France, Switzerland, the Netherlands, and communist Poland, as she reveals in her remarkable and extensive correspondence of the time.[4] It came to be accepted in several countries that the principles of hospice care could be practised in many settings—in specialist inpatient units, but also in homecare and daycare services. Hospital units and support teams were established that brought this new thinking on care of the dying and those suffering with advanced disease into the very heartland of acute medicine. By the 1980s, a growing cadre of doctors was developing an interest in the care of this group of patients and their families. While many had transferred into this work in mid-career or later, others were beginning to dedicate their entire professional lives to it. However, without formal recognition, the pathways into, and routes through a training programme for specialized work in the care of the dying remained unclear.

Specialization in the United Kingdom and Ireland

In the United Kingdom, beginning in the early 1980s, three factors conjoined to build a platform for the wider development of this new field of activity: a medical association was formed to support its practitioners; a scientific journal was established; and, in due course, recognition was given to palliative medicine as an area of specialization.[5]

By 1985, plans were being developed in the United Kingdom for an association to represent the interests of physicians working in palliative care. Cicely Saunders wrote enthusiastically about it to Derek Doyle (Figure 6.1)[6] who, together with Robert Twycross and Richard Hillier, made up a key group of early protagonists. All three were physicians employed in hospices. Following medical missionary work in South Africa, Derek Doyle had been instrumental in establishing St Columba's Hospice in Edinburgh, which opened in 1977 and where he was its first medical director. Robert Twycross had joined St Christopher's as a medical research fellow in 1971, and in 1976 was appointed consultant physician at the NHS hospice Sir Michael Sobell House in Oxford. Richard Hillier was a former GP who had been drawn into hospice care in the 1970s and became the medical director of Countess Mountbatten House in Southampton in 1977.[3] Robert Twycross describes the context.

> We didn't have a 'palliative care association' and I guess round about 1983/1984 Cancer Relief Macmillan Fund was playing a major part and was bringing people from the NHS units together in an annual weekend in November, not far from Oxford, and we'd meet and talk. And I remember talking, particularly with Richard Hillier, about, should we have some national organization? But we were also living under the shadow of Cicely Saunders and we didn't want to do anything to offend her, which I think is fair enough, and she didn't come forward and say: 'Here is the national organization.' So I think there was a reticence. And by the time we got to '84, or thereabouts, Richard was certainly of the opinion we should set up a 'palliative care association'. But I felt we should, as doctors, get *our* act together, and then as a doctors' group go to the nurses, go to the social workers, and say: 'Let's come together as a national organization.' But if we set up a national organization for all-comers, it would be medically dominated, and I think this was not what I wanted. So I won the argument, and Richard Hillier backed down on the multi-professional association. And, I think I'm right in saying, in Birmingham, October 1985, we had an inaugural meeting of what was to become the Association for Palliative Medicine. Obviously by now we had drawn in Derek Doyle and, not surprisingly, Derek Doyle was elected inaugural Chair Person, and Richard was Secretary, and I was Treasurer. It was skillfully led by Derek ... And the fascinating thing was that, once we got a letterhead and people could see that there was such a thing as palliative medicine, within two or three years we were a recognized specialty ... Now I know people like Gillian Ford did much of the spadework, because she was on secondment from the Ministry and knew how to deal with the powers that be. I think it must have made her task much, much easier that we had a coherent professional organization ... A very important landmark.[7]

Following some early discussion about whether the term *hospice* should appear in the name, the group soon came to be known as the Association for Palliative Medicine for Great Britain and Ireland. The executive committee of the new association quickly became aware of a paper written by the then deputy chief medical officer for England, Gillian Ford, in which she outlined the potential for this new field of medicine to gain recognition as a specialty in its own right. Dr Ford was an important ally in the process. She and Cicely Saunders had shared a flat as medical students, and she had taken up a volunteer role providing medical cover at St Christopher's Hospice on weekends as well as later taking up a secondment there. She describes her position there in some detail.[8]

I was part of the management team for the hospice, and I started looking at things like training for medical staff in palliative care, as well as the things which were precisely St Christopher's interests. And I did some studies. . . for instance, a survey on the qualifications and experience of those medical staff who were in career grades, what their background had been, what their qualifications had been; and I presented this to the Association of Palliative Medicine at one of its earlier meetings. I sent out a questionnaire to something like 800 general practitioners asking them what they would identify, if anything, as their needs in this field. And I think I had replies back from about 150, or 160, saying they were interested, and then I sent them a detailed questionnaire about pain and symptom control, support of families, communications and those things. *Almost all* of them wanted pain and symptom control, and so I put on a conference for them. So looking at what people's backgrounds were, finding out more and more about training needs, realising that the hospice movement needed to do things like appoint its senior staff in conformity with the National Health Service, the value of joint contracts or at least honorary contracts, the need for the sort of principles and attitudes to get back into mainstream medicine, suggested that there needed to be specialist training in the specialty in order for the people to be listened to.

Well, the Association for Palliative Medicine was set up in about October/November '85, and . . . I was a member of the executive of that, and I think that the paper I wrote about establishing palliative medicine (it wasn't called that) . . . establishing a specialty in this work; hospice terminal care, I think that was seen by the executive and it was certainly [based on] the material I had derived from the surveys I'd done about what people's backgrounds were. At the same time Derek Doyle had . . . I think he'd been talking to the juniors who were in the Association, and asking what they needed. But, as I say, the driving force for this was really the need for this expanding group of people to be recognized for the work that they were doing, and for the teaching that they were doing.[9]

Discussions got underway with a number of key groupings within the Royal Colleges, including the Intercollegiate Committee on Oncology, and ideas were subsequently developed about how a training programme for the field could be put together. The most influential group in this regard was the Joint Committee on Higher Medical Training (JCHMT). At the time, a growing number of universities and medical schools were calling on those working in hospices to teach students about pain control and physician–patient/physician–family communication, though as yet no formal curriculum on palliative medicine existed. Gillian Ford prepared a paper for the JCHMT and, at the same time, encouraged the chair of the Specialty Advisory Committee in General Medicine and other senior medical colleagues to visit St Christopher's for an appreciation of the work being done there. These senior medical colleagues found themselves impressed by the research of Robert Twycross on the actions of morphine and diamorphine,[9] and by the evaluations that Colin Murray Parkes had conducted on the impact of hospice care.[10] There was also considerable interest in the multidisciplinary approach adopted at the hospice and the way team efforts were focused on the *total pain* of the patient, seen in a multifactorial light. Yet there was still a sense that the constituent elements of what came to be called specialist palliative care had not yet been teased out. This made for difficulty in devising a training programme for what were known then as the senior registrar years within medical training. It was also necessary to determine the specific prior experience that would be required for entry into the new field.

The outcome of these deliberations was enormously important for the history of palliative care in the United Kingdom and Ireland and, arguably, much further afield too.[11] In 1987, palliative medicine was established as a subspecialty of general medicine, initially on a seven-year 'novitiate', which once successfully concluded led to it being a specialty in its own right. In 1987, all UK doctors working full-time in hospices were granted specialist registration. Thereafter, entrants into higher medical training for the new specialty were required to be members of the Royal Colleges of Physicians, general practitioners, or psychiatrists, or fellows of the Royal College of Surgeons. This was modified in 2002 to include members of the Irish College of General Practitioners and fellows of the Royal Colleges of Radiologists and Anaesthetists. Initially, membership in the Royal College of General Practitioners was not a recognized mode of entry; however, considerable protest and further campaigning led to its recognition within a few years.

In a 1988 article in the *British Medical Journal*, Richard Hillier celebrated the achievement. After 21 years of pioneering work from Cicely Saunders, the breakthrough had been achieved. As Hillier put it, 'the Royal College of Physicians recognised terminal care as a subspecialty of general internal medicine and called it palliative medicine'.[12] William Munk would have been astonished, and we must assume, delighted.

The four-year training programme in the United Kingdom was designed to equip trainees with skills to practice palliative medicine in any setting. It was heavily supported by the Cancer Relief Macmillan Fund, which provided pump-priming grants to set up new senior registrar training programmes. There were 10 posts funded in its first wave of development.[12] The training generally included spending at least two years working within hospice or hospital-based specialist palliative care teams, to gain a range of experience in chronic pain management, oncology, community services, or paediatric palliative care. Importantly, UK programmes also required competence in a range of essential management skills including recruiting, managing staff, and service development. In 2005, it was noted by Doyle that 'in practice, most recruits into the specialty today have had several years' experience in general medicine, oncology, or radiotherapy after gaining their higher qualification, but only a few have had experience of specialist palliative medicine as an SHO [senior house officer]'.[13] In 2007, Professor John Tooke's inquiry into medical careers recommended that medical training in the United Kingdom should consist of one foundation year (similar to the house officer year), three years of general training in a broad mix of specialities, followed by four to five years in higher specialist training. Progression through the three stages would require achievement of competencies and a rigorous selection process, and this was to become the new framework for training in palliative medicine.

As the initial developments about the specialty were taking place in the 1980s, discussions were also underway about the creation of a journal to publish research, reviews, and debate relating to the work. Following some discussion about its name and orientation, the first issue was published in 1987, bearing the title *Palliative Medicine*, under which a 'strap line' appeared on the cover stating: A MULTI-PROFESSIONAL JOURNAL. The wording was crucial and did a fair amount to antagonize colleagues in other professions, but the message was clear—medical practitioners had seized hold of the new field of caring for those with advanced disease at the end of life and, over time, the medical model would exert a growing influence on thinking and practice. Enigmatically, the first issue contained a paper by Cicely Saunders entitled 'What's in a name?'[14] Designed to clarify, her observations may have further muddied waters that were already being stirred up by the debate on definitional matters. The particular discussion about which point in the disease trajectory should trigger the entry of palliative care would continue to unfold over the next quarter century.

> Although all palliative care aims to improve the quality of life remaining for patients whose disease cannot be eliminated, somewhat confusingly it is also used to refer to different stages of disease and its treatment. This is particularly obvious in malignant disease . . . It is unrealistic to aim for cure in over half the patients at the stage when they present with this diagnosis and they need what is termed 'palliative' treatment from the beginning. However, those working in units or services designated as palliative do not normally treat patients at the stage when the *disease* itself can be mitigated or controlled; their skills are focussed on alleviating the *symptoms* and general suffering associated with uncontrollable disease in its final stages, although a regression of the disease process has still to be watched for and exploited . . . This journal is concerned with the second phase of palliative rather than the more 'active' stages of treatment for cancer (or other persistent disease) which are well covered elsewhere.[15]

Despite these questions, progress towards specialty recognition was getting underway elsewhere. Developments in Ireland took a similar path. In 1989, the first post of consultant physician in palliative medicine was created in the form of a joint appointment between the long established Our Lady's Hospice and St Vincent's University Hospital, Dublin. Then in the mid-1990s, the Irish Medical Council considered the inclusion of palliative medicine in its list of recognized specialities. Such recognition required evidence of a significant corpus of knowledge specific to palliative medicine, over and above that which would be within the competence of any registered medical practitioner, as well as the existence of a reputable body to oversee developments in the new specialty, including training and education. The Minister for Health and Children approved the inclusion of palliative medicine among the list of recognized Irish medical specialities in June 1995.[15]

Within an intensive period of activity lasting just a few years, both the United Kingdom and Ireland had succeeded in establishing the specialty of palliative medicine with a training programme leading to consultant status. Arrangements for representing the interests of the field were now in place and an appropriate scientific journal had been created. Subsequently, considerable expansion in the palliative medicine workforce would follow.

A survey of the membership of the Association of Palliative Medicine (APM) in 2004[16] revealed that 58.1 per cent were in full-time appointments in palliative medicine and 70.4 per cent of the workforce was female. There were 325 consultants, 49 associate specialists, and 78 staff grade post-holders, as well as 160 specialist registrars, of which 83 per cent were female. Some 60 consultants held honorary NHS contracts, but despite an APM recommendation, there were very few NHS consultants holding honorary contracts with hospices. In Ireland specifically, there were seven consultant physicians in palliative medicine in 2005, with a further seven consultant posts in the process of being filled.[17]

Such growth in the palliative medicine establishment had been made possible by wider service developments and policy changes. During the 1970s and 1980s, a major programme of hospice expansion had taken place in the United Kingdom, gaining wide geographic coverage. The expansion in charitable hospices was also reflected in a growing number of NHS inpatient units, though the ratio between the two remained fairly constant at roughly 3:1. Indeed, it was the 'mixed economy' of care between the non-government and government sectors that became a distinct hallmark of the palliative care developments in the United Kingdom and Ireland. From the later 1980s onwards, hospice and palliative care services in the United Kingdom also benefited from special government funding streams that enabled consolidation and expansion, initially providing ring-fenced monies for independent hospices, and then for palliative care more generally.[18]

There were also some specific policy innovations at this time. In 1992, an expert group of physicians and nurses reporting to the UK Minister of Health was instrumental in making a case for palliative care to be provided based on need, rather than diagnosis. The report called for wider education in palliative care for all health professionals and greater emphasis on matching services to the needs identified at the population level.[19] Three years later, the Expert Advisory Group on Cancer produced what came to be known as the Calman Hine Report on the commissioning of cancer services in England and Wales.[20] It was crucial in giving a prominent place to palliative care within the different tiers of cancer care provision and in giving guidance on staffing levels required in relation to population. The report was seized upon by the palliative medicine community as an opportunity for development. Demand for palliative medicine was growing and there were more jobs on offer than candidates to fill them.

In early 1989, the United Kingdom also saw the creation of its first university chair in the palliative care field at the United Medical and Dental Schools of Guy's and St Thomas' Hospitals, London. Dr Geoffrey Hanks was appointed as the first professor of palliative medicine in Europe, and this set the tone for subsequent academic developments in the field, which tended to focus on the clinical disciplines. After graduating from University College Hospital Medical School in 1970, Hanks had completed his clinical training and spent a year in general practice. He then explored his interest in clinical pharmacology, working from 1975 until 1979 in senior positions within the pharmaceutical industry. In 1979, he was appointed Research Fellow and Honorary Senior Registrar at Sir Michael Sobell House, Oxford, where he collaborated with Robert Twycross, and also had a base in the Oxford Regional Pain Relief Unit. He kept a foot in both the palliative care and the pain communities and was instrumental in bringing a searching medical rationality to the management of pain in the palliative care setting. In 1983, he was appointed to the first hospital consultant post in palliative medicine in the United Kingdom, at the Royal Marsden Hospital, a stronghold of acute cancer medicine. Here, he started the new clinical service at the Sutton branch of the hospital, and he was also responsible for developing the unit at Fulham Road, and bringing them together as a single functional service. He forged a particular interest in the benefits of the emerging modified-release morphine formulations, which came to have a huge influence on the practice of palliative medicine.[21] As professor of palliative medicine, he quickly set about working to raise the banner of palliative care and, in particular to influence medical thinking about the new specialty.

In 1993, Hanks moved to Bristol for a new position and a department created for his team, all of whom moved with him. It was a significant year for the field, as well as for Hanks himself, with the 1993 publication of the first edition of the *Oxford Textbook of Palliative Medicine*, which he edited alongside his Scottish and Canadian colleagues, Derek Doyle and Neil Macdonald.[22] The work contained 18 major sections furnished by 103 authors, with 43 of them from North America. Derek Doyle describes how it came about.

> Why did we do it? Well the answer's an obvious one, because we had to say to the non-palliative medicine doctors . . . 'Will you take us seriously?' There was a certain urgency about producing a major 860-page book and saying: 'Now do you take us seriously?' Oxford University Press insisted that it must not be a British book and it must not be for British readership; it must be 'world' and, therefore, they insisted that it should be approximately equal both sides of the Atlantic. And, as we know, in North America, what they call palliative medicine is not what we call palliative medicine . . . Why did we choose the authors that we did? We must have a major lot of contributors, and big contributions, from the UK, but after that we'd have to be diplomatic. The next question was; would we go to people that are only in palliative medicine? I don't think we spent five minutes talking about this because we looked around and said, 'we haven't enough'. We have not enough people that are authoritative, highly enough qualified, experienced enough, and have got a track record of writing as opposed to being super at the bedside and, do we possess all the knowledge? And the three of us said straightaway: 'No.' And there's a message that's important here; we may be the full-time specialist practitioners of it, but we wouldn't be here if it wasn't for the others to whom we can turn, who advise us, guide us, inspire us, challenge us, kick us up the backside. And they have things to contribute, and so that's why you've got people who are all totally sympathetic to what we are doing . . .
>
> The next big question was, would this be a textbook of palliative 'care'? There was no doubt about that, the answer was: 'No, not at all.' We felt that we needed a textbook of palliative 'medicine' for the following reasons—we needed medical respectability and credibility. We had to stand up and say to the College of Physicians and Surgeons, and others all over the world, and I mean *all over the world* . . . The other thing was that we felt that it was going to be too big, and too nebulous, and far too difficult for us to edit if it was to be everything in palliative care. And the more we looked at 'medical only' the more we realised that was, in fact, a major book—medicine only. How to make it relevant for the world was another issue, and we failed. There is no doubt, we failed. The book has, in that way, I think, taught Geoff and me a lot. It has helped the people in the medically sophisticated first world, where palliative medicine started and is growing. Whereas what we wanted to say in that book was that palliation applies to everybody in the world . . . We felt we wanted all that. Now that was difficult, of course; we were producing a book for the generalist as well as for the specialist; we were producing a book for the researcher as well as for the ordinary doctor. But, of course, it turned out to be a book which seemed the *pièce de résistance* of the best that could possibly be offered in a medical first world. It has made a contribution, there's no question about this.[23]

These challenges of developing palliative medicine in the global context had been building up in the decade before the publication of the Oxford textbook. Jan Stjsernswärd at the World Health Organization (WHO) had been a key player in this regard. In writing the final chapter of the first edition of the textbook, he had an opportunity to summarize developments by 1993, and in particular to highlight the role of the WHO.

Global dimensions—the World Health Organization

As we already discussed in Chapter 5, in 1973 John Bonica hosted the first international pain meeting, providing a forum for debate, discussion, and the development of pain relief in cancer and other fields.[24] Interaction between pain and terminal care experts began to increase. A crucial change came when Stjernswärd was appointed to work at the WHO, as he recalls in this memoir.

> When I left the Ludwig Institute in 1980 to become chief of cancer at the World Health Organization, I applied the principle of finding out what is already known, organising services to reflect this knowledge, and research to address continuing uncertainties. My philosophy was that nothing would have greater impact in global cancer control than being able to deliver the knowledge that already existed in the developed world. Out of the eight most common cancers globally, five were more common in developing than in developed countries. Three of these were preventable; early diagnosis increased survival in three; therapy is curative in three, but only if the diagnosis is made at an early stage; and pain relief and palliative care are needed for most.[25]

Driven by this orientation, as described in Chapter 5, a meeting was convened by Stjernswärd in 1982 to tackle the problem of cancer pain at the population level.[26] It established the principle that drugs would be the mainstay of cancer pain relief and that an inexpensive and easily applicable approach to this should be developed. Four years later, the WHO published a guide to cancer pain relief [27] with a view to relieve cancer pain worldwide by the early twenty-first century. In this guide, pain relief was conceptualized as a 'ladder', with the regular giving of oral morphine as the linchpin of clinical practice for all involved in the care of patients experiencing pain from advanced malignancy. Field testing of the ladder took place in several locations. 'WHY NOT FREEDOM FROM CANCER PAIN?' became its advocacy slogan. The 1986 document was translated into 22 languages and, by 1996 when a second edition appeared, it had sold half a million copies.

The approach was predicated on three foundation or *process* measures that were deemed low-cost but capable of producing big effects, and prioritized above the goal of establishing *outcome* measures. The three elements consisted of education (of the public and professionals); drug availability (requiring changes to legislation and prescribing practices); and governmental policy (to give support to the other measures). By 1993, Stjernswärd could report that 11 countries had adopted such policies: Canada, France, Australia, Japan, Sweden, Finland, Italy, Mexico, Netherlands, Vietnam, and the Philippines.[28]

Over time, the WHO broadened its interest beyond the specific issue of cancer pain relief. A 1990 publication[29] maintained the focus on cancer, but now engaged more widely with the question of palliative care. It considered more broadly what could—and should—be done to comfort patients suffering from the distressing symptoms of advanced malignant disease. Prepared by a group of nine experts in oncology, neurology, pain management, hospice and nursing care, the booklet drew together the evidence and arguments needed to define clear lines of action, whether on the part of the medical and nursing professions, or in the form of national legislation. It marshalled arguments for palliative care based on the magnitude of unrelieved suffering borne by the majority of terminally ill patients. Although methods for the relief of pain were emphasized, other physical, psychological, and spiritual needs for comfort were also included in the report's recommendations.

The conceptualization of palliative care pivoted on its concern with quality of life and comfort before death, emphasizing the family as the unit of care, dependence on teamwork, and its relationship to curative interventions. The WHO's booklet contained sections on measures for the relief of pain and other physical symptoms, the psychosocial needs of the patient and family, and the need for spiritual comfort. A section devoted to ethics provided several important statements concerning the legal and ethical distinction between 'killing the pain' and 'killing the patient', and the need to recognize the limits of medicine. The work, fully endorsed by the WHO, was a landmark moment in the history of palliative care, which had now been fully defined, moreover as a global, public health issue.

The definition was the product of a large expert group, although Stjernswärd[25] states that the drafting skills and penmanship of Robert Twycross played a big part. It framed palliative care as:

> ... the active total care of patients whose disease is not responsive to curative treatment. Control of pain, of other symptoms, and of psychological, social and spiritual problems, is paramount. The goal of palliative care is achievement of the best quality of life for patients and their families. Many aspects of palliative care are applicable earlier in the course of the illness in conjunction with anti-cancer treatment ... Palliative care ... affirms life and regards dying as a normal process ... neither hastens not postpones death ... provides relief from pain and other distressing symptoms ... integrates the psychological and the spiritual aspects of care ... offers a

support system to help patients live as actively as possible until death ... offers the family a support system to help the family cope during the patients illness and in their own bereavement.[29]

Many elements here might have been recognized by William Munk. The WHO booklet was certainly endorsed by Cicely Saunders and welcomed by the emerging cadre of palliative care leaders around the world. It achieved a broad consensus and was widely used to advocate, to teach, and to lobby governments for recognition.

Twelve years later, a new definition of palliative care appeared from the WHO. The field was becoming better known, debates about its mission and scope were proliferating, there was an increasing interest in not limiting its vision simply to terminal care or to oncology, and instead make it available to patients and families where the disease was not so far progressed, or where the distinction between curative and palliative approaches might not be so clear cut. This time, however, the process of producing a definition appeared to be different. The work was published in a journal article, rather than in a WHO publication, and seemed to be not the product of a multinational expert group, but rather of the named authors, who were each employed by WHO and included Stjernswärd's successor as head of cancer and palliative care. Published in 2002, the second WHO definition saw some critical changes.

Palliative care is an approach that improves the quality of life of patients and their families facing the problems associated with life-threatening illness, through the prevention and relief of suffering by means of early identification and impeccable assessment and treatment of pain and other problems, physical, psychosocial, and spiritual.[30]

The definition went on to state that palliative care

- provides relief from pain and other distressing symptoms;
- affirms life and regards dying as a normal process;
- intends neither to hasten or postpone death;
- integrates the psychological and spiritual aspects of patient care;
- offers a support system to help patients live as actively as possible until death;
- offers a support system to help the family cope during the patient's illness and in their own bereavement;
- uses a team approach to address the needs of patients and their families, including bereavement counselling, if indicated;
- will enhance quality of life, and may also positively influence the course of illness;

◆ is applicable early in the course of illness, in conjunction with other therapies that are intended to prolong life, such as chemotherapy or radiation
therapy, and includes those investigations needed to better understand
and manage distressing clinical complications.[30]

Some clinical experts in the field disliked the 2002 reference to palliative
care as an 'approach', seeking instead to make a claim for its specialist status.
Nevertheless, those with a more public health orientation welcomed the new
language.

> Two important revisions are incorporated in WHO's new definition. First, 'terminal
> illness' is replaced by 'life threatening illness'. Superficially, this modification may
> appear to be slight, but its implication is nothing short of revolutionary, broaden-
> ing the reach of palliative care to all people suffering from chronic illnesses. By so
> doing, the WHO's definition has been brought into line with recent medical ad-
> vances. Diseases formerly considered to be 'death sentences', such as cancer, cardiac
> disease, and infection with HIV, are now manageable. Second, 'relief of suffering
> by means of early identification' has been added. Thus, palliative care is envisioned
> as *pre-emptive*, as well as responsive. In one bold stroke, the WHO affirms that end
> of life problems have significantly earlier origins, and that treating them early en-
> hances management though the course of illness.[31]

These were large and complex claims, not least when major concerns existed
about the extent to which palliative care services were achieving them, either
due to a lack of coverage, or because the services did not have the capacity to
deliver multidisciplinary care at this level of sophistication. Despite emerging evidence about increased palliative care development around the world,
progress remained uneven, with many regions and populations underserved.

A second edition of the WHO work on the pain ladder, with the addition of
a guide to opioid availability, was published in 1996.[32] Two years later, another
expert document was published on pain relief and palliative care in children
with cancer.[33] In the 1998 publication *Symptom Relief and Terminal Illness*,[34]
it was stated that more than 60 countries of the world had developed national
strategies on cancer pain management. Here, and again drawing on the contributions of Twycross, MacDonald, Ventadfridda, and others, the focus
shifted to the management of symptoms other than pain. It placed a strong
emphasis on constant evaluation of the patient's condition (by both doctor
and nurse) to 'build a picture of the disease itself, the patient as a whole, and,
in particular to build a picture of the effects of the illness on the patient's
quality of life'.

A key aspiration within the emerging palliative care community had been
to engender interest in and support for palliative care on the part of intergovernmental agencies, and particularly those with a major influence on global

policy making. In this context, WHO stands out as the first key agency of this type to take an active interest in international palliative care development.[35] Undoubtedly, in many resource-poor countries, the input of WHO was significant in promoting cancer pain relief and palliative care developments. Less clear was the enduring relevance of the WHO's approach in the more affluent nations, where its influence seemed less visible and less central to processes of advocacy and development. Of more significance is the question of whether the WHO's public health model of palliative care was fully adequate to tackle the barriers to development that existed. The 'foundation measures', for example, are persuasive in their descriptive power, but did not seem to offer an adequate model for action and change. Meanwhile, other organizations had inserted symbolic language about palliative care into their policies—for example, the World Health Assembly's statement on cancer prevention and control, 2005; and the United Nations Programme on Ageing, 2002 (updated 2008). However, the effect of such endeavours was difficult to gauge, other than in relation to general awareness-raising. If the WHO established a platform for recognition, undoubtedly there remained many opportunities for other intergovernmental organizations and professional networks working in an international context.

Global networks and organizations

From the 1980s, pioneers of hospice and palliative care worked to promote their goals in many countries, building increasingly on international networks of support and collaboration.[36] Many of these were medical doctors, often working with colleagues from nursing, social work, allied health professions, community activism, and academia. Over time, local groupings expanded, made connections elsewhere, and international cooperation became a striking feature of many palliative care innovations.

In 1976, the First International Congress on the Care of the Terminally Ill was held in Montreal and organized every two years thereafter by Balfour Mount and colleagues. It quickly became a celebrated meeting, with attendance from all over the world. It also became known for its own particular orientation and culture—something different from, and going beyond, the more standard format of a medical meeting. Balfour Mount describes the process and the impact.

> The first conference was in the fall of 1976 and it featured Cicely and Elizabeth Kübler-Ross among others, and it was meant to mark the end of our two-year pilot project. In essence Cicely told about St Christopher's and what was done there, Elizabeth talked about her work, and I talked about the pilot project. And that was the first one. We decided that it was sufficiently successful in terms of generating

discussion and interest and positive experience that we'd have another one. And so the next one was then in '78. The idea behind them was to put together a conference that was of the highest possible standard in terms of content and speakers, and that the programme—again taking a note from Cicely—reflected patient/family care research and teaching, and in the clinical aspects reflected all domains of human experience, so physical, psychosocial, spiritual, existential, whatever ... and with as nearly as possible equal weighting in each of those areas. And I think that's been the guiding principle in putting together the programmes ... We've had some really memorable times and speakers: we've often ... been most successful when we've incorporated lateral thinking when it's somebody from another field or another area ... something that touches on some aspect of our work can give us a fresh perspective from a different vantage point, you know. And that has often worked well ... Part of it is out of respect for staff stress and so we tried to build in things that will be nurturing and positive things for the people who are there. And some of the things we've just sort of stumbled onto, but others were sort of planned that way. One of the most interesting examples is the little part of the meetings we call 'Reflections' ... my sense was we needed to do something to produce an experience of community that would be fairly intense and focused and yet brief ... and so we'd select around the theme of a piece of music, and then select visuals that work with that music and then we have a reading or something that is said to introduce it beforehand and the whole thing has to be under five minutes. And we call these 'Reflections', and the first time we did it, we did it two or three times, and to my astonishment there were people who wrote in on their evaluation form that the best part of the meeting were the 'Reflections', and I thought, 'Gee, I'm not sure that's want I want to hear', you know. But it said something about our need, that part of what we go to conferences for is a sense of community ... because it certainly produces a powerful experience of community.[37]

North America

If the Montreal meetings were fostering a sense of international community, there was also much that needed to be done on the domestic front of North America. Philippines-born physician Josefina Magno[38] graduated from the University of Santo Tomas, Manila, in 1943. Her husband died of cancer in 1955, and from the late 1960s, she based herself in the United States. In 1975, she took up a fellowship in medical oncology at Georgetown University Hospital, which was where she came across the hospice approach. She describes here how she came to visit St Christopher's in 1976.

I realised we were treating those patients until they were dead, you know. Georgetown is a research institution, so of course we have all of these sophisticated new drugs, and these sophisticated protocols, and I watched those patients spending the last days of their lives throwing up because of this chemotherapy. And I talked to my boss and I said, 'Why are we doing this? Why are we treating them and they are not curable?' And his answer sort of changed my life because he said, 'Jo, it's easier to go on treating them than to say there's nothing more that we can do.' Very good, OK.

I had read a little paragraph in a book written by Cicely and I said, 'Well, hospice!' I wrote to her, I didn't even know who she was, I didn't know her address, I just said 'Cicely Saunders, London.' I said, 'May I come to see what you are doing?' And she wrote back and she said, 'Come.' So I went to St Christopher's prepared for the worst. I said, 'My God, they have a place where everybody's dying, it must be horrible.' Anyway, you know how it is, they were dying, but they were dying painlessly, they were dying peacefully. And I said, 'We can do all this in the United States because we have the expertise, we have the caring attitude, and we have the resources, maybe more than England has.' So I learned everything I could there.[39]

She came back determined to promote hospice in the Georgetown area of Washington. She quickly created a pilot hospice programme, and the following year she established the Hospice of Northern Virginia. Determined to get wider support for the hospice ideal, by 1980 she was the first executive director of the National Hospice Organization and was soon extensively involved in the move for Congress to support hospice care under Medicare.[40] In 1984, she established the International Hospice Institute (IHI) to promote physician involvement in hospice and four years later, she founded the Academy of Hospice Physicians, leaving IHI to take on an increasing interest in the developing world.

By 1996, as the IHI and College, it was under the leadership of Edinburgh-based Derek Doyle and, subsequently, as the International Association of Hospice and Palliative Care (IAHPC), it had a string of medical doctors as president of its board, all of them specialists in palliative medicine.[41] These included an Australian, Roger Woodruff (1997–1999); two Argentinians, the US-based Eduardo Bruera (2000–2004) and Roberto Wenk (2008–2013); as well as the American Kathleen Foley (2005–2007); and the German Lukas Radbruch (2014–).[42]

Europe

In 1988, the European Association for Palliative Care (EAPC) was formed in Milan, Italy, and Vittorio Ventafridda, who had been involved in the early discussions and shaping of the WHO approach to cancer pain relief, became its first president the following year.[43] Ventafridda was well established as a pain specialist with expertise in cancer. He had been a founding member of the International Association for the Study of Pain in 1973 and had served on some of its committees in the 1980s. Born in the northern Italian city of Udine, he graduated at Pavia's Medical University in 1952 before spending four years in the United States where he did his internship, and then took a residency in anaesthesiology at the Research and Educational Hospital of the University of Illinois, Chicago. On returning to Milan, he took charge of the anaesthesiology department at the Istituto Nazionale dei Tumori and began to get interested in palliative care. He also forged a close friendship with the industrialist Virgilio Floriani and his wife Loredana, and together, in 1977, they established the Floriani Foundation to promote care of the terminally ill in Italy.[44] When discussions began about the creation of a European coordinating society for palliative care, the Foundation offered to assist.

The British social work academic Frances Sheldon describes the process of formation, the key players, and the explicitly multidisciplinary approach that was taken.

> Elisabeth Earnshaw-Smith, who was the principal social worker at St Christopher's and a very well-respected figure, was unable to go to a meeting that was called in Milan to discuss setting up the European Association of Palliative Care ... which was called by Vittorio Ventafridda ... so I sort of went along in her stead ... so there was this fascinating meeting in Milan at Christmas-time when ... they had red carpets down the street and bay trees outside the shops because it was Advent and Christmas-time; it was a very magical sort of time in Milan. And there was this group of people from all over Europe gathered, with me and Richard Hillier and probably Robert Twycross and someone else from the UK—there must have been a senior nurse and I can't remember who it was—and with people from all over, gathered by Vittorio Ventafridda on his sort of network and contacts, to set up this European group. It was really absolutely fascinating to be trying to put this organization together over that weekend. So I was very lucky to be part of that grouping and I hung on in there because I wished to be part of it because I thought it was interesting, and I thought there should be a voice for social care and I was the only voice for social work and social care in that group. Yes, there was a sort of constitution drawn up ... I remember sitting in this very, very elegant lawyer's office in Milan on the Sunday morning as we all had to sign endless Italian legal documents about this and people's planes were coming and going and we somehow felt we were locked into this office until we'd all signed these documents setting up the EAPC ... there was something fascinating, in a sense, you know, watching the different European perspectives, watching Vittoria Ventafridda and Derek Doyle negotiating from their very, very different personalities and different perspectives on the world, [it] was absolutely fascinating to be a *player* in that, although a rather small player.[45]

Starting in 1990, the EAPC held regular congresses, soon alternating with the meeting in Montreal, across western and eastern European capital cities. The first of these, in Paris, was a milestone event, and saw palliative care in Europe operating on a new scale. The guests included French president François Mitterrand, as well as Her Royal Highness the Duchess of Kent. There was simultaneous translation in English and French. Some 1 630 participants from 23 countries and about 50 journalists were present. During the three days of the congress, more than 30 French and European journals and magazines published articles about palliative care, and all French television channels and several radio stations reported the event. Sixty-five invited speakers from different countries participated in the Scientific Programme, and 105 'posters' on research, clinical activity and on service provision were presented by teams from numerous European countries and also from outside Europe. Nurses made up half of the participants, followed by physicians (27 per cent). In addition, there were volunteers, psychologists, social workers, auxiliaries, pastoral counsellors, professional trainers, physiotherapists, chemists, hospital administrators, dietitians, and speech therapists. The joint chairs of the organizing committee were Professor Maurice Abiven and Dr Michèle Salamagne from France, and the chair of the scientific committee was Professor Geoffrey Hanks from the United Kingdom.[46] Some 14 years after the first Montreal congress, Europe had put down a marker of its interest in the newly formed specialty. Its influence was to increase rapidly, and in time the EAPC meetings were branded as 'world congresses' of palliative care.

By the mid-1990s, EAPC was producing important clinical guidelines for palliative care. Hanks exerted significant leadership in this regard, and had been one of its 42 founding members in 1988 in Milan. In addition to chairing the scientific committees of the first congress in Paris, he was EAPC vice president (1989–1995) and then president (1995–1999). He participated in and led a number of research and study groups and was the main author of the EAPC guidelines on morphine and opioids for cancer pain, first published in 1996, and updated in 2001 and 2012.[47]

Palliative care in Western Europe made rapid progress from the early 1980s, but by the late 1990s there were still striking differences in provision across states.[48] After the foundation of St Christopher's in England in 1967, it was 10 years until the first services began to appear elsewhere—in Sweden (1977), Italy (1980), Germany (1983), Spain (1984), Belgium (1985), France (1986), and the Netherlands (1991). In all of these countries, the provision of palliative care moved beyond isolated examples of pioneering services run by enthusiastic founders. Palliative care came to be delivered in a variety of settings (domiciliary, quasi-domiciliary, and institutional), though these were not given uniform priority everywhere.

In 1989 and 1992, the European Parliament adopted resolutions on the counselling and care of the terminally ill but, thereafter, showed little interest in related issues until January 2005, when the question was put to the parliament concerning what action the Commission had taken to prepare a strategy for palliative care. Meanwhile, the Council of Europe had published a set of European guidelines on palliative care in 2003, which described palliative care as an essential and basic service for the whole population. Its recommendations were used quite actively in countries with less-developed palliative care systems, particularly in Eastern Europe, where they served as a tool for advocacy and lobbying, but they seemed to resonate less in the countries of Western Europe.

Policy issues relating to palliative care in Europe were also raised by the EAPC and other organizations. At conferences in 1995 (Barcelona)[49] and 1998 (Poznań),[50] exhortatory declarations were made, calling for government action on palliative care on a national level and drawing attention to key issues facing palliative care as it developed internationally. By 2003, the European Society for Medical Oncology was giving greater recognition to palliative care.[51] In 2004, the European Federation of Older Persons launched a campaign to make palliative care a priority topic on the European health agenda.[52] The same year, the European office of WHO produced an important document, *Better Palliative Care for Older People*, with an aim 'to incorporate palliative care for serious chronic progressive illnesses within ageing policies, and to promote better care towards the end of life'.[53] A companion volume, *Palliative Care: The Solid Facts*, became a resource for policymakers in a context where 'the evidence available on palliative care is not complete and ... there are differences in what can be offered across the European region'.[54] Despite the advocacy potential of these and other publications however, evidence of their impact remained unclear.[55]

Eastern Europe

By the late 1990s, interest in palliative care was also growing among healthcare workers and volunteers in the countries of Central and Eastern Europe that were emerging from communist rule. Some of these were active in establishing hospice and related services in their own local communities and were also taking part in study visits and exchanges with hospice and palliative care units elsewhere in Western Europe. In 1999, and supported by the international outreach of George Soros's Open Society Institute, the Eastern and Central European Palliative Task Force came into being at an EAPC congress held in Geneva. Mary Callaway of the Open Society Institute describes how it came about.

> We had the [Open Society] Foundations identify two potential leaders, or two people in their country that were interested in hospice and palliative care and we brought these people together for two and a half days in Geneva, in advance of the European Association for Palliative Care meeting, and we met with them to try to find out what their needs were in their country. So they said that they had an enormous need for professional education; that their doctors and nurses and social workers, if they had social workers, weren't receiving training on end-of-life care in medical schools and nursing schools; that the public wasn't *aware* of end-of-life care; and they weren't *aware* that they were entitled to pain management or decision-making at end of life, so there was an enormous need for public education; that drug availability was a

huge issue in all of these countries, that there weren't opioid analgesics available for basic pain management; and then the last area was that there needed to be changes in health care policy and in systems in each of these countries. So we went back and basically developed a programme to address those issues and announced . . . areas that we were going to develop: fund resource training centres; develop hospice and palliative care national and regional education programmes; translation grants because there is an enormous need for available educational materials in the native languages; and travel grants and scholarship grants for professionals to receive training outside; and then a series of national education programmes.[56]

The Task Force aimed to gather data on hospice and palliative care in the region, share experiences of achievements and obstacles, influence the institutions of government, set standards to meet local needs, and raise awareness. A key leader within the group was Professor Jacek Luzack who had graduated from the medical faculty of the Academy of Medical Science, Karol Marcinkowski, in Poznań in 1959. He specialized in cardiology and then anaesthesiology, and held a number of academic appointments. By the early 1980s, with civil unrest heightening in Poland around the *Solidarity* movement, and in an atmosphere of change and foment, he became familiar with a few activists who were becoming interested in the idea of establishing a hospice in Poznań. This was a major spur to hospice development in Poland. By the mid-1980s, he was in contact with Jan Stjernswärd at WHO and Vittorio Ventafridda in Milan, and was running his own small cancer pain service at the University Hospital in Poznań. In 1988, with help from Robert Twycross, he and his nursing colleagues went to Milan for training, and this was quickly followed by the first palliative care symposium in Poland. By 1991, and working closely with Twycross, he was offering palliative care training programmes and also beginning to engage in discussions with the Ministry of Health. He talks about these influences on his thinking.

My meeting with Robert Twycross was important in '88. When I was starting with palliative care, I started with pain treatment, and I met in one conference with Robert Twycross, and he asked me: 'You are paying attention to the pain, but it is not all, it is only a small thing in all the problems to providing appropriate holistic care.' And it was obviously that . . . yes. I am thinking that I am only on the *pain* concerned, it is not enough. Yes, he told me this, and he told me also: 'You are probably also now paying big attention to pain, but it is not sufficient. It must be widened, extended, your point of view of the patient as a person.' And I also very much appreciated meeting with Professor Corr, and he sent me Eric Cassell's book on *The Nature of Suffering and the Goals of Medicine*,[57] and it helped me very much talking with him about death and dying. I think some persons helped me very much to develop my philosophy. And also co-operation and influences made in Poland. How the people are taking care, how enthusiastic they were, how they sacrificed their time. It is like some movement which helps other people to understand what this means. We also organise every week meetings with our volunteers' group. We are talking about what is the hospice? What is the approach? What is death and dying? What is our feeling? We started this in '89.[58]

Across the former communist countries of Eastern Europe and Central Asia, there were few palliative care developments in the years of Soviet domination. Most initiatives can be traced to the early 1990s, after which many projects got under way. These were documented in detail,[59] and in 2003, there was evidence of some service provision in 23 out of 28 countries in the region. Poland and Russia had the most advanced programmes of palliative care, with considerable achievements also made in Romania and Hungary. Nevertheless, in a region of over 400 million people, there were just 467 palliative care services, more than half of which were found in a single country, Poland.

Latin America

Eduardo Bruera was born in Argentina in 1955. The son of a cardiologist, he went to medical school in Rosario, and gained his MD in 1979 before moving to Buenos Aries for further training, qualifying in internal medicine and medical oncology in 1984. It was during this residency training that he noted the need of terminal cancer patients for symptom control and supportive care. However, despite finding other sympathetic medical students and publishing material himself in the American medical literature, there were no posts in palliative care in Argentina, and he moved to Canada to pursue his interest. In 1984 he began a fellowship in supportive care at the National Cancer Institute of Canada at the University of Alberta, and by 1988, he had become the director of the palliative care programme in Edmonton, Alberta. This was a clinical and academic post. Then in 1993, Bruera became Canada's second professor of palliative medicine. He describes his early palliative care awakening in Buenos Aires.

> So I became progressively disappointed by the fact that while we were making so much emphasis on success, that success was really helping a very small proportion of the patients we came to see. And for those who we didn't have much to offer to, we were not really doing any emphasis in trying to learn more about symptom control and supportive care. The prevailing feeling in oncology was that it was just a matter of time before adequate therapy developed, and therefore we could not be distracted from looking at the issues of the cancer treatment and cancer cure, because once that was achieved then the suffering associated with terminal illness would disappear automatically. On the other hand, looking at the evidence, that wasn't clear to me; it wasn't as clear to me how we were going to make such an enormous difference in such a short time. So I became progressively disappointed of the fact that we were not focusing on pain, malnutrition, nausea, dyspnoea, confusion, those things that I was seeing daily.

> I remember having gone to hear lectures, by Ventafridda, for example, on the concepts of palliative care, to an almost empty auditorium of the faculty of medicine in Buenos Aires. The books from Robert Twycross were not translated, but they were available. I read some of his material, but I would say that the concepts were completely unknown, both at the pre-graduate and postgraduate ... areas of medical education. And to my knowledge no other disciplines at all, like nursing, psychology, sociology were aware of the issues related to the care of the terminally ill. So in my case I came across some of this literature out of frustration with the *status quo* as far as literature, and looking for something else within the area of oncology, I couldn't find it ... of course, there was no association of palliative care, there was not a single palliative care programme or service in the country, there was no forum for dissemination of these, or discussion, or debate, or anything like that.[60]

In the late 1980s, however, Argentinean doctors such as Roberto Wenk and Gustavo de Simone began to organize training programmes and palliative care services, mainly in the hospital setting. One who was taught by them, Dr Jose Eisenchlas, describes the context by 2001.

> In Buenos Aires for instance there are more or less I think 14 or 15 public hospitals and there are palliative care teams in six of them. In two or three main cities there are palliative care teams too. And nowadays it looks like the media has gained some insight into the palliative care field too and they release more information about this. You know, Latin culture is quite different from Saxon culture, and people in Argentina, it seems don't want to hear nothing about death. So it's a great difficulty to continue running more and more palliative care, but I believe too that the hyper-technology in medicine is rising to the top and declining, they are in crescendo for instance about human rights in Argentina ... support from the Church too, is increasing the palliative care field nowadays: really it's good for us who are working there. Day by day there is more knowledge from the public over palliative care and day by day there are younger people who become involved in palliative care and that reinforces us who are working from perhaps longer times there. Really, I am very enthusiastic about what palliative care can be in Argentina.[61]

The turn of the millennium in 2000 saw the creation of the Latin American Association of Palliative Care.

Asia

Asia: Korea, Japan, and China

The first evidence of hospice developments in the Asia Pacific region came with a service for dying patients in Korea at the Calvary Hospice of Kangung, established by the Catholic Sisters of the Little Company of Mary in 1965—two years before the opening of St Christopher's; such services had increased to 60 in Korea by 1999.[62] In Japan, the first hospice was also Christian, established in the Yodogwa Christian Hospital in 1973. By the end of the century, the country had 80 inpatient units.[63] Protocols for the WHO three-step analgesic ladder were first introduced into China in 1991, and there were said to be hundreds of palliative care services in urban areas by 2002.[64] In 2001, the Asia Pacific Hospice Palliative Care Network was founded; representing 14 countries where hospice and palliative care services had become available.[65]

Asia: India

An extensive review of hospice and palliative care developments in India in 2006 mapped the existence of services state by state and explored the perspectives and experiences of those involved, with a view to stimulating new development.[66] The study found that 135 hospice and palliative care services existed in 16 states. These were usually concentrated in large cities, with the exception of the state of Kerala, where services were much more widespread. Non-government organizations and public and private hospitals and hospices were the predominant sources of provision. Palliative care provision could not be identified in 19 states or union territories. Nevertheless, successful models existed in Kerala for the development of affordable, sustainable, community-based hospice and palliative care services,[67] and these seemed to have potential for replication elsewhere.

Dr M. R. Rajagopal and Dr Suresh Kumar had both been instrumental in initiating palliative care developments in Kerala, working closely with a friend, P. K. Ashok Kumar. Rajagopal studied at Trivandrum Medical College, qualifying in 1971, and did postgraduate work in anaesthetics at the All Indian Institute of Medical Sciences. In 1976, he returned to Trivandrum as an anaesthesiologist in the government service and, a decade later, in 1986, he became professor and head of the department of anaesthesiology at Calicut Medical College. As a result of conversations with Suresh Kumar and Ashok Kumar following a lecture given by the English nurse, Gilly Burn, founder of Cancer Relief India, Rajagopal began to take an interest in palliative care. The three founded the Pain and Palliative Care Society in Calicut, Kerala, in 1993 and began seeing patients at the beginning of 1994. Cancer Relief India provided early financial support and opportunities for training in Oxford. Rajagopal describes the motivations and the context.

> One turning point for me was one patient. That was a college professor, I think he was 42, he came to me with a cancer of the tongue and it was spreading to his lower jaw. He'd had some treatment already but it was incurable, and I gave him a mandibular nerve block. The next day he was pain-free and I was patting myself on my back: I was very happy. He didn't look very happy but I hardly noticed that, in retrospect. The man committed suicide the next day. One of his cousins was a colleague of mine, so he told me later that the fact that I did a nerve block was the first thing that indirectly communicated to him that his disease was incurable. While I was patting myself on my back, I didn't check to see what his level of knowledge

was; I didn't bother to find out how he *felt*: I just looked at his nerve block. I wasn't bothered about anything else. Obviously my nerve block was successful and the patient died—but that was a very nebulous idea, it was a disquieting thought, nothing more than that. It's not as if that gave me a sense of direction or anything, it didn't. It just told me that what I was doing was not right enough. But what actually had happened was a few years prior to that, when I had a little bit of money on me, I ordered a couple of books out of a catalogue. One of them was *Treatment of Cancer Pain*[68] by Twycross and Lack. I thought the book—from the title, I didn't know who Twycross or Lack were—from the title I thought it would tell me all sorts of things about nerve blocks. When it came, and I read the book, it was about one paragraph on nerve blocks: I was disgusted and I kept it in the cupboard, I didn't bother to read it. But after this incident I went back to the book and some things started making sense.

But even then I must admit that things were very nebulous, but a few things changed it. One was my association with Suresh and one of his friends, Ashok. Suresh was a member of our department of anaesthesiology and Ashok was a friend of his and we used to exchange ideas and thoughts. They were very vibrant, young people—unlike me!—with their large circle of friends and a lot of ideas and they had their own experiences. Like Suresh has experience of his friend's mother who once told Suresh—she was a cancer patient—when he was talking to her, supporting her, she said, 'Suresh, you are interested only in the drugs, you are not interested in me' . . . which was something that struck him tremendously. Ashok similarly had a lot of experience with friends and relatives who were treated like machines by the medical system. So they used to think about all this and much of what we have now developed came out of our conversations between the three of us.

But another major influence was Gilly Burn. In those days when we used to talk about a lot and say things like how absurd the medical system was and how we were not doing the right thing with the patients, we still didn't have a sense of direction, but I went to attend a workshop in Trivandrum which was conducted by Miss Gilly Burn of Cancer Relief India. All of a sudden several things became clearer to me. That was, though I had some sort of nebulous idea from Robert's book, it was then that the concept of palliative medicine became a bit clearer to me. And then we continued to talk it over between us and we decided to do what we could. We decided to form the Pain and Palliative Care Society and registered charitable organisation. And then Gilly again helped: she took me on a course to Oxford which was very helpful for me—a ten-weeks course—and she also gave some money. She gave us around 100 000 rupees, with no tax attached. She said use it on what you think best, and that's something that kicked the ball, and that was one of the beginnings of our organisation.[69]

Southeast Asia: Malaysia

Dr Ednin Hamzah studied medicine in Britain and practised in the northern city of Newcastle, before returning to Malaysia in 1997. The previous year, a chance meeting with the chairman of Hospis Malaysia (Kuala Lumpur) had brought to his attention that the post of medical director with this service had been vacant for two years. He applied for and accepted the appointment and, while still in England, prepared himself through an attachment to St Oswald's Hospice, Newcastle. After seeking advice from Australasia experts Dr Cynthia Goh and Dr Rosalie Shaw, he presented a new vision to the Hospis Malaysia board in which palliative care was perceived 'as a needs-based care not a prognosis-based care'. The board approved this shift in emphasis and a rigorous development programme followed. Key changes were to result: a new approach to care; different patterns of work; public awareness initiatives; a focus on cultural issues; family conferences; data collection and evaluation; and a comprehensive programme of education and training. He describes the context for the development of palliative care in Malaysia.

> The concept of hospice started in 1991, it came out of an international meeting in Singapore not long before that I think it was '88 or '89, a lot of people from Malaysia attended that meeting and I think Kathy Foley and quite a few others in palliative care attended that meeting and a number of the participants from Malaysia came back and thought 'Wow this is something really, really profound and it needs to happen here'. In Kuala Lumpur it was basically led by an Australian GP working in a family medicine department in the university . . . and she put together a group of people—a couple of doctors, a couple of nurses, some business people and others, lawyers and whatever else, and they decided to form this organisation 'Hospis Malaysia'. Similarly, a different group was working in Penang to set up another hospice service there. So this was the start of things and they worked initially in someone's house and then eventually one of these people that were involved with this thing was chairman of a local hospital and he enabled a room at this hospital to be used as the headquarters for this fledgling hospice and there they stayed until I came by in '97.[70]

Africa

The African Palliative Care Association (APCA) was founded in 2004, seeking to represent all palliative care interests across the whole continent. Its first chief executive was Faith Mwangi-Powell, who had come from working as an advocacy officer for the Diana, Princess of Wales Memorial Fund. No stranger to palliative care in the African context, she describes her goals at the time of taking up her new position.

> And my role is really to take the leadership in APCA in really enhancing, our mission statement is to promote and support culturally acceptable and affordable palliative care across Africa, and I think that's really what we are hoping to do by supporting countries which do not have any services to start up; supporting countries which have palliative care to scale up; and really through training trying to help them fund-raise; trying again to really raise their profile, you know, being the spokesman of people who really have nobody to speak on their behalf, and just be the resource for palliative care in Africa. And being maybe much more the link between what is happening in Africa and what is happening

internationally so we have very big plans for APCA: it's a huge job, it's a huge challenge, but at the same time I think it's much needed and I think there is hunger for APCA and I think there is so much commitment and we've got such a fantastic board, who are very, very committed to APCA, and we just hope that it will go from strength to strength.[71]

A 2006 review[72] of hospice and palliative care developments in Africa mapped the existence of services country by country and explored the perspectives and experiences of those involved. The 47 countries studied were grouped into four categories of palliative care development: no identified hospice or palliative care activity (21); capacity-building activity under way to promote hospice and palliative care delivery (11); localized provision of hospice and palliative care in place, often supported by external donors (11); hospice and palliative care services achieving some measure of integration with mainstream service providers and gaining wider policy recognition (4).

Major difficulties included opioid availability; workforce development; ability to achieve sustainable critical mass; absorption capacity in relation to major external funding initiatives; ability to cope with the scale of HIV/AIDS-related suffering. The authors concluded that models existed in Uganda, Kenya, South Africa, and Zimbabwe for the development of affordable, sustainable community-based hospice and palliative care services, and that the newly formed APCA had significant potential to promote innovation in a context where interest in the development of hospice and palliative care in Africa had never been greater. A small number of studies also appraised the development of palliative care in sub-Saharan Africa[73,74,75] and stimulated interest in the evaluation of services.

Global organization and activism

During these years, there was evidence of a growing spirit of collaboration between activists interested in the global development of palliative care. In 2003, a world summit held in The Hague led to the creation of the first World Hospice and Palliative Care Day, which ran annually thereafter. The following year, the Venice Declaration of 2006 brought forward by IAHPC and EAPC called for strategies and resources to support research activity on palliative care in developing countries.[76] In 2007, palliative care associations at the Budapest congress of the EAPC entered into a set of commitments for palliative care improvement.[77] The same year, in collaboration with 25 other organizations, the IAHPC developed a list of essential medicines for palliative care in response to a request from the Cancer Control Programme of the WHO.[78] During this period, debates also began to emerge in which access to palliative care was considered as a human right,[79] and access to palliative medication was incorporated into a United Nations Commission on Human Rights resolution—'[calling on states] to promote effective access to such preventive, curative or palliative pharmaceutical products or medical technologies'[80]—reflecting a growing interest in the relationship between palliative care services and their accessibility to the populations of individual countries.

There were also many developments at the country level, and a substantial literature on national developments in hospice and palliative care recorded important achievements and successes in the face of adversity, as well as the barriers to development.[81] A comprehensive review of palliative care growth in some of the English-speaking countries where progress had been most significant (the United Kingdom, United States, Canada, Australia, and New Zealand) acknowledged that each had different starting points for palliative care development but 'in the longer run most countries tend to develop a mix of independent, hospital-based, and community-based services'.[82] By the end of the twentieth century, the published literature contained a small but growing comparative perspective on hospice and palliative care developments in different regions of the world.[83]

Before the turn of the millennium, there was little systematic understanding of how palliative care was emerging in the global context. While activists in the field did occasionally comment on international links and initiatives, there was almost no evidence from research studies to shed systematic light on the state of service development, policy recognition, or the general vitality of palliative care in different settings around the world. Some countries had established national associations for palliative care, occasionally with directories of services, but in the main, it remained difficult to access any useful information about resources and infrastructure other than through local contacts. Despite some green shoots of growth, the idea of collaborative endeavours in policy innovation, service development, or research to promote palliative care in the international context was still in its infancy. Accordingly, the evidence base for palliative care provision and the notion that it might be rooted in public health approaches—a view to which WHO was strongly committed—were both weakly developed, and often not considered by palliative care activists to be a high priority.[82]

The start of the new millennium, however, was a key time in the development of palliative care globally. All around the world, palliative care leaders seemed to bemoan the same problems: a lack of public recognition and understanding of their work; professional indifference on the part of many health and social care providers; a lack of third party funding to set up demonstration projects; poor recognition of palliative care within the architecture of both national and international health policy; weakly developed training programmes, with few routes for accreditation and professional recognition; and a limited evidence base about the overall development of palliative care and its efficacy, costs, and benefits.

Following that first summit on international palliative care development that had taken place in 2003 in The Hague, others followed—in Seoul in 2005, Nairobi in 2007, and Vienna in 2009—leading that year to the creation of the Worldwide Palliative Care Alliance (later the Worldwide Hospice and Palliative Care Alliance). These meetings brought together the existing organizations with international palliative care interests, as well as other 'outward facing' national associations from specific countries, together with funders, activists, and researchers. As the first decade of the twenty-first century closed, the international palliative care community appeared organized as never before, with growing levels of commitment to development issues, but major challenges still in prospect.

In 2011, two separate declarations emphasized the importance of palliative and end-of-life care. The United Nations referred to the need for palliative care provision in its statement about the care and treatment of people with non-communicable disease.[84] In addition, the World Medical Association made its case for end-of-life care improvement, stating that receiving appropriate palliative medical care must not be considered a privilege but a true right, independent of age, or any other associated factors.[85] At the same time, calls for the legalization of assisted dying and euthanasia were growing in several jurisdictions, and public debate for and against continued to flourish, often stimulated by high profile examples of key cases and endorsement by leading opinion formers.

Significantly, studies were also emerging that could underpin palliative care development with the beginnings of an evidence base. Despite being limited by the methodological and practical challenges of research on an international scale, new studies began to describe the key issues and to map an agenda for scientific collaboration in a rapidly developing field.

Key international studies

Early projects

The first research study to explore the development of palliative care in a comparative manner across jurisdictions focused on seven western European countries.[86,87] It showed two variations in the delivery of palliative care.[88] First, palliative care services were found in a variety of settings: domiciliary, quasi-domiciliary, and institutional. Second, these forms were not prioritized equally in every country. Allowing for population differences, there were great variations in the numbers of palliative care services across nations, and the number of specialist palliative care beds per head of population varied from 1:c18 000 persons in the United Kingdom to 1:c1.9 m persons in Italy.

This work led directly to another study that successfully mapped the development of palliative care across 28 former communist countries in Eastern Europe and Central Asia.[60] Only Poland and Russia had more than 50 palliative care services, and five countries had none. Homecare was the form of service most commonly found, followed by inpatient provision. There was a great absence of hospital mobile teams, as well as services in nursing homes and daycare provision. Only 48 paediatric palliative care services were identified, covering just nine of the 28 countries.

Using a related approach, a team at the University of Giessen carried out a study covering 16 countries across Eastern and Western Europe. This incorporated a comprehensive analysis of demographics: the history of hospice and palliative care; the number of current services; funding; education and training of professional staff; and the role of volunteers—with an in-depth portrayal of particular services.[89]

In the period 2003–2009, the International Observatory on End of Life Care (IOELC), based at Lancaster University in the United Kingdom, became the key source of palliative care mapping studies around the world, constructing national reports for over 60 countries.[90] In particular, it carried out major reviews of palliative care development in Africa (26 countries),[73] the Middle East (six countries),[91] and South East Asia (three countries),[92] as well as a study covering the whole of India.[67] These reviews had several features in common. They established the number and character of palliative care services existing in a given country, funding arrangements, the level of policy support, and the specific context of opioid availability. They also contained rich narratives of experience, based on accounts from local activists in palliative care.

Global comparison of palliative care development

Emerging from this series of studies was an ambitious attempt in 2006 to measure and classify palliative care development in every country in the world. The IOELC built on a basic description that had been produced earlier by Avril Jackson at the Hospice Information Service, St Christopher's Hospice, but which had not been tested or published. An attempt was now made to add more depth into the analysis by developing a four-part typology depicting levels of hospice and palliative care development across the globe, an idea which had first been developed in the review of services in Africa.

Group 1: Countries with no known hospice/palliative care activity

Group 2: Countries with capacity-building activity

Group 3: Countries with localized hospice and palliative care provision

Group 4: Countries where hospice and palliative care services were reaching a measure of integration with the mainstream healthcare system[93]

By presenting a world map of hospice and palliative care development, the study sought to contribute to the debate about the growth and recognition of palliative care services—in particular, whether or not the four-part typology reflected sequential levels of palliative care development. The typology differentiated levels of palliative care development in both hemispheres and in rich and poor settings. It showed that only half the world's countries had some form of designated palliative care service.

In 2011, the analysis was updated with a refined six-point typology.[94] Now 136 of the world's 234 countries (58 per cent) had established one or more hospice/palliative care services—an increase of 21 countries (+9 per cent) from 2006. By 2011, although there were indications of growing interest in palliative care on the part of national governments and policymakers, *advanced* integration of palliative care with wider health services (the highest category in the typology) had been achieved in only 20 countries globally (8.5 per cent).

Global Quality of Death Index

Building on this approach, a study commissioned by the Lien Foundation in Singapore and carried out by the Economist Intelligence Unit was published in 2010.[95] This also attempted a ranking of palliative care development in 40 countries, with a more complex set of indicators. The Quality of Death Index scored on 24 indicators in four categories, each with a separate weighting, as follows:

(1) Basic end-of-life healthcare environment (20 per cent)

(2) Availability of end-of-life care (25 per cent)

(3) Cost of end-of-life care (15 per cent)

(4) Quality of end-of-life care (40 per cent)

The study ranked the United Kingdom first, with the best quality of death, owing to its advanced hospice care network and a history of state involvement in end-of-life care. Some advanced nations rank poorly—for instance, Finland at 28 and South Korea at 32. The report noted the high position of Hungary (11) and Poland (15). The United States, however, with the largest spending on healthcare in the world, ranked at just 9 in the index, principally due to limited public funding for end-of-life care, the costs to the patient, and the restriction of government-funded reimbursements through Medicare only for patients who give up curative treatments.

The report noted that across the world, public healthcare funding often prioritizes conventional treatment and provides only partial support for end-of-life care services, meaning such care must rely on philanthropy and community help. It took the view that a widespread cultural belief in affluent countries that governments should provide and pay for healthcare services has hampered private sector provision for end-of-life care services. At the other end of the scale were developing countries, such as China and India, where state funding levels for end-of-life care were very low, provision-sparse and localized, and private payment was the norm. The revised and expanded 2015 Index evaluated 80 countries using 20 quantitative and qualitative indicators across five categories: the palliative and healthcare environment (20 per cent); human resources (20 per cent); the affordability of care (20 per cent); the quality of care (30 per cent); and level of community engagement (10 per cent).[96]

Prospects for global improvement

Taken together, internationally there was by the early decades of the twenty-first century a growing nexus of funders, intergovernmental organizations, philanthropic bodies, and non-profit organizations devoting some or all of their interests to palliative care development. The decade after 2000 saw a great burst of international activity from within the palliative care community. New associations came into being; interchange and information flow between key players increased; and high-level declarations resonated from palliative care congresses intent on raising the profile of end-of-life issues. For the first time in its short history, palliative care became the focus of international and comparative research studies, and an evidence-based picture emerged of palliative care provision around the world. Greater interest in palliative care was also seen on the part of philanthropic and intergovernmental donors. It was a time of considerable achievement. Nevertheless, at the same time it exposed specific problems.

For some, palliative care remained limited by an inward-looking culture. This manifested itself in several ways. Major conferences rarely featured key figures from outside the specialty. (The International Congress on Palliative Care held biannually in Montreal was an exception.) Research collaborations were similarly constrained. There was a striking absence of senior figures from oncology, old age medicine, psychiatry, and primary care working towards the development of palliative care and making appropriate connections. Even public health showed little engagement, despite the efforts of some palliative care leaders to champion their work within a public health model.

Such observations, it might be argued, could seem consistent with the emergence of a new field and with a still-small number of countries in which policy integration and specialty recognition (see the next section 'Further progress in achieving specialty status') had been attained. There was much to do to build up internal critical mass—in service provision, education, and research programmes. Yet, the field also appeared preoccupied with questions of definition and there was much argument about differences between hospice, palliative, supportive, and end-of-life care.

The appetite for these debates within the palliative care world seemed incommensurate with the interest of external colleagues. Indeed, when others did look in from the outside, they were prone to ask some simple but challenging questions: what is palliative care doing for people with HIV disease? How is it responding to the growing needs of ageing populations with high levels of comorbidity at the end of life? What can it teach primary care and the specialities of hospital medicine? How can it be mainstreamed into general health and social care? And what is the evidence for its cost-effectiveness? Certainly, there were achievements in all of these areas, but the scaling up of activity in education, research, and service delivery continued to challenge the resources of the palliative care community.

For such reasons, palliative care remained poorly framed within evidence-based global policymaking. The discourse surrounding the global development of palliative care was still weakly articulated and relatively sparse. Within the palliative care field, especially among clinical academics and researchers, there was an understandable and strong focus on demonstrating the efficacy of palliative care interventions. This concentrated efforts in characterizing syndromes, clusters of pain and other symptoms, and on measuring the relative impact of differing therapeutic regimes on outcomes of care. A smaller group focused on the economic costs and benefits of good palliative care—for the healthcare system, as well as for patients and families. Far less effort was expended on understanding how palliative care could be positioned within the language of global policymaking. Palliative care was not one of the Millennium Development Goals. It was hard to find in the priorities of the United Nations, UNESCO, and other global organizations. It had only the most tentative recognition in the frameworks of the World Bank, the Global Fund, and in the concerns of the world's largest philanthropic donors and foundations. Much more needed to be done to demonstrate the links between primary care and palliative care; to explore the role of palliative care in poverty reduction and community cohesion; and to examine how palliative care could reduce social, economic, and gender inequalities.[97]

Nevertheless, by 2010, the global palliative care community could claim some significant successes. With a growing global infrastructure for advocacy, fundraising, and collaboration, the next decade would be crucial in achieving a higher level of policy recognition. A significant breakthrough came in 2014. First, the World Health Organization, with the Worldwide Palliative Care Alliance, published the first ever Global Atlas of Palliative Care,[98] which was endorsed by the WHO executive board.[99] A few months later, the World Health Assembly passed a resolution requiring all governments to recognize palliative care and make provision for it in national health policies.[100] It was a powerful moment and celebratory statements followed from around the world. However, recognition alone, heavily informed by rights-based reasoning, seemed unlikely to overcome the challenges that palliative medicine continued to face.

Further progress in achieving specialty status

In 2007, Carlos Centeno and colleagues[101] reported on a survey of palliative medicine specialization in the WHO European region, covering 52 countries. They found that palliative medicine had official certification in just seven European countries. In five countries, palliative medicine had become a subspecialty following certification in a full specialty—Poland (1999), Romania (2000), Slovakia (2005), Germany (2006), and France (2007). In 10 other countries—Czech Republic, Denmark, Norway, Sweden, Finland, Iceland, Spain, Malta, Israel, and Latvia—there was evidence of action in progress relating to certification in palliative medicine. Professor Stein Kaasa, chair of palliative medicine in Trondeim, Norway, and at the time also president of the EAPC, describes in 2004 some of the struggles to gain recognition for the field in his own country.

> I think the development has been extremely interesting the last four to five years. We have seen a fast development. First of all, recently, all the health regions in Norway got permanent funding for having centres of expertise within all the health regions and that is established now. These are not clinical centres but centres which shall promote palliative care within their health regions and that do research. Then, secondly, palliative medicine was recently acknowledged as a . . . field within the medical community in Norway, so now our palliative medicine society is part of the Norwegian Medical Association. And now we see also that, in a couple of years, I think that all health regions in Norway will have a university-based unit. And recently, we got the second chair in palliative medicine in Bergen, here in Norway . . . We've just started a Nordic course in palliative medicine. It's a two-year course. We meet six times over one week for two years and there are working assignments

in-between. And it has been very successful so far, I think, with two courses in Norway, two in Sweden and one in Denmark and one in Finland, and we are starting with a second round in half a year from now. I think there are several challenges. One is related to skills and competence and, from a medical point of view, I think the only solution to do, to formalise competence and skills, is that palliative medicine is officially recognised as a specialty. But we need to do something about it.[102]

By 2010, around 18 countries worldwide had established palliative medicine as a specialty or subspecialty,[103] with considerable diversity in the procedures governing specialty status. Palliative medicine, whether described as a specialty or subspecialty, did not constitute a uniform 'currency' of specialization for the field. Healthcare systems differed significantly in their accreditation of medical practitioners and especially in their accreditation of specialist training, and this was reflected in the recognition of palliative medicine in different places. There were also resource implications affecting support for training, though these did not explain the wide variations in length of training that could be observed.

In 2014, more information was available on the European context[104] when Centeno and colleagues reported that specialty recognition for palliative medicine had been obtained in 18 out of the 53 countries in the WHO European region. The report described the main features of the specialization process in each country and the date of certification. Eleven countries had now joined the list since the previous European study: Malta, Czech Republic, Finland, Georgia, Latvia, Norway, Israel, Italy, Hungary, Portugal, and Denmark. Ten of these countries had recognized the specialty, subspecialty, or field of competence status within the five previous years. A high level of heterogeneity in the training processes and programmes was again acknowledged.

Beyond the WHO European region, there was no well-documented assessment of countries with palliative medicine accreditation; however, one addition to the 2010 list was Lebanon (2013).[105] Taking this into account, it was estimated that in 2014 there were at least 26 countries around the world that had recognized some form of accreditation for the specialty or subspecialty of palliative medicine: Argentina, Australia, Czech Republic, Denmark, Finland, France, Georgia, Germany, Hong Kong, Hungary, Ireland, Israel, Italy, Latvia, Lebanon, Malaysia, Malta, New Zealand, Norway, Philippines, Poland, Portugal, Romania, Slovakia, United Kingdom, and the United States.[106]

Australia had what was widely accepted as the first professor of palliative care in the world with the chair of Dr Ian Maddocks in 1988 in Adelaide. He describes here how his appointment came about, and the slender and opportunistic edifice upon which it was built.

That interest in palliative care came about first, I think, through the article that Victor Zorza wrote, I think it was in *The Guardian*, about 1980,[107] that described the death of his daughter in a hospice. And it was beautifully written, with great feeling, and it described how this young woman, dying, I think, of lymphoma, how she had helped her parents through the terrible distress of losing her. How she, given the comfort and support of that hospice situation, had really looked after them. And I found that very moving. And I went to the chief of the hospital and said, you know, 'Read this, because we really don't do death at all well here. Why don't we do something about it? You've got some empty space there, you know, why don't we set up a little hospice in the hospital? You know, do something'. So we set up a little working group. We didn't know much about hospices anywhere else in the world. We set up a working group that consisted of people from the Anti Cancer Fund, the community nurses, domiciliary care agencies, general practitioner representatives, people from the hospital itself, and we explored: What shall we do about this? What do we know about what can be done? And we started off by getting some 'soft' money to employ a research worker to say, 'What are the gaps in care of people who are dying in Southern Adelaide?' And she went around and asked different providers, patients' relatives, GPs and so on: 'What are the problems that you are having with the care of dying people?' And she identified about seven or eight gaps in the care of dying people: There were no volunteers available, the GPs didn't know much about palliative care, there were no respite beds, there were no specific hospice beds. Those sorts of things. We wrote this up and submitted it to the Health Authorities with recommendations that something should be done to establish a hospice programme, that would not duplicate any existing service, but would seek to introduce some additional resources that would work alongside, and network with, existing district nursing services, existing oncology and pain management services, and so on.

The Director of Nursing at the hospital was captured by this, and she actually gave us a very good senior nurse, a woman who had been in charge of the oncology ward and who was very interested in moving in this direction, and she became the first appointment. One single nurse to serve Southern Adelaide. And later she was joined by two sessions, one full day's equivalent of a doctor, who happened to be an anaesthetist. And I had become the Chairman of this group that was organising this (I was still just doing my own thing; I wasn't involved in palliative care, but I was promoting it, I was talking about it, I was advocating for it, I was encouraging it, looking for funds, making the submissions to government and so on), and we gradually added to this team. And, at that time, there was some funding for good ideas. And so, gradually we built it up, and we were able to take on a half-time doctor, and a social worker, and so on. Then came this conversation: 'Why don't we ask the Minister for a Chair in Palliative Care?' And they said, 'well, you know, you know about this stuff; palliative care'. And I thought, 'I haven't been practising it all, I'm still just being a generalist physician'. So I wrote a proposal for a Chair of Palliative Care, and the Minister at that stage . . . the idea of a hospice appealed to him. So the next thing was to write a job statement for a Chair of Palliative Care, and an advertisement for a Chair of Palliative Care. And I did all of those, and then I wrote an application for a Chair of Palliative Care. And of course there was nobody else in Australia that was trained in palliative care, there was nobody trained in palliative care. So I didn't really have very much opposition for the job, and so I was appointed in the middle of 1988, and started to establish a hospice.[108]

This came some 20 years before formal specialty recognition in Australia. The Royal Australasian College of Physicians (RACP) established a pathway for subspecialty training in palliative medicine in 1991, with a three-year training programme. But as palliative medicine was not on the federal government's list of medical specialities, the fellows emerging from the programme were classified as specialists in general medicine. In 1999, a chapter of palliative medicine was created within the Adult Medical Division of the RACP, again with its own training pathway and, in order to create a second entry point to specialist training, this one with a two-year training programme. The result was that all doctors, whether new graduates or specialist practitioners, had a defined route into specialized training in palliative medicine. This quickly led to specialty recognition in New Zealand, which was achieved in 2001. In Australia, the process proved longer and more complex, culminating in recognition of the new specialty by the Minister for Health in 2005.[109]

The development of palliative medicine in the United States happened in three phases:[110] (1) the period before the work of Elizabeth Kübler-Ross and Cicely Saunders became known; (2) the period of development of hospice programmes across the country, when services in the United States grew dramatically from the founding organization in New Haven in 1974, to some 3000 providers by the end of the twentieth century; and (3) the development of a distinct and officially recognized subspecialty of medicine. Within this scheme, the path to subspecialty recognition for palliative medicine in the United States began in 1988 with the creation of the Academy of Hospice Physicians, later known as the American Academy of Hospice and Palliative Medicine. Further progress was made in the 1990s when the Institute of Medicine, the American College of Physicians, and the American Board of Internal Medicine all highlighted the need for greater physician competency in the care of persons with terminal illness.

Several key developments occurred in the 1990s. National representative bodies appeared to take a more professionalized approach to their activities, giving greater emphasis to palliative care as a specialized field of activity (the National Hospice Association became the National Hospice and Palliative Care Association; the American Academy of Hospice Physicians became the American Academy of Hospice and Palliative Medicine). At the same time, two major foundations developed extensive programmes concerned with the improvement of end-of-life care in American society (the Robert Wood Johnson Foundation created the Last Acts initiative; and the Open Society Institute established the Project on Death in America). An influential report by the Institute of Medicine (IoM), published in 1997, sought to strengthen popular and professional understanding of the need for good care at the end of life.[111] This was followed in 2001 by a further report from the IoM, listing ten recommendations addressing the role of the National Cancer Institute in promoting palliative care.[112] In 2004, the National Institutes of Health held a 'State-of-the-Science' meeting on Improving End-of-Life Care that brought together prominent clinicians and researchers to focus on defining end of life, understanding major considerations related to end-of-life care, and developing interventions for symptom management, social and spiritual care, and caregiver support.[113]

The American Board of Hospice and Palliative Medicine (ABHPM) was formed in 1995 to establish and implement standards for certification of physicians practising hospice and palliative medicine and, ultimately, for accreditation of physician training in the discipline. The ABHPM created a certification process that paralleled other member boards of the American Board of Medical Specialities (ABMS). A paper published in 2000 by Charles von Gunten and colleagues[114] showed that in the first three-and-a-half years of the ABMS, and over the administration of seven examinations, 623 physicians achieved board certification in hospice and palliative medicine. The authors concluded that there was significant physician interest in seeking professional recognition of expertise in caring for terminally ill persons and their families through the creation of a specialty in hospice and palliative medicine, with certification of physicians and accreditation of training programmes as key elements in the process.

There were three challenges:

1. To develop a consensus within medicine on the appropriate organizational base for a subspecialty in palliative medicine;

2. To seek ABMS approval for such a subspecialty within one or more existing specialities of medicine;

3. To seek formation of a residency review committee within the Accreditation Council of Graduate Medical Education (ACGME) to implement accreditation guidelines for palliative medicine fellowship programmes.[114]

Those seeking to promote the recognition of palliative medicine were aware that modern medical specialities are built around the twin pillars of accreditation of education and certification of competency. For the subspecialty of hospice and palliative medicine to be taken seriously as a mature medical discipline, it required credible accreditation and certification processes. Institutionalizing the specialty (through ABMS recognition and ACGME accreditation) would help assure that the achievements of palliative medicine were passed on to the next generation of physicians and that knowledge in the field continued to grow.

In the three-year period from the end of 2000 through to the close of 2003, the number of diplomates almost doubled from 779 to 1 538. Another critical concern to the ABMS was whether there would be a sufficient number of graduates of fellowship training programmes to sustain the field at a steady state. In fact, the number of fellowship programmes quickly expanded from just a handful to approximately 45, and it was anticipated that close to 100 fellows would graduate annually in the coming years.

Throughout these years, ABHPM staff and trustees carried out a strategic campaign to educate both leaders and grassroots professionals in the palliative medicine field about the steps needed to bring about formal recognition. It was considered important to build support that would be tangible and visible to the leadership of the other specialty disciplines. It was a huge challenge, but in 2006, the ACGME and the ABMS approved and recognized a new specialty in hospice and palliative medicine.[115]

This involved a transition in the physician certification process from the independent ABHPM to the ABMS and, thereafter, in the accreditation of training programmes from another independent organization to the ACGME.[116] In this process, hospice and palliative medicine became a subspecialty of no less than 11 primary specialities, a first in the history of the ABMS. Formal certification of physicians and accreditation of training programmes began in 2008.

Meanwhile, in neighbouring Canada, where Balfour Mount first coined the term *palliative care* in 1974,[117] a Senate report in 2000 stated that no extension of palliative care provision had occurred in the previous five years, and it set out recommendations for further development among the country's 600 services.[118] In Canada, following serious and detrimental delays in the eyes of one commentator,[119] specialty status for palliative medicine was not attained until 2014.

Anomalies, variations, and discontents about specialization

There are some major anomalies in how palliative medicine has gained recognition and accreditation, with widely differing standards, timescales, and expectations in the specialist training programmes of different countries. It has been noted that 'the original heated debate that accompanied the development of palliative medicine as a medical specialty in the United Kingdom in 1987 has continued in all other countries where the effort has been made to develop the specialty'.[120] At the same time specialty recognition can be seen as a turning point in hospice and palliative care history, opening up the field to formal recognition, scrutiny, and greater public awareness.[121]

For some, specialization was key to palliative care's integration into the mainstream health system, and a major platform upon which to develop an *evidence-based* model of practice crucial to long-term viability. Others balked at the undue emphasis of physical symptoms at the expense of psychosocial and spiritual matters. Just a few years after it achieved specialist recognition in the United Kingdom, Michael Kearney, a St Christopher's-trained, Irish palliative medicine physician, raised concerns about a specialty narrowly bounded by the practice of 'symptomatology', and thereby failing to create the conditions for deeper, personal 'healing'.[122] In a later work, he emphasized the need for palliative medicine to draw upon Greek traditions associated with Aesculapian healing and for these to be integrated with the modern science of symptom control.[123] Likewise, questions were raised about whether palliative medicine was really *specialist* territory and not, more properly, the domain of the generalist. Why had there been so little discussion on why specialization in palliative medicine came about, whether it was the most appropriate way to address acknowledged deficiencies in care, and whether it could be sustained in the long term? Examining the factors that contributed to the evolution of palliative medicine as a specialty, some even declared that its future was in doubt.[121] As the specialty developed, its attention tended to focus on pain and symptom management as a set of problems within the relief of suffering, giving weight to the charge of creeping medicalization.[124] There was a sense that the only aspect of Cicely Saunders's concept of total pain that received full attention was that concerned with physical problems.

One theme that can be identified across all these developments is the recognition that palliative care is an area of medicine for which the healthcare system as a whole should take responsibility. This found its most articulate expression in the concept that palliative care should be seen as a *public health issue*,[125] and that the knowledge and skills of palliative care must be translated into evidence-based, cost-effective interventions that can reach everyone in the population. This would require governments to adopt policies in support of palliative care at all appropriate levels of the healthcare system, and for these policies to have community support and endorsement. The WHO was the most powerful advocate of this approach, although it later found favour with palliative care experts in many contexts.

By the early twenty-first century, a growing commitment to the evidence base was emerging in palliative medicine, though several reviewers still found this a rather fragile enterprise and made claims for the particular problems faced by palliative care in assessing its practice by such means.[126], [127] Two forces for expansion were, however, clearly visible. First was the impetus to move palliative care further upstream in the disease progression, thereby seeking integration with curative and rehabilitation therapies, and shifting the focus beyond terminal care and the final stages of life. Second was a growing interest in extending the benefits of palliative care to those with diseases other than cancer in order to make 'palliative care for all' a reality. The new specialty was delicately poised. For some, such integration with the wider system was a *sine qua non* for success; for others it marked the entry into a risky phase of new development in which early ideals might be compromised.

It had been suggested that palliative medicine had the advantage of being a new and emerging specialty. It was relatively unencumbered by vested interests and capable of avoiding the mistakes made in other areas of medicine—in particular, the risk of achieving a lot for a few, while the needs of the majority remain unmet.[28] For such an approach, it was important to develop a worldwide perspective, accompanied by specific knowledge of local problems and issues and how they might be overcome. Careful thought also needed to be given to the contribution that specialization in palliative medicine could make to the global need for appropriate care of those with advanced disease and those facing death. The fate of palliative medicine would be only one of the factors to determine how dying people were cared for in the future.

Notes

1. **Durkeheim E** (1893 [1964]). *The Division of Labour in Society*. New York, NY: Free Press.
2. **Weisz G** (2006). *Divide and Conquer: A Comparative History of Medical Specialization*. Oxford, UK: Oxford University Press.
3. **Clark D** (2007). From margins to centre: A review of the history of palliative care in cancer. *Lancet Oncology*, 8(5):430–8.
4. **Clark D** (2002). *Cicely Saunders: Founder of the Hospice Movement, Selected Letters 1959–1999*. Oxford, UK: Oxford University Press.
5. **Clark D**, interview with Dr Gillian Ford, 6 June 1996; Clark D, interviews with Dr **Derek Doyle**, 28 December 1995 and 13 February 1996.
6. **Derek Doyle**, letter to Cicely Saunders, 15 October 1985. In: Clark D (ed.) (2002). *Cicely Saunders. Founder of the Hospice Movement. Selected letters 1959–1999*, p. 262. Oxford, UK: Oxford University Press.
7. Hospice History Project: David Clark interview with Robert Twycross, 25 October 1996.

8. Hospice History Project: David Clark interview with Gillian Ford, 6 June 1996.

9. **Twycross RG** (1977). Choice of strong analgesic in terminal cancer: Diamorphine or morphine? *Pain*, 3:93–104.

10. **Murray Parkes C, Parkes J** (1979). Hospice versus hospital care—re-evaluation after ten years as seen by surviving spouses. *Postgraduate Medical Journal*, 60:120–4.

11. **Hillier R** (1988). Palliative medicine, a new specialty. *British Medical Journal*, 297:874–5.

12. **Overy C, Tansey EM** (2013). *Palliative Medicine in the UK c1970–2010.* Wellcome Witnesses to Twentieth Century Medicine, vol. 45. London, UK: Queen Mary, University of London.

13. **Doyle D** (2005). Palliative medicine: The first 18 years of a new sub-specialty of general medicine. *Journal of the Royal College of Physicians of Edinburgh*, 35:199–205.

14. **Saunders C** (1987). What's in a name? *Palliative Medicine*, 1(1):57–61.

15. **O'Brien T, Clark D** (2005). A national plan for palliative care—the Irish experience. In: **Ling J, O'Siorain L** (eds.). *Palliative Care in Ireland*, pp. 3–18. Maidenhead, UK: Open University Press.

16. Association for Palliative Medicine of Great Britain and Ireland (2004). *Reports from Medical Workforce Database 2004.* Southampton, UK: APM.

17. Report of the National Advisory Committee on Palliative Care. Department of Health and Children. Available at http://health.gov.ie/wp-content/uploads/2014/03/nacpc.pdf, accessed 27 July 2015.

18. **Clark D, Seymour J** (1999). *Reflections on Palliative Care. Sociological and Policy Perspectives.* Buckingham, UK: Open University Press.

19. Standing Medical Advisory Committee/Standing Nursing and Midwifery Advisory Committee. *The principles and provision of palliative care.* London, UK: HMSO.

20. Expert Advisory Group on Cancer (1995). *A policy framework for the commissioning of cancer services.* London, UK: Department of Health and Welsh Office.

21. **Hanks GW, Twycross RG, Bliss JM** (1987). Controlled release morphine tablets: A double blind trial in patients with advanced cancer. *Anaesthesia*, 42:840–4.

22. **Doyle D, Hanks GWC, MacDonald N** (1993). *Oxford Textbook of Palliative Medicine*, 1st ed. Oxford, UK: Oxford University Press.

23. Hospice History Project: David Clark interview with Derek Doyle, 13 February 1996.

24. **Seymour J, Clark D, Winslow M** (2005). Pain and palliative care: The emergence of new specialities. *Journal of Pain and Symptom Management*, 29(1):2–13.

25. **Stjernswärd J** (2013). Personal reflections on contributions to pain relief, palliative care, and global cancer control. The James Lind Library. Available at http://www.jameslindlibrary.org/articles/personal-reflections-on-contributions-to-pain-relief-palliative-care-and-global-cancer-control/, accessed 11 June 2015.

26. **Meldrum M** (2005). The ladder and the clock: Cancer pain and public policy at the end of the twentieth century. *Journal of Pain and Symptom Management*, 29(1):41–54.

27. **World Health Organization** (1986). *Cancer Pain Relief.* Geneva, Switzerland: World Health Organization.

28. **Stjernswärd J** (1993). Palliative medicine—a global perspective. In Doyle D, Hanks GWC, Cherny N, MacDonald N (eds.). *Oxford Textbook of Palliative Medicine*, 1st ed., pp. 805–16. Oxford, UK: Oxford University Press.

29. **World Health Organization** (1990). Cancer Pain Relief and Palliative Care. WHO Technical Report Series 804. Geneva, Switzerland: WHO.

30. **Sepúlveda C, Marlin A, Yoshida T, Ullrich A** (2002). Palliative care: The World Health Organization's global perspective. *Journal of Pain and Symptom Management*, 24(2):91–6.
31. **Gifford D** (2009). Palliative care—evolution of a vision. *Medicine and Health Rhode Island*, 92(1):35.
32. World Health Organization (1996). *Cancer Pain Relief—with a guide to opioid availability*, 2nd ed. Geneva, Switzerland: World Health Organization.
33. World Health Organization (1998a). *Cancer pain relief and palliative care in children.* Geneva, Switzerland: World Health Organization.
34. World Health Organization (1998b). *Symptom Relief in Terminal Illness.* Geneva, Switzerland: World Health Organization.
35. **Stjernswärd J, Clark D** (2003). Palliative medicine: A global perspective. In: Doyle D, Hanks GWC, Cherny N, Calman KC (eds.). *Oxford Textbook of Palliative Medicine*, 3rd ed., pp. 1199–224. Oxford, UK: Oxford University Press.
36. **Clark D** (2004). History, gender, and culture in the rise of palliative care. In: Payne SS, Seymour J, Ingleton I (eds.). *Palliative Care Nursing. Principles and Evidence for Practice*, pp. 39–54. Maidenhead, UK: Open University Press.
37. Hospice History Project: David Clark interview with Balfour Mount, 14 March 2001.
38. **Magno J** (2007). *Hospice in America.* New York, NY: iUniverse.
39. Hospice History Project: David Clark interview with Josefina Magno, 9 December 1995.
40. **Buck J** (2014). Ideals, politics, and the evolution of the American hospice movement. In: Jennings B, Kirk TW (eds.). *Hospice Ethics.* New York, NY: Oxford University Press.
41. **Bruera E, de Lima L, Woodruff R** (2002). The International Association for Hospice and Palliative Care. *Journal of Pain and Symptom Management*, 24(2):102–5.
42. International Association for Hospice & Palliataive Care. IAHPC History. Available at http://hospicecare.com/about-iahpc/who-we-are/history/, accessed 3 June 2015.
43. **Blumhuber H, Kaasa S, de Conno F** (2002). The European Association for Palliative Care. *Journal of Pain and Symptom Management*, 24(2):124–7.
44. **Fondazione Floriani.** Vittorio Ventafridda. Available at http://www.fondazioneflori-ani.eu/vittorio-ventafridda, accessed 9 June 2015.
45. Hospice History Project: David Clark interview with Frances Sheldon, 25 June 2003.
46. European Association for Palliative Care. Report 1st Congress of the EAPC—Paris, France, October 1990. Available at http://www.eapcnet.eu/Corporate/Events/EAPCMainCongresses/PreviousMainCongresses/1990ParisReport.aspx, accessed 3 June 2015.
47. **Caraceni A** et al. (2012). Use of opioid analgesics in the treatment of cancer pain: Evidence-based recommendations from the EAPC. *Lancet Oncology*, 13(2):e58–68. doi:10.1016/S1470-2045(12)70040-2.
48. **ten Have H, Clark D** (2002). *The Ethics of Palliative Care. European Perspectives.* Buckingham, UK: Open University Press.
49. Barcelona Declaration on Palliative Care (1995). *European Journal of Palliative Care*, 3(1):15.
50. **Poznań Declaration** (1998). *European Journal of Palliative Care*, 6(2):61–5.
51. **Cherny NI, Catane R, Kosmidis P** (2003). ESMO takes a stand on supportive and palliative care. *Annals of Oncology*, 14(9):1335–7.

52. **Eurag-Europe.org**. European Federation of Older People in Organisations, available at http://www.foragenetwork.eu/en/database/item/97-eurag-european-federation-of-older-people/, accessed 27 July 2015.

53. **Davies E, Higginson IJ** (2004). *Better Palliative Care for Older People*. Copenhagen, Denmark: World Health Organization.

54. **Davies E, Higginson IJ** (2004). *Palliative Care: The Solid Facts*. Copenhagen, Denmark: World Health Organization.

55. **Clark D, Centeno C** (2006). Palliative care in Europe: An emerging approach to comparative analysis. *Clinical Medicine*, 6(2):197–201.

56. Hospice History Project: David Clark interview with Mary Callaway, 22 July 2003.

57. **Cassell EJ** (1982). *The Nature of Suffering and the Goals of Medicine*, 2nd ed. Oxford, UK: Oxford University Press.

58. Hospice History Project: David Clark interview with Jacek Luczak, 17 March 1996.

59. **Clark D, Wright M** (2003). *Transitions in End of Life Care: Hospice and Related Developments in Eastern Europe and Central Asia*. Buckingham, UK: Open University Press.

60. Hospice History Project: David Clark interview with Eduardo Bruera, 9 November 1995.

61. Hospice History Project: Michelle Winslow interview with **Jorge Eisenchlas**, 2 October 2001.

62. **Chung Y** (1999). Palliative care in Korea: A nursing point of view. *Progress in Palliative Care*, 8(1):12–16.

63. **Maruyama TC** (1999). *Hospice Care and Culture*. Aldershot, UK: Ashgate.

64. **Wang XS, Yu S, Gu W, Xu G** (2002). China: Status of pain and palliative care. *Journal of Pain and Symptom Management*, 24(2):177–9.

65. **Goh CR** (2002). The Asia Pacific Hospice Palliative Care Network: A network for individuals and organizations. *Journal of Pain and Symptom Management*, 24(2):128–33.

66. **McDermott E, Selman L, Wright M, Clark D** (2008). Hospice and palliative care development in India: A multi-method review of services and experiences. *Journal of Pain and Symptom Management*, 35(6):583–93.

67. **Shabeer C, Kumar S** (2005). Palliative care in the developing world: A social experiment in India. *European Journal of Palliative Care*, 13(2):76–9.

68. The actual reference is: Twycross RG, Lack SA (1983). *Symptom Control in Far Advanced Cancer: Pain Relief*. London, UK: Pitman.

69. Hospice History Project: David Clark interview with MR Rajagopal, 24 January 2003.

70. Hospice History Project: Michael Wright interview with Ednin Hamza, 22 September 2004.

71. Hospice History Project: Jenny Hunt interview with Faith Mwangi-Powell, 14 November 2004.

72. **Wright M, Clark D** (2006). *Hospice and Palliative Care Development in Africa. A Review of Developments and Challenges*. Oxford, UK: Oxford University Press.

73. **Harding R, Stewart K, Marconi K, O'Neill JF, Higginson IJ** (2003). Current HIV/AIDS end-of-life care in sub-Saharan Africa: A survey of models, services, challenges, and priorities. *BMC Public Health*, 3 (Oct.):33.

74. **Sepulveda C et al.** (2003). Quality care at the end of life in Africa. *British Medical Journal*, 327:209–13.

75. **Harding R. Higginson IJ** (2005). Palliative care in sub-Saharan Africa. *Lancet,* 365 (9475):1971–7.
76. International Association for Hospice and Palliative Care (2007). The Declaration of Venice: Palliative care research in developing countries. *Journal of Pain & Palliative Care Pharmacotherapy*, 21(1):31–3. Available at http://www.ncbi.nlm.nih.gov/pubmed/17430827, accessed 7 July 2014.
77. **Radbruch L, Foley K, De Lima L, Praill D, Fürst CJ** (2007). The Budapest Commitments: Setting the goals, a joint initiative by the European Association for Palliative Care, the International Association for Hospice and Palliative Care, and Help the Hospices. *Palliative Medicine* 21(4):269–71.
78. International Association for Hospice and Palliative Care. IAHPC List of Essential Medicines for Palliative Care. Available at http://hospicecare.com/resources/palliative-care-essentials/iahpc-essential-medicines-for-palliative-care/, accessed 27 July 2015.
79. **Harding R** (2006). Palliative care: A basic human right. *id21 Insights Health* 8 (Feb.):1–2. Available at http://r4d.dfid.gov.uk/PDF/Outputs/IDS/insights_health8.pdf, accessed 27 July 2015.
80. Commission on Human Rights Resolution 2004/26, Item 7c. United Nations Human Rights. Available at http://www.un.org/en/terrorism/pdfs/2/G0414734.pdf, accessed 27 July 2015.
81. *Ibid.* note 35.
82. **Lewis M** (2007). *Medicine and the Care of the Dying. A Modern History*, p.157. Oxford, UK: Oxford University Press.
83. **Saunders C, Kastenbaum R** (1997). *Hospice Care on the International Scene.* New York, NY: Springer.
84. General Assembly of the United Nations. High-level meeting on non-communicable diseases. Available at http://www.un.org/en/ga/president/65/issues/ncdiseases.shtml, accessed 1 December 2013.
85. World Medical Association. WMA declaration on end-of life medical care. Available at http://www.wma.net/en/30publications/10policies/e18/index.html?World%20Medical%20Association%20declaration%20on%20end%20of%20life%20medical%20care, accessed 1 December 2013.
86. **ten Have H, Janssens R** (2001). *Palliative Care in Europe, Concepts and Policies.* Amsterdam, Netherlands: IOS Press.
87. **ten Have H, Clark D** (2002). *The Ethics of Palliative Care: European Perspectives.* Buckingham, UK: Open University Press.
88. **Clark D, ten Have H, Janssens R** (2000). Common threads? Palliative care service developments in seven European countries. *Palliative Medicine*, 14(6):479–90.
89. **Gronemeyer R, Fink M, Globisch M, Schuman F** (2005). *Helping People at the End of Their Lives: Hospice and Palliative Care in Europe.* Berlin, Germany: Lit Verlag.
90. **Clark D, Wright M** (2007). The international observatory on end of life care: A global view of palliative care development. *Journal of Pain and Symptom Management*, 33(5):542–6.
91. **Bingley A, Clark D** (2009). A comparative review of palliative care development in six countries represented by the Middle East Cancer Consortium (MECC). *Journal of Pain and Symptom Management*, 37(3):287–96.
92. **Wright M** (2010). *Hospice and Palliative Care in South East Asia.* Oxford, UK: Oxford University Press.

93. **Wright M, Wood J, Lynch T, Clark D** (2008). Mapping levels of palliative care development: A global view. *Journal of Pain and Symptom Management*, 35(5):469–85.

94. **Lynch T, Connor S, Clark D** (2013). Mapping levels of palliative care development: A global update. *Journal of Pain and Symptom Management*, 45(6):1094–106. doi:10.1016/j.jpainsymman.2012.05.011.

95. The Economist Intelligence Unit (2010). *The Quality of Death: Ranking end-of-life care across the world*. Available from http://graphics.eiu.com/upload/eb/quality-ofdeath.pdf, accessed 27 July 2015.

96. The Economist (2015). Quality of Death Index. Available at http://www.economistinsights.com/healthcare/analysis/quality-death-index-2015, accessed 21 November 2015.

97. **Clark J** (2010). Terminally neglected? The marginal place of palliative care within global discourses on health. Unpublished master's thesis. Sheffield, UK: University of Sheffield.

98. Worldwide Palliative Care Alliance. WHO global atlas on palliative care at the end of life. Available at http://www.thewpca.org/resources/global-atlas-of-palliative-care/, accessed 7 July 2014.

99. World Health Organization. Strengthening of palliative care as a component of integrative treatment within the continuum of care. Available at http://apps.who.int/gb/ebwha/pdf_files/EB134/B134_R7-en.pdf, accessed 7 July 2014.

100. International Association for Hospice and Palliative Care (2014). Policy and advocacy: Palliative care in the 67th World Health Assembly. Newsletter 15, no. 6 (June). Available at http://hospicecare.com/about-iahpc/newsletter/2014/6/policy-and-advocacy/, accessed 7 July 2014.

101. **Centeno C, Noguera A, Lynch T, Clark D** (2007). Official certification of doctors working in palliative medicine in Europe: Data from an EAPC study in 52 European countries. *Palliative Medicine*, 21:683–7.

102. Hospice History Project: David Clark interview with Stein Kaasa, 5 November 2004.

103. **Clark D** (2010). International progress in creating palliative medicine as a specialized discipline. In: Hanks G et al. *Oxford Textbook of Palliative Medicine*, 4th ed., pp. 9–16. Oxford, UK: Oxford University Press.

104. European Association for Palliative Care. Specialisation in Palliative Medicine for Physicians in Europe 2014. A supplement of the EAPC Atlas of Palliative Care in Europe. Available at http://www.eapcnet.eu/Portals/0/Organization/Development%20in%20Europe%20TF/Specialisation/2014_SpecialisationPMPhysicianInEurope.pdf, accessed 27 July 2015.

105. Syndicate of Hospitals. Palliative Medicine: A New Specialty in Lebanon. Available at http://www.syndicateofhospitals.org.lb/Content/uploads/SyndicateMagazinePdfs/7564_28-29%20Eng.pdf, accessed 27 July 2015.

106. University of Glasgow. End of Life Studies. Palliative medicine as a specialty. Available at http://endoflifestudies.academicblogs.co.uk/palliative-medicine-as-a-specialty/, accessed 7 July 2014.

107. **Zorza V, Zorza R** (1978). Death of a daughter. *The Guardian Weekly*, 118(7), 12 February.

108. Hospice History Project: David Clark interview with Ian Maddocks, 8 December 1995.

109. **Cairns W** (2007). A short history of palliative medicine in Australia. *Cancer Forum*, 31(1):6–9.
110. **Ryndes T, von Gunten CF** (2006). The development of palliative medicine in the USA. In: **Bruera E, Higginson IJ, Ripamonti C, von Gunten C** (eds.). *Textbook of Palliative Medicine*, pp. 29–35. London, UK: Hodder Arnold.
111. **Field MJ, Cassel CK** (1997). *Approaching Death: Improving Care at the End of Life.* Washington, DC: National Academy Press.
112. **Foley KM, Gelband H** (2001). *Improving Palliative Care for Cancer. Summary and Recommendations from the National Cancer Policy Board, Institute of Medicine, and National Research Council.* Washington, DC: National Academy Press.
113. **Grady PA** (2005). Introduction: Papers from the National Institutes of Health State-of-the-Science Conference on Improving End-of-Life Care. *Journal of Palliative Medicine,* 8(Suppl 1):s1–s3.
114. **von Gunten C, Sloan PA, Portenoy RK, Schonwetter RS**, Trustees of the American Board of Hospice and Palliative Medicine (2000). Physician board certification in hospice and palliative medicine. *Journal of Palliative Medicine* 3(4):441–7.
115. **Lupu D, Moga DN, Portenoy R, Radwany S** (2009). Hospice and palliative medicine in the USA: The road to recognition. *European Journal of Palliative Care,* 16(3):136–41.
116. **Schonwetter R** (2006). Hospice and palliative medicine goes mainstream. *Journal of Palliative Medicine*, 9(6):1240–2.
117. **Mount B** (1997). The Royal Victoria Hospital palliative care service: A Canadian experience. In: Saunders C, Kastenbaum R (eds.). *Hospice Care on the International Scene.* New York, NY: Springer.
118. **Carstairs S, Chochinov H** (2001). Politics, palliation, and Canadian progress in end-of-life care. *Journal of Palliative Medicine*, 4(3):396–9.
119. **Macdonald N** (2006). The development of palliative care in Canada. In: Bruera E, Higginson IJ, Ripamonti C, von Gunten C (eds.). *Textbook of Palliative Medicine*, pp. 22–8. London, UK: Hodder Arnold.
120. **Bruera E, Pace EA** (2006). Palliative care versus palliative medicine. In: Bruera E, Higginson I, Ripamonti C, von Gunten C (eds.). *Textbook of Palliative Medicine*, pp. 64–7. London, UK: Hodder Arnold.
121. **Fordham S, Dowrick C, May C** (1998). Palliative medicine: Is it really specialist territory? *Journal of the Royal Society of Medicine*, 91:568–72.
122. **Kearney M** (1992). Palliative medicine—just another specialty? *Palliative Medicine*, 6:39–46.
123. **Kearney M** (2000). *A Place of Healing. Working with Suffering in Living and Dying.* Oxford, UK: Oxford University Press.
124. **James N, Field D** (1992) The routinization of hospice: charisma and bureaucratisation, *Social Science and Medicine*, 34 (12):1363–75.
125. **Stjernswärd J, Foley KM, Ferris FD** (2007). The public health strategy for palliative care. *Journal of Pain and Symptom Management*, 33(5):486–93.
126. **Higginson I** (1999). Evidence based palliative care. *British Medical Journal*, 319:462–3.
127. **Keeley D** (1999). Rigorous assessment of palliative care revisited. Wisdom and compassion are needed when evidence is lacking. *British Medical Journal*, 319:1447–8.

Chapter 7

Palliative medicine: Historical record and challenges that remain

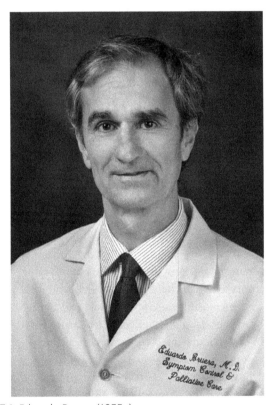

Figure 7.1 Eduardo Bruera (1955–)

Born and trained in medicine in Argentina, Bruera moved to North America in the mid-1980s to pursue a developing interest in palliative medicine. From positions in Alberta and then Texas, he supported an unprecedented range of clinical studies, which helped establish the initial evidence base for the new specialty. He also took on a strong international leadership role and became one of the few palliative care physicians who seemed equally at ease in the clinic, the research conference, or the policy forum.

Reproduced by kind permission of Eduardo Bruera. Copyright © 2016 The University of Texas MD Anderson Cancer Center.

Assessing the past and contemplating the future

In concluding this work, it is time to do two things.

First, we must assess the progress that palliative medicine made over the period of 100 years—from the publication of William Munk's key work in 1887, to the first recognition of the specialty in the United Kingdom, in 1987. This chapter will return to cover that ground, highlighting key forces, determinants, and opportunities, leading us to an assessment of what was achieved and the implications for further development.

Second, the chapter will go beyond this time period to consider some of the practical and conceptual challenges identified into the early decades of the twenty-first century, and the prospects for overcoming them. Some of these issues have already been explored in Chapter 6. Here the record is less clear, as the issues and debates are still underway and have not yet been resolved. For this later period, therefore, judgements are not so easy to formulate. As we come closer to the present day, critical reflection may be all the prudent scholar has to offer. But while writing this in the summer of 2015, when interest in hospice and palliative medicine worldwide is achieving greater interest and recognition than perhaps ever before, it would be inconsiderate to not at least touch further—if not exhaustively—on this period and the issues raised by it.

A century of development

We have seen that the field of palliative medicine was forged in a crucible of wider changes, not only in medicine but affecting society as a whole. Its origins coincided with the era of modernization, urbanization, population growth, and increasing mobility. We are still living with the consequences and out-workings of such changes. Care of the dying began to crystallize as an area of particular medical interest at a time when the epidemiological transition was transforming the social circumstances of death; from that of a visitor who came unawares, to one where protracted dying came to be both anticipated and more commonplace. In this context, fears shifted from religious and existential concerns about what might lie beyond the grave, to more direct material anxieties about the process of dying itself.

For medicine, this created interesting possibilities. If ministers of religion were retreating from the deathbed, doctors may then become more active there. A space was opening up that could prove congenial to medical discourse and practice, and provide fertile ground for innovation and expansion. First, however, 'dying' must be diagnosed and its signs and symptoms described. Nineteenth-century physicians created a nosology of dying. They began to treat dying as if it were a disease, with its own onset, progression, and natural history. This could then lead to estimates of prevalence, trends, and population characteristics—not of those dying, but of the conditions and characteristics they exhibited. It could also form the basis for clinical judgement and knowledge to be shared with others. The nineteenth-century doctors described in Chapter 1 were at the forefront of such developments. They reflected on their clinical experience with the dying and wrote about it for the benefit of fellow physicians.

However, as they did so, they encountered problematic aspects of clinical judgement. These touched on moral and religious matters. What was the role of medicine at the bedside? Should medicine always seek to relieve suffering, or might the endurance of pain and other symptoms be, in some instances, a necessary evil in order to attain a greater good? We have seen that pain in the dying process was, in the earlier nineteenth century, presumed to be a route to quicker entry into heaven. But if pain-relieving formulations were at hand, might their use lead to a different perception of the meaning of suffering, something that could be overcome by human agency, wisdom, and knowledge—but therefore having no intrinsic merit? Over time, this came to be the settled view of medicine. Pain was unnecessary, dysfunctional, and an enemy to be overcome. Nevertheless, by the closing of the nineteenth century, this had already crystallized into a fundamental question. Are there certain circumstances in which medicine should intervene to end suffering and, in so doing, end life itself?

William Munk's foundational text, which forms the conceptual, if not exactly chronological, starting point for this book, appeared when the term *euthanasia* was about to change significantly in meaning. His work was the high watermark for euthanasia as the idealized easeful death. For him, it meant safe passage from the world with the accompanying ministrations of physician, family, and friends. Soon it would come to mean intervention by doctors deliberately to end life when suffering had become unbearable. Others shared Munk's goals relating to easeful death, albeit a limited circle. His work was met with positive reactions in Britain and America. In both these countries, homes for the dying were also coming into existence. However, they did not have much in the way of material resources and they seem to have been rather cut off from the professional world of academic and elite medicine. Usually run by religious orders of nuns or by religiously inspired women, they nevertheless created the first concentrated institutional focus on the care of those approaching death. It is unclear why these places elicited so little in the way of innovative medical interest in the late nineteenth and early twentieth centuries. Certainly, they had on their own dedicated staff doctors, a few in full-time positions, and most as attending physicians. An example was Howard Barrett, who documented his activities assiduously in a series of annual reports, which were later to be read by and to influence others. However, generally doctors in the homes for the dying were preoccupied with their day-to-day clinical responsibilities, mindful of the charitable status of the places in which they worked, and perhaps temperamentally not disposed to personal aggrandizement or influence. Moreover, patients at the end of life were neglected by the charitable hospitals, which wanted little to do with the care of the dying and sought to project themselves as modern centres for innovative practice, unwilling to admit the terminally ill and moribund, and focused more on goals of treatment and rehabilitation.

At the same time, the terminal care homes were well documented, as they kept careful records that have endured. Their annals and reports were written for particular institutional or fundraising purposes, which adopted certain stylistic conventions. They tended to highlight idealized examples of good care, as well as of spiritual enlightenment reached against the odds, but they provide a basis for understanding the approach adopted—and this was one readily accepted by twentieth-century innovators like Cicely Saunders, who saw in them much to emulate and adapt.

It remains unclear why there was such a dearth of medical writing about the end of life in the final years of the nineteenth and the early decades of the twentieth centuries. From the publication in Britain of Munk's work in 1887, it was a very long pause before Alfred Worcester's lectures appeared in the United States on the care of the ageing, the dying, and the dead in 1935.[1] Worcester offers some explanation for why this might be the case. The care of the aged and dying, he states, had not become an area for specialist interest; rather it was one left to general practitioners, who in the main had ceased to communicate to the wider profession the results of their experience, with the result that 'neither medical science nor the art of practice advances'. Likewise, the medical literature on 'senescence', he opined, was dreary, dated, and largely repetitious. In the care of the dying, he judged medical practice to have deteriorated in the half century preceding the publication of his book. Doctors had abandoned their dying patients to the care of nurses and sorrowing relatives: 'This shifting of responsibility is un-pardonable. And one of its bad results is that as less professional interest is taken in such service less and less is known about it.'

Extrapolating from such a perspective, we might infer that in the first half of the twentieth century the medical care of the dying was deteriorating. Neglected in medical schools, devoid of leaders and champions, unduly associated with religious associations, and focused mainly on patients who could make little improvement, the judgement of early twentieth-century medicine was that 'nothing more can be done' for the obviously dying patient. At best, such pessimism could be tempered by a paternalistic benevolence on the part of family doctors who did remain with their dying patients. For them, the liberal, if clumsy, use of morphine was the last resort of treatment. A collection of medical writings on the care of the dying published in Britain in 1948 could therefore amount to little more than an assemblage of anecdotes and aphorisms. Poor care at the end of life, at least by omission if not by intention, must have prevailed for many dying people in Britain—and elsewhere in the western world—in the first half of the twentieth century.

The 1950s gives us our first systematic look at the nature of the problems. The abject social condition of those dying from a stigmatizing disease like cancer was first investigated in Britain in the period after World War II. The strategic direction of this work initially came from outside the National Health Service. However, the quickening interest of doctors and of some researchers began to attract attention. Major journals produced editorials on terminal care; their editors published new studies that threw light on late diagnosis of cancer, the care of older people at the end of life, and the prospects for new ideas and approaches began to take hold. There was also a growing interest in pain relief, the understanding of the mechanisms of pain and the wider skills required for appropriate pain management. The prominent voice in much of this—achieved against the odds of her gender, her late entry into medicine, her overtly Christian stance, and her resolve to set up a charitable institution to further her goals—was that of Cicely Saunders.

Saunders galvanized interest and support from like-minded people in Britain, America, and elsewhere. She created a model that was widely emulated and adapted. She stood out in the field for her energy, determination, global reach, and above all, her ability to define an aspect of care that had become lost to modern medicine, but which resonated with the western *zeitgeist* of the 1960s and 1970s. This vision and local action, however, as developed by Saunders and her contemporaries, were not enough to take forward 'at scale' the work of caring for people at the end of life. This would require the development of a new field of medicine. The particular character of the work had to be demonstrated in its clinical dimensions, and in relation to research and teaching. This was incremental, empirical activity, through which pioneering physicians, services, patients, and families, by their direct involvement, demonstrated the claims and practices of hospice and palliative medicine.

The origins of modern palliative care lie in a movement to improve care of the dying that configured first around notions of hospice care. Pioneers emerging from within the healthcare system would not come until later. From the 1950s and 1960s, activists such as Cicely Saunders and Florence Wald looked to a hospice tradition that had got underway in the late nineteenth-century religious homes for the dying, which had developed in France, Britain, America, and Australia. Nevertheless, these were a mixture of people with and without religious inspiration. They sought to reinvent older hospice traditions in a new guise and in so doing to challenge the growing western tendency to deny death and to sequestrate the dying. The 'hospice movement' was a small revolution against prevailing 'death-ways' in western culture. In some instances, it was a reaction against meddlesome medicine and futile interventions. In others, it was stimulated by the medical neglect of the dying in healthcare systems that prioritized cure and rehabilitation over the needs of those close to death. In time, it became a recognized area of specialization and indeed a career pathway.

The development of modern hospice care had many of the characteristics of a new social movement. It was associated with a single issue and fostered by strong advocacy, as well as charismatic leadership. It grew out of communities of interest, communities of practice, and communities of place. In many instances, services were initiated without the endorsement of the formal healthcare system, but with strong local support. This often led to tensions and confrontation as the hospice pioneers sought recognition for their cause in the face of scepticism, indifference, and bureaucratic inertia.

To succeed more widely, and thereby meet population level needs, it became increasingly clear that hospice ideas and practice would need to find a place within the mainstream of healthcare systems and structures. This was recognized in the early 1970s by the Canadian surgeon, Balfour Mount, who also took the view that the work needed a different nomenclature. He coined the term *palliative care*, drawing not only on established medical notions of palliation, but also on wider meanings of the word in relation to 'cloaking' or 'shielding'. The first named palliative care services soon began to appear. As we have seen, the 1980s were a period of intense development in many countries, during which journals, training programmes, and major conferences came to be dedicated to palliative and hospice care. New services were being founded, international links were forged, and new organizations came into existence to take forward the work of promoting palliative care to the wider public, to fellow professionals, and to policymakers, and people of influence. The United Kingdom was on the leading edge of this curve, and in 1987, seemingly with great alacrity, it was the first country to recognize palliative medicine as a specialist area of activity.

The new services were also diversifying and palliative care began to be delivered not only in specialist inpatient units and hospices, but also in the wards and outpatient clinics of acute hospitals, in the community, in residential care settings, and in people's own homes. Commensurate with this was a growing interest in research, evaluation, and attempts to develop policies and strategies for palliative care delivery for whole jurisdictions. Palliative care was taking on the characteristics of a field, which could be recognized alongside other specialities in health and social care and bore the recognizable hallmarks of an evidence base, standards and guidelines, codes of training and practice, and professional accreditation.

Professional bodies proliferated and emphasized the multidisciplinary aspects of palliative care as a specialism that involved medicine, nursing, social work, psychology, spiritual and religious support, and the involvement of allied health workers and volunteers. Some of these developed their own subspecialized journals, in nursing and social work, which might seem contradictory in a field that was so committed to multidisciplinary and multi-professional approaches. From the mid-1990s, research studies were conducted that mapped the differential development of palliative care in specific regions of the world, and also globally. Understanding grew of the common elements that united the palliative care ethos, but also of internal differences, the variations in local practice cultures and assumptions, and the specific ethical challenges to which they gave rise. As the global palliative care landscape became more richly articulated, so too it became possible to see the variations in approach, the struggle to adopt a common language for the specialism, and the requirement for medicine to articulate its particular role within it.

Twenty-first-century issues

Palliative care in its modern guise seeks to prevent and alleviate suffering associated with life-limiting illness, and it is particularly associated with care at the end of life and in bereavement. Its principles are holistic and multidisciplinary, focusing on physical, social, psychological, and spiritual concerns in the context of serious illness. To these ends, it engages the skills of medicine, nursing, social work, psychology, allied health professions, family members, and often volunteers and wider communities. It has developed specific expertise in the understanding and management of pain associated with advanced disease, and it provides expertise in relation to other, often complex, symptoms that may occur across the trajectory of illness. As we have seen, within the broader multidisciplinary landscape of palliative care, there also exists the specific area of specialization called palliative medicine. The purpose of this book has been to better understand the history and character of this field of medicine.

Palliative care has attracted the interests and commitments of those well beyond the world of healthcare delivery, albeit focused around a specific aspect of care. It is much spoken about, debated, and commented on in the mainstream and social media, among policymakers and politicians, as well as in popular writing and debate. *Public engagement* has become a key element in the palliative care 'project', as it seeks to use social marketing and other techniques to promote its interests and get its message to wider audiences. In turn, the work of palliative care has captured the interests of artists and writers, film-makers, and photographers, who see in it a crucible of contemporary debates around the meaning of illness and care in society and, in particular, the issue of how we die.

However, palliative care is also a multifaceted field of specialization, along with associated academic endeavours in teaching and research, with a growing recognition among professional societies, scientific funders, universities, and training establishments. It has been drawn to a public health paradigm when considering levels of need and appropriate policies and services for delivery, together with suitable quality assurance and evaluation. It also makes an expanding claim for recognition as a human right. Increasingly, the reach of palliative care extends to health policymakers, politicians, global health organizations, and related discourses.

Palliative care has a close but sometimes complex relationship with hospice care, and this differs across countries of the world. Many varieties of hospice and palliative care delivery can now be observed in a wide range of settings. While few of these are supported by proven evidence of success, they do testify to the rich field of activity and the imaginative and diverse approaches that have been developed in different resource, cultural, and healthcare contexts. Palliative care is also seeking to develop an appropriate relationship with other areas of the healthcare system, in particular those primarily focused on curative treatments, rehabilitation, or the management of long-term conditions. It faces specific challenges in the light of changing demographics, epidemiology, and patterns of symptomatology.

Countries and cultures are at varying points on the epidemiological transition away from infectious disease as the primary cause of death, to the slower trajectory of death from non-communicable and chronic conditions. Healthcare systems vary enormously in their levels of preparedness for the care of people at the end of life. There are different ethico-legal systems in which jurisdictions approach the issue of dying. There are differing local moral worlds of dying, death, and bereavement; often in flux due to wider social forces and sometimes creating tensions over the body of the dying person. In addition, there is little unanimity about appropriate interventions at the end of life and the correct role of medicine within them. The evidence to better understand these issues is emerging, but often policy and practice are developed without appropriate foresight and reflection.

The distribution and availability of palliative care globally is known to be highly inequitable, being concentrated in a small number of countries, and this has led the World Health Assembly to call on all governments to give it higher priority. It has been estimated that less than 10 per cent of those who might benefit from palliative care currently have access to it worldwide. Only 20 countries have achieved a significant degree of palliative care development as demonstrated by levels of service provision, education, drug availability, research, financing, and policy recognition. Palliative *medicine* is recognized as a specialist field of activity in around 25 countries worldwide.

For some years the United Kingdom has been seen as the benchmark country that heads the league table in these developments. By 2005, there were some nine chairs in medicine and nursing related to palliative care in the United Kingdom, as well as three chairs occupied by social scientists with a major interest in the field. It was also home to significant research centres, such as the Cicely Saunders Institute, led by Professor Irene Higginson—a leading figure in the move to establish an evidence base for the specialty. By 2014, there were 13 chairs in British universities in *palliative medicine* alone. Yet, a study of the research outputs from these facilities for the years 2001–2008 found that there were less than 40 UK-based academics with a sustained commitment to the field.[2]

Definitional issues and wider understanding

There has been significant debate—and no lack of disagreement—about the various definitions and models of palliative, end-of-life, and hospice care that now exist. The World Health Organization (WHO) has produced two definitions, in 1990 and in 2002, but many more are described in the subsequent literature. These definitional problems continue to inhibit clarity of thought and action in the field.

For example, a paper focusing on definitions of the term *palliative medicine* and *palliative care* in two languages found a total of 37 English and 26 German versions, confirming a lack of a consistent meaning about key terms and approaches.[3] This also applied to cognate areas. In 2004, a National Institutes of Health State-of-the-Science Conference statement noted: 'There is no exact definition of end of life; however, research supports the following components: (1) the presence of a chronic disease(s) or symptoms or functional impairments that persist but may also fluctuate; and (2) the symptoms or impairments resulting from the underlying irreversible disease that require formal either paid, professional, or informal unpaid or volunteer care and can lead to death.[4] Surprisingly, a 2012 volume offering an international public health perspective on the subject offered no clarification, often using end-of-life care interchangeably with palliative care.[5]

In 2011, the *Washington Post* [6] reported on the findings of a recent opinion poll in the United States.[7] At that time and by a wide margin, Americans believed it more important to enhance the quality of life for the seriously ill, even if this meant a shorter life (71 per cent), rather than to extend life through every medical intervention possible (23 per cent). More than half of all Americans (55 per cent) believed that the healthcare system has the responsibility, technology, and expertise to offer treatments and to spend however much it takes to extend lives. This compared to 37 per cent who thought the healthcare system spends far too much trying to extend the lives of seriously ill patients. Americans, however, were largely unfamiliar with the term palliative care (only 24 per cent said otherwise), especially compared to end-of-life care (known by 65 per cent) and hospice care (86 per cent). Yet, nearly two out of every three Americans (63 per cent) have had personal or family experience with palliative care, end-of-life care, or hospice care. A strong majority believe there should be a more open debate about public policies regarding palliative care options (78 per cent). Respondents also agreed that educating patients and their families about these issues is important (97 per cent) and think a public dialogue will provide more information about care options (86 per cent). Yet roughly half (47 per cent) of respondents across all political affiliations say they worry that emphasizing palliative and end-of-life care options could interfere with doing whatever it takes to help patients extend their lives as long as possible.[8] These contradictions seem to be at the heart of the modern orientation to end-of-life care. They constitute the fragmented moral terrain on which palliative medicine—at least in the rich world—must operate.

In the same year, 2011, a similar study was conducted on the other side of the Atlantic in Northern Ireland. While the majority of respondents (83 per cent) reported that they had heard the term palliative care, most revealed they had little or no knowledge of its meaning: over half claimed to have little knowledge, while a fifth stated they had no understanding of the concept of palliative care at all. Women, however, reported higher levels of knowledge than men. Those with the most knowledge tended to work in the healthcare system. The majority defined palliative care as pain relief for people with terminal illness at the end of life with the aim of achieving a peaceful death. Although participants were not asked to specify conditions, many associated palliative care with cancer and care of older people. When respondents were asked to reflect on the aims of palliative care, the majority cited the delivery of comfort (82 per cent), pain relief (81.3 per cent), and dignity (76.3 per cent) as priorities.[9]

Back in the United States, another study conducted in the same year found similar results.[10] The term palliative care appears to have little or no meaning to American healthcare consumers. Yet, once informed, they seem extremely positive about it and want access to this care if they need it: 95 per cent of respondents agree that it is important that patients with serious illness and their families be educated about palliative care; 92 per cent of respondents say they were likely to consider palliative care for a loved one if they had a serious illness; 92 per cent of respondents say it is important that palliative care services be made available at all hospitals for patients with serious illness and their families. The study was particularly important in that it developed and tested a 'new language' definition of palliative care and suggested it should be used when defining or describing palliative care for consumers.

> Palliative care is specialized medical care for people with serious illnesses. This type of care is focused on providing patients with relief from the symptoms, pain, and stress of a serious illness—whatever the diagnosis. The goal is to improve quality of life for both the patient and the family. Palliative care is provided by a team of doctors, nurses, and other specialists who work with a patient's other doctors to provide an extra layer of support. Palliative care is appropriate at any age and at any stage in a serious illness, and can be provided together with curative treatment.[10]

It is a paradox, therefore, that while the field of palliative care, and of palliative medicine within it, has been growing, and expanding its reach, it remains poorly understood by the wider public. An interesting attempt to address this came from the United States in 2014 when the film *You Are a Bridge* appeared on YouTube, supported by the group Get Palliative Care,[11] itself a public arm of the Center to Advance Palliative Care[12] led by Dr Diane Meier, one of the leading US figures in palliative care. Aimed at the general public, the short animated film explains what palliative care is and where it is relevant.

> Palliative care is a specialised form of medical care specifically designed for people with serious illness. Its main goal is to improve your quality of life by relief from the symptoms, pain, and stress that are an inevitable bi-product of both the disease and the medical intervention.[13]

Such a definition should not be seen as having, and is perhaps not intended to have, universal relevance. It appears to be one crafted specifically for the American healthcare industry and to have the modern healthcare consumer as its target audience. Nevertheless, in the context of the history described in this book, it seems to have travelled a long distance from the goals of both Munk and Saunders. It contains no mention of suffering in any wider existential way, and strikingly, the language of death and bereavement is completely absent. Highly instrumental in its orientation, it appears the converse of Saunders's famous (but unreferenced) aphorism: 'Don't just do something, *sit there.*'

The clinical realm

As palliative care developed into a recognized field of practice, it sought to define and circumscribe its areas of interest and competency. This has remained a matter for debate and contestation.

As we have seen, in the nineteenth century, medical writers such as William Munk focused their attention on easeful death as their principal objective, when efforts to prolong life were no longer productive. Munk, in common with his predecessors from earlier in the century, used the term *euthanasia* to describe this. He was referring to the relief of suffering through judicious use of pain medication, to the management of the sick room and deathbed in order to achieve dignity and comfort, and to the role of religious solicitude in preparing the dying person for a life to come, surrounded by family and friends. By such means, the idealized *good death* was to be realized.

However, as the nineteenth century came to a close, the meaning of euthanasia quite quickly began to change. If suffering might be relieved by the administration of strong opiates, such as morphine and diamorphine, which had been synthesized and put into commercial production in earlier decades, might suffering also be *prevented* by more direct intervention? Moreover, might indeed death be hastened deliberately by the physician in order to achieve this? Now some doctors began to take a serious interest in this issue, which also became a matter of public debate and controversy. As the public influence of religion in western culture moved into a phase of decline, attention focused less on the meaning of death and the afterlife, and more on the process of dying and the ability to exert control over it. Medicine had become the central influence over the deathbed.

Therein developed a struggle; for if some doctors endorsed the new definition of euthanasia and supported its legalization, others were opposed to this on religious and moral grounds and sought to direct their efforts to improving care in advanced illness and, thereby, to thwart the need for medicalized killing. This ethical divide became an increasingly marked feature of western medical culture during the twentieth century, and by the start of the twenty-first century, was also in evidence in some low and middle-income countries. It fuelled an ethical debate significantly influenced by Christian ideas about the sanctity of life, but over time, it was taken up in other religious and cultural contexts. By the second decade of the twenty-first century, it appeared to have become a matter of global interest.

Perhaps the strongest voice in opposition to euthanasia and in support of palliative care was that of Cicely Saunders herself. A lifelong opponent of euthanasia, she argued consistently that demand for assisted death diminishes wherever the principles of good palliative care are in evidence. Her central instrument in support of this claim was the concept of *total pain*, which recognized that the suffering of a person at the end of life can be multifaceted—physical, emotional, social, psychological, and spiritual. It was to suffering at this level that she addressed her attention, with notable success. However, for Saunders, the practice of hospice and palliative care was not simply a medical service; it was enriching of society and a measure of its moral worth. This enabled palliative care to find a wide audience, beyond that of healthcare workers and specialists. It attracted volunteers, fundraisers, and well-wishers convinced that the ability to control pain and other symptoms and the determination to give dignity to the dying and bereaved were skills and values worth promoting across the whole of society.

After the death of Cicely Saunders in 2005, it is possible to discern a contracting of this broader vision. New mantras emerged about choice in dying, neo-liberal policies served to lessen collective responsibility for the care of those at the end of life in favour of individualist and consumerist orientations as to how we should die. Within the field itself, expansive thinking about the meaning of care gave way to more reductionist efforts to measure effectiveness, assess cost-benefits and 'roll-out' strategies through guidelines and policies. The world of palliative medicine seemed to turn its attention to a number of discrete questions. Its leaders were mainly visible when responding to crises of care, such as those associated with the Liverpool Care Pathway, and less in evidence in setting an agenda for development and improvement. They were however attentive to some key ethical issues relating to clinical practice, where medical interventions at the end of life can be challenged by pervasive moral dilemmas.

Double effect, refractory symptoms, and sedation

The control of pain in palliative care has been the topic of much scrutiny and debate. The principle of double effect has been used to justify the administration of proportionate medication to relieve pain, even though it may lead to the unintended, albeit foreseen, consequence of hastening death; for example, by causing respiratory depression. Some have argued that there is little evidence to support the view that such analgesics carry this risk. From this perspective, the belief in the double effect of pain medication perpetuates the under-treatment of physical suffering at the end of life. At the same time, the concept of double effect in the use of opioids has also been used to support the legalization of physician-assisted suicide and euthanasia. This position typically takes one of two forms. First, it is argued that, as hastening death by drugs is already being done and is ethical, medical practice should be extended to allow physician-assisted suicide. The second argument is that because physicians are already hastening death, euthanasia should be legalized in order to provide safeguards, checks, and appropriate controls.[14]

Clinical practice in palliative care has acknowledged that at times refractory symptoms, often highly distressing to patients, family members, and staff, can be difficult to manage. Interest has grown in using deep sedation (variously termed) as an approach to this problem. Comparative studies show how rates of sedation at the end of life vary between settings and countries. The notion developed that dying for many had come to involve a set of decision-making processes, some of which result in the option to sedate the patient. This might be on a temporary basis, or until such time as death ensues. It might also be at the request of the patient. Palliative care was then called on to produce definitions, guidelines, and studies of this practice in order to give clarity and transparency to its procedures. In this context, the focus was not on the use of opioid drugs, but rather on benzodiazepines, such as midazolam. There was also the need to distinguish the practice from euthanasia, usually explained by the process of titrating the drugs to achieve sedation while maintaining respiratory function and not hastening death.

A *Cochrane Review* appeared in 2015 addressing the issue of terminally ill people who experience a variety of symptoms in the last hours and days of life, including delirium, agitation, anxiety, terminal restlessness, dyspnoea, pain, vomiting, and psychological and physical distress.[15] It noted that in the terminal phase of life, these symptoms may become refractory and unable to be controlled by supportive and palliative therapies specifically targeted to these symptoms. Palliative sedation therapy is one potential solution to providing relief from these refractory symptoms. Sedation in terminally ill people is intended to provide relief from refractory symptoms that are not controlled by other methods. Sedative drugs, such as benzodiazepines, are titrated to achieve the desired level of sedation, which can be easily maintained and the effect is reversible. The goal of the review was to assess the best evidence for the benefit of palliative pharmacological sedation on quality of life, survival, and specific refractory symptoms in terminally ill adults during their last few days of life. The results show some of the clinical and research challenges that exist in this area of modern medicine.

There was insufficient data for pooling on any outcome, so no meta-analysis was possible, and the authors were reduced to reporting a narrative of the outcomes. The searches resulted in 14 relevant studies, involving 4 167 adults, of who 1 137 received palliative sedation. More than 95 per cent of the participants had cancer. No studies were randomized or quasi-randomized. All were consecutive case series, with only three having prospective data collection. Risk of bias was high due to lack of randomization. No studies measured quality of life or participant well-being, which was the primary outcome of the review. Only five studies measured symptom control, and each used different methods. The results demonstrated that even when sedation was practised, delirium and dyspnoea were still troublesome symptoms for these people in the last few days of life. Control of other symptoms appeared to be similar in sedated and non-sedated people. Thirteen of the 14 studies measured survival time from admission or referral to death, and all demonstrated no statistically significant difference between sedated and non-sedated groups. The authors concluded that there was insufficient evidence about the efficacy of palliative sedation in terms of a person's quality of life or symptom control. There was evidence that palliative sedation did not hasten death, which had been a concern of physicians and families in prescribing this treatment. However, this evidence comes from low quality studies, so should be interpreted with caution.

Other challenges—changing trajectories

As the clinical practice of palliative care developed through the last quarter of the twentieth century, other issues began to challenge its orientation. Defined from the outset as a *multidisciplinary* endeavour, nevertheless the role of medicine appeared to be *primus inter pares*. There was a tendency for medical perspectives, medical assumptions and cultural practices, and medical solutions to frame the debate about how palliative care should develop. This was often because palliative physicians were looking over their shoulder at other specialities and seeking to keep pace with developments in cognate fields—oncology, geriatrics, cardiology, and respiratory medicine. It led some external commentators to argue that a process of 'medicalization' was at work within palliative care that would quickly dissipate its early, more holistic intentions. There were also detractors from within, who cautioned against palliative medicine becoming 'just another specialty', and for whom an over-emphasis on pain and symptom management seemed to be at the expense of attending to the whole person—including not only a person's physical problems, but also social issues, spiritual, religious, or existential matters, as well as the needs of family caregivers, and matters of psychological and mental health. It was as if the specialty of palliative *medicine* might make progress at the expense of the early goals of palliative *care*.

Palliative care began with an unequivocal focus on patients and families affected by cancer. It seemed that the widespread stigma associated with the disease, the poor prognosis that existed in many instances, the fairly predictable progression, and the possibility of severe pain and other debilitating symptoms all combined to make a perfect testing ground for the palliative care ethos. This came to be known as the 'rapid decline' trajectory, and it appeared to fit well with the perspective of hospice care, primarily focused on the final months and weeks of life. Palliative medicine at first locked onto this paradigm and gave particular focus to alleviating the challenging problems associated with specific pain syndromes, as well as breathlessness, anorexia and cachexia, anxiety, and depression—all of which came to be seen as key determinants of quality of life in patients with advanced cancer.

Over time, there were calls to extend the perceived benefits of palliative care, beyond patients with cancer to those dying from—and living with—other conditions. This meant two things. First, patients started to be seen for whom the medical context was less familiar. Initially, this involved people with neurological conditions, such as multiple sclerosis and motor neurone disease, but in time it was extended to those with heart failure, stroke patients, people with dementias, as well as those affected by HIV/AIDS. Second, there was pressure to move palliative care interventions further upstream in the disease progression to earlier stages of the illness, where palliation might sit alongside curative treatments and interventions. Now palliative care began to uncouple from the paradigm of terminal illness and eventually to reframe itself as an extra layer of support for patients, right across the treatment trajectory, with its various consequences and side effects.

The distinction between cancer and non-cancer palliative care was in evidence for a period starting in the 1990s, but became less commonly used over time. This was driven by the growing recognition of multiple morbidities and symptom burdens that occurred in medicine, which seemed particularly relevant to palliative care. At the same time, cancer was in many western countries making the transition into a treatable disease, associated with the new phenomenon of cancer survivorship, and of cancer as a chronic and/or 'social care' issue. Palliative care, therefore, had to focus on patients with complex multiple problems, which might endure for potentially long periods. Attempts were made to characterize these into specific trajectories of dying, but if these seemed to make sense conceptually, they were found difficult to map onto any empirical reality. In the West at least, the epidemiology of many cancers migrated into that of a chronic disease and, at the same time, the concept of multiple morbidities became increasingly recognized clinically, meaning that the care of patients became more complex and protracted in a setting where patterns of decline associated with frailty, dementia, and impoverishment became more prevalent.

This shift was also associated with an ageing population. The baby boom-ers drew attention to the growing reservoir of care needs in later life that resulted from the heightened birth rate in the two decades before the mid-1960s. Moreover, at the same time these people were set to live longer lives, as the improved healthcare and public health measures of the twentieth cen-tury increased life expectancy. This in turn became a global issue. Around 58 million deaths occur in the world every year and this number may rise to 90–100 million by mid-century and beyond. This increase in the number of deaths will be caused by a combination of population growth and population ageing. The likely demand this will place on caregivers and services suggests a humanitarian issue—if not crisis—of enormous scale and complexity.

If modern palliative care had begun in the 1960s and 1970s with the cer-tainties of cancer as a terminal disease of predictable course, by the second decade of the twenty-first century it was located in far less predictable set-tings. It now sat alongside curative interventions, closely tied in with the needs of older people, but also subspecialized in paediatrics as well as in other medical specialities. When accreditation for hospice and palliative medicine was achieved in the United States, it was formalized as a subspecialty of no less than 11 fields of specialist care. In each case, new knowledge would be required to build a palliative care orientation matched to a specialist field of medical intervention, as well as to the social dimensions of the underlying disease type or the complexities of multiple morbidity. In short, the medical landscape in which palliative care is required to operate has become far more complex and nuanced in 2015 than it was 50 years earlier, when the first col-laborations were developing between the early pioneers.

Assisted dying and palliative care

Like palliative care, the territory of assisted dying has its own problems of definition. Some use the term to encapsulate events that might otherwise be described as (physician-) assisted suicide or voluntary euthanasia; although mechanically they differ, at the heart of each is the positive choice for death.[16] *Assisted dying* and *euthanasia* are terms that have proven notoriously difficult to define and are subject to multiple interpretations.[17] In these specific areas, carefully crafted definitions produced by philosophers are often roughly han-dled by the public and by protagonists who use distinct and separate terms interchangeably, or with a lack of clarity of meaning. This is a sociological reality that can undoubtedly create a gulf between formal conceptual work and the living world of disputation, action, and decision-making. It is easily witnessed in the inexact drafting of bills to legalize assisted dying that come before parliaments around the world.

Nevertheless, in the same period that palliative care gained traction, so too did debates and arguments in favour of the legalization of assisted dying—particularly in affluent countries. In the Netherlands, euthanasia was practised by physicians in a decriminalized context from the early 1990s onwards, using a procedure of notification. The first legal case of euthanasia in the world occurred in the Australian Northern Territories in 1995, although the legislation was quickly reversed. Assisted suicide was approved by voters in the US state of Oregon in 1994 and legalized in 1997; subsequent endorsements occurred in Washington state (2008), Vermont (2013), New Jersey (2014), and California (2016). In Switzerland, where the subject of *suicide tourism* has attracted considerable debate, assisting a person to die is not an offence in certain circumstances. Full legalization of euthanasia and assisted suicide was passed in the Netherlands in 2001—the first national legislation to do so. Belgium followed in 2002 with legalization of euthanasia only. In Luxembourg, euthanasia and assisted suicide were legalized in 2009. The institution of active euthanasia has been legal in Colombia since 2015.

Across many other countries, parliamentary debates have taken place, laws have been drafted, and wider public discussion gains momentum around the theme of assisted dying—how, in what circumstances, and with what safeguards might some form of legislation be framed that permits *choice* in dying—allowing persons a measure of control over the manner and timing of their death? Nevertheless, as the European Court of Human Rights has noted, there is no consensus in Europe on the ethics of assisted suicide and indeed, the Council of Europe (2012) has stated: 'Euthanasia, in the sense of the intentional killing by act or omission of a dependent human being for his or her alleged benefit, must always be prohibited.'[18]

The mainstream orientation of palliative care towards assisted dying is essentially oppositional. It is rare to see palliative care practitioners endorsing such practices and unusual for them to be viewed as a part of the delivery of palliative care.

In the public consciousness, there might not be so much 'clear water' between the two positions however. The furore in the United Kingdom over the widespread use of the Liverpool Care Pathway (LCP),[19] for example, revealed that from the perspective of relatives and patients themselves, 'best palliative care practice'—withdrawing interventions, closely monitoring symptoms, and aiming for the minimization of suffering and discomfort—were seen as a form of backdoor euthanasia. Indeed, the public discussion on this, the review of the LCP, and its eventual withdrawal in 2013 may well have brought to an end the era of what we might call 'unconditional positive regard for palliative care' in the public consciousness.

The ideological orientation of palliative care practitioners has been to oppose assisted dying because it is not needed when palliative care is fully available. Moreover, of course, a subset opposes it on moral or religious grounds. Supporters of assisted dying, who claim that palliative care can never be the sole solution in all cases and contexts, challenge this thinking. They argue for choice and self-determination, suggesting that even the best palliative care cannot always eliminate suffering. They also point out that some consumers of healthcare services may not be attracted to the ethos of palliative care for various reasons, such as its religious connections, its desire to delve into spiritual and existential areas where it does not belong, or its unwelcome associations with charity or volunteer involvement.

The protagonists have been engaged in a struggle where 'dignity' has become the contested space, with each side claiming to provide it. Key to the palliative care ethos in its early days was dignity of the patient. But organizations practising or promoting assisted dying have adopted dignity within their names, for example, Dignitas (Switzerland), Dignity in Dying (United Kingdom), and the Association for the Right to Die with Dignity (Spain). These groups also have in common an emphasis on quality of life. For those in favour of assisted dying, quality of life is a key element in the argument. When it is poor and likely to deteriorate further, then the case for *choice* in dying must be advanced. Nevertheless, from the palliative care side, poor quality of life is seen as a clinical challenge to be overcome and remedied through the skills and involvement of a multidisciplinary team.

In Belgium, the two viewpoints have been encouraged to sit side by side. Not only is euthanasia legal in Belgium, but also at the time of its enactment, palliative care services were already well developed in the country. Indeed, some palliative care teams see euthanasia as a part of the service they offer—the so-called 'integral' model of palliative care. Bernheim[20] found that in Belgium the movement for legalization of euthanasia promoted the improvement of palliative care, and the existence of sufficient palliative care was instrumental in making the legalization of euthanasia ethically and politically acceptable. However, this reciprocal approach may only be prevalent in one part of the country. One study aimed to find out how Flemish palliative care nurses and physicians think about euthanasia.[21] An anonymous questionnaire was sent to all physicians (147 total, with 70.5 per cent response) and nurses (589 total, with 70.5 per cent response) employed in palliative care teams and institutions in Flanders, Belgium. Analysis of the questionnaire responses identified three clusters: (moderate) opponents of euthanasia (23 per cent); moderate advocates of euthanasia (35.2 per cent); and staunch advocates of euthanasia (41.8 per cent). A majority in all clusters believed that as soon as a patient experiences the benefits of good palliative care, most requests for euthanasia disappear and that all palliative care alternatives must be tried before a euthanasia request can be considered. Since most Flemish palliative care nurses and physicians were not absolutely against voluntary euthanasia, their attitudes may differ from those of their palliative care colleagues elsewhere. However, the attitudes of the Flemish palliative care nurses and physicians are largely contextual. For a very large majority, euthanasia is an option of last resort only.

Another study has looked at the interplay between the legalization of assisted dying and euthanasia and the level of development of palliative care, in specific countries, taking as its staring point the claim such legislation can hold back the development of palliative care and stunt its culture.[22] Seven European countries with the highest level of palliative care development, and which included the three 'euthanasia-permissive' Benelux countries and four 'non-permissive' countries were compared, using structural service indicators for 2005 and 2012 from successive editions of the *European Atlas of Palliative Care*. The rate of increase in structural palliative provision was the highest in the Netherlands and Luxembourg, while Belgium stayed on a par with the United Kingdom, the benchmark country. The hypothesis that legal regulation of physician-assisted dying slows the development of palliative care was, therefore, not supported by the Benelux experience. On the contrary, regulation appears to have promoted the expansion of palliative care in these jurisdictions.

In the US state of Oregon, where assisted dying has been legal since 1997, and where the number of cases remains low at around 0.21 per cent of all deaths per annum, claims have been made that there exists an ideal and comprehensive system for end-of-life care. Around one-third of those issued with the lethal prescription to end their own lives never use it. Moreover, in a context where hospice and palliative care services are well developed, some 90 per cent of those availing themselves of the assisted dying legislation are on hospice programmes. Could this prove a model for other jurisdictions? A study by Goy and colleagues[23] found the majority of hospice nurses and social workers noted positive changes in the provision of palliative care by physicians since the introduction of the Oregon Death with Dignity Act, apart from a level of apprehension when prescribing opioid medications.

In the Netherlands, a rather different picture is evident. Here palliative care developed in the context of a country that had decriminalized euthanasia and where the majority of the population accepted such a practice. This is the reverse of the situation in many other countries. It meant that palliative care in the Netherlands developed at first in isolation from the wider palliative care community, which, paradoxically, was often intensely interested in the practice of euthanasia in Holland. It was not until 1991 that the first hospice was established in the Netherlands. Later, in the 1990s, significant government funds were invested in centres of excellence for the promotion of palliative care. Meanwhile, problems with the legal framework of euthanasia were in evidence: insecurity for physicians in following legal requirements that were sometimes unclear; a growing sense of the right of euthanasia-on-demand among the public; and a sense of normalization surrounding its practice.[24] The high-level care hospices in the Netherlands remain centres of opposition to euthanasia; elsewhere the practice is not criticized, but there is a clear moral argument from the palliative care community that greater availability of their services would reduce the demand for assisted death. Despite this, and the growth of palliative care in the Netherlands, the number of cases of euthanasia each year has been increasing.

The *slippery slope* argument continues to underpin some of the debates about whether or not assisted dying should be legalized. Jose Pereira, a professor of palliative medicine based in Canada, has argued that in all jurisdictions that have legalized euthanasia or assisted dying, there has been disregard for the laws and safeguards that were put in place to prevent abuse and misuse of these practices.[25] Prevention measures have included, among others, explicit consent by the person requesting euthanasia, mandatory reporting of all cases, administration only by physicians (with the exception of Switzerland), and consultation by a second physician. Pereira provides evidence that these laws and safeguards are regularly ignored and transgressed in all the jurisdictions, and that increased tolerance of these transgressions in societies with such laws represents a social slippery slope, as do changes to the laws and criteria that followed initial legalization. Although the original intent was to limit euthanasia and assisted suicide to a last-resort option for a very small number of terminally ill people, some jurisdictions now extend the practice to newborns, to children, and to people with dementia. A terminal illness is no longer a prerequisite. In the Netherlands, euthanasia for anyone over the age of 70 who is 'tired of living' is now being considered. Legalizing euthanasia and assisted suicide, Pereira argues, places many people at risk, affects the values of society over time, and does not provide controls and safeguards.

From the still-small number of countries where euthanasia and assisted dying are legal or decriminalized, it does not seem possible to find evidence that the development of palliative care has been compromised. Nevertheless, the two remain in an uneasy relationship. It seems that within the community of palliative care practitioners, there remains higher resistance to legalizing assisted dying than is found among healthcare workers in particular, and the wider society as a whole. As the extent of legalized assisted dying increases, this may precipitate a significant practical and moral challenge to the field.

Public health, equity, and human rights in palliative care

The years after the turn of the millennium gave birth to the twin ideas that palliative care is both a public health and a human rights issue. Both are contentious. The first assumes the insertion of palliative care into the public health system, thereby positioning it within a discourse of need, supply, and resource allocation. The second assertion, that palliative care is a human rights issue, may prove challenging to progress.

Public health

It was only a matter of time before end-of-life care would come to be seen as a concern of public health. Across the 100-year span from William Munk to the recognition of a new specialty, progress was made in the classification of the terrain of palliative medicine. Knowledge was accumulated and codified, and practices were scrutinized for their consequences and efficacy. Estimates were established of the value of interventions and their potential to benefit, not just individual patients, but also whole populations of people at the end of life. This made it possible to focus on pain relief and palliative care as matters affecting communities and societies, in need not only of clinical knowledge and research, but also of the tools of population science, policy, and planning. The seeds of this are quite visible in Saunders's writings. In the twenty-first century, a whole cadre of other physicians began to contribute to the development.

In 2015, at the European Association for Palliative Care's world congress in Copenhagen, the sociologist Professor Luc Deliens gave a plenary lecture that underlined the need for palliative care to engage with the model of public health. This is an often-repeated statement—but what is the link between palliative care and public health? First, there is concern that palliative care is still not well understood; it requires integration within healthcare systems, and it needs measurable outcomes. This public health articulates closely with that of the WHO and is the stuff of the World Health Assembly resolution of 2014.

In palliative care terms, it has four components—the so-called WHO foundation measures: drug availability, education, policies, and (added later[26]) implementation. Against these measures, there is still much progress to be made in establishing palliative care provision and making it fully available at the population level through the healthcare systems of individual countries. Over 30 years since the measures were first articulated, one wonders whether the paradigm is right.

Second, there is a view that palliative care has a different starting place. This begins with communities and capacity, rather than services and deficits. It has been widely articulated by Professor Allan Kellehear, another sociologist, but his notion of public health is rather different. Kellehear begins from the perspective that for much of our lives, including at the end of them, most of us are not face to face with healthcare professionals and services. Rather, we encounter illness, loss, and mortality as social experiences that are shaped primarily by culture, by geography, by beliefs, by communities and relationships. Within this, medicine and medical care can be quite small elements. When he calls for a public health model of palliative care, he is therefore talking about something rather different. For Kellehear, palliative care seldom embraces public health ideas about community engagement, community development, and citizenship. He points us to the significance of community and ideas about prevention, harm-reduction, and early intervention strategies to address the social epidemiology of death, dying, bereavement, and long-term caregiving. This outlook has a health-promoting dimension, sees the main source of end-of-life care as families and communities (not specialists and services), and argues for a societal reappraisal of death, dying, and bereavement.[27, 28] The goal in this version is to achieve a greater measure of compassion and dignity in all aspects of dying and death, in whichever aspect of society they are manifested, and certainly not within the healthcare system alone.

We might take the plurality of debate around these issues as either a sign of strength or an indication of weakness. A willingness to discuss openly the aims, boundaries, and contours of the field is for many an indicator of insight and reflexivity. For others it denotes confusion, mission creep, and an inability to articulate to others the core message of palliative care. However, it is curious that a palliative care that is uncertain about its boundaries and definitions is seeking alliances with another part of health discourse—public health—around which so many similar debates revolve and swirl. As Erika Blacksher wrote in 2014: 'There is no settled account or definition of public health.'[29] It seems important, therefore, to clarify with which 'public health' it would be desirable for palliative care to align, and to what ends.

Equity

The need for palliative care has been heavily defined by the disease status of patients and their particular associated needs. Nevertheless, as the field matures, a new front of exploration opens up associated not with the diagnosis, organs of the body, or disease severity, but with the particular places, settings, and social groups that might benefit from palliative care. From the 1990s on, specialist interest began to develop in palliative care for prisoners, for homeless people, and for those identifying as lesbian, gay, bisexual, or transgender. Palliative care availability and access were increasingly framed as matters of *equity* and then of *human rights.*

After 2000, a number of key developments took place globally in end-of-life care, including a series of important summit meetings on international palliative care development and the creation of the Worldwide Palliative Care Alliance. In the autumn of 2011, two separate declarations emphasized the importance of palliative and end-of-life care. The United Nations (2011) referred to the need for palliative care provision in its statement about the care and treatment of people with non-communicable disease. Then, the World Medical Association (2011) made its case for improvement in end-of-life care, stating that receiving appropriate end-of-life medical care must not be considered a privilege but a true right, independent of age, or any other associated factors.

The palliative care community itself has also been active in producing exhortatory charters and declarations, usually promoted at specialist international conferences.[30] These call on governments to develop health policies that address the needs of patients with life-limiting or terminal illnesses, and to promote the integration of palliative care alongside other health services. They promote the need for access to essential medicines, including controlled medications, for all who require them, and they focus on the identification and elimination of restrictive barriers that impede access to strong opioids for legitimate medical use. These pronouncements also emphasize the importance of the supply line for such drugs, along with appropriate rules and laws governing their distribution and prescription, by properly trained practitioners. Such calls underline the need for appropriate initial and undergraduate education programmes for healthcare providers to ensure that basic knowledge about palliative care is widely disseminated and can be applied wherever the need should arise in the healthcare system. They also highlight the need for postgraduate and specialty palliative care programmes, so that patients with complex problems can receive appropriate care. Key to all this—and at the heart of the public health orientation—is the requirement that palliative care is properly integrated into wider healthcare systems with services designed in relation to need and demand.

Human rights

Recognition of palliative care as a human right[31] has been developing, and access to palliative medication has been incorporated into a resolution of the United Nations Commission on Human Rights;[32] but the goals of such work are difficult to define and the likelihood of reaching them is highly unpredictable. The claim that palliative care is a human right seems to be but partially founded.[33] The United Nations Committee on Economic, Social and Cultural Rights has stated that it is critical to provide attention and care for chronically and terminally ill persons, sparing them avoidable pain, and enabling them to die with dignity. Also, under article 12 of the International Covenant on Economic, Social, and Cultural Rights, and article 7 of the International Covenant on Civil and Political Rights, countries are obliged to take steps to ensure that patients have access to palliative care and pain treatment.

Likewise, according to the United Nations Committee on Economic, Social, and Cultural Rights, states are under the obligation to respect the right to health by refraining from denying or limiting equal access for all persons to preventive, curative, and palliative health services. Access to palliative care is a legal obligation, as acknowledged by UN conventions, and has been advocated as a human right by international associations, based on the right to the highest attainable standard of physical and mental health. In cases where patients face severe pain, government failure to provide palliative care can also constitute cruel, inhuman, or degrading treatment. However, of course, governments of many different stripes can flout the law and ignore human rights. There are problems with framing palliative care as a human rights issue from a western perspective and thereby setting standards that low and middle-income countries will find hard to attain. Nevertheless, there have been legitimate interests in palliative care from organizations like Human Rights Watch, and these seem set to continue.[34]

Conclusions and final reflections

Palliative care developed strongly in the early decades of the twenty-first century and came to have a global reach, albeit with patchy coverage. As it grew into a recognizable field of activity, discernible fissures opened up in its approach and orientation. Palliative care grew out of a hospice-type response to the needs of dying cancer patients. Its model of care fit a particular trajectory of treatment and its associated illness experience. Within that model, it identified an ethical and moral space in which to promote the holistic care of the patient and family, and it adopted particular strategies for pain and symptom management. Now, in many countries, it seeks to meet the complex needs of ageing populations characterized by multiple morbidities in situations where demand for end-of-life care is growing. This requires it to adopt an ethics of public health and to champion the claim that access to palliative care is a human right. In addition to these clinical and service level challenges, palliative care has to find an appropriate orientation to contexts where assisted dying is legalized. This may require it to modify its historic opposition to assisted death. As increasing numbers of jurisdictions enshrine this in law, so the oppositional stance of the palliative care community will become more difficult to maintain.

In 2014, Atul Gawande's book *Being Mortal—Illness, Medicine, and What Matters in the End*, and his accompanying British Broadcasting Company (BBC) Reith Lectures offered a compelling analysis of what is happening with end-of-life care, what palliative care has to contribute, and what needs to change.[35] A surgeon at the Brigham Young Women's Hospital in Boston, a health policy and public health analyst, and former advisor to President Bill Clinton, Gawande read politics, philosophy, and economics at Oxford before embarking on medical training in the United States. *Being Mortal* set out the complexities, challenges, and dilemmas of modern medicine and brought a clear-eyed perspective to the innovations required to improve things—not just in the author's home country, but also globally.

Gawande's project has a history, going back almost 50 years. He reached a large public audience in his writing about mortality, dying, and death, just as the psychiatrist Elizabeth Kübler-Ross did from the Billings Hospital in Chicago, where she started working in 1965 and from where, in 1969, she published her book *On Death and Dying*. Like *Being Mortal*, Kübler-Ross's book quickly became a best seller. It was followed by other popular books on the failings of American medicine in the face of human mortality. The surgeon Sherwin Nuland's *How We Die: Reflections on Life's Final Chapter* (1992) was a *New York Times* best seller, won the National Book Award for nonfiction, and was shortlisted for the Pulitzer Prize. Ten years later, Canadian physician David Kuhl's *What Dying People Want* (2002) took him onto the *Oprah Winfrey Show* and out to a wide audience with a work based on conversations and interviews with dying people and their families. He followed it in 2006 with *Facing Death, Embracing Life*. And, over the years, the well-known palliative care doctor Ira Byock has reached a large readership with works such as *Dying Well* (1997), *The Four Things That Matter Most* (2004), and *The Best Care Possible* (2012). These general readership books on end-of-life issues sold in quantities that most academic authors and their publishers can only dream about.

Yet, it is a genre completely absent from other parts of the Anglo-Saxon world. Cicely Saunders wrote widely on these topics but aside from the occasional newspaper article, she never found a popular audience. None of the British palliative care doctors reached out to engage with the public in the fashion of their North American counterparts. British medicine seemed to have failed to produce a popular writer of serious thought concerned with the broad perspective on ageing, mortality, and care at the end of life. Gawande deals with these topics superbly. His book is packed with stories about patients and families, and full of memorable observations across many individual cases, in which the vital questions are frequently the same.

> What is your understanding of the situation and its potential outcomes? What are your fears and what are your hopes? What are the trade-offs you are willing to make and not willing to make? And what is the course of action that best serves this understanding?[34]

Translated out of baby-boomer talk and into any local vernacular, these last four questions are pertinent, telling, and enormously consequential for individualized care at the end of life.

At the end of 2014, Gawande delivered the annual set of Reith Lectures for the BBC's *The Future of Medicine*. The third lecture was called 'The Problem of Hubris'. It is an extended account of one person's experience of hospice care in the United States. Gawande introduces us to his daughter's piano teacher, Peg. We learn of Peg's struggles with advanced illness and its treatment, her painful decision to 'transition to hospice', and the benefits that flowed in the weeks that followed. In the discussion, the story of Peg was contextualized in what we know about the reach of hospice in America, but also the limits of its funding model, the tensions between the hospice approach and the wider concept of palliative care, and the thorny topic of assisted dying. Atul Gawande was only now echoing the thesis set out by Ivan Illich almost 40 years earlier: that we have lost the capacity to accept death and suffering as meaningful aspects of life; that there is a sense of being in a state of 'total war' against death at all stages of the life cycle; that there has been a crippling of personal and family care, and a devaluing of traditional rituals surrounding dying and death; and that a form of social control exists in which a rejection of 'patienthood' by dying or bereaved people is labelled as deviance. Gawande revisits all of this and puts it firmly in a twenty-first century context of ageing and the struggle to provide dignified care at the end of life.

The present book has shown how the orientation of medicine to those with life threatening illness, particularly those close to death, has been changing since the late nineteenth century. In that time, a special field of medical practice has emerged that not only defines a key area of care, but must also advocate for it and gain recognition within the broader discourse of medical thinking and practice. In this context, it seems appropriate to give the final word to a physician. Not one who was a member of the first generation of palliative medicine pioneers, nor one who was exposed early to their work. Rather, Dr Eduardo Bruera (Figure 7.1), a doctor who came to the world of palliative care from the poor and public hospitals of Latin America, who saw the need for medicine to change, and then dedicated his career to the new specialty, working within the medical rule book to gain recognition for it. Over a long career[36] he gained a global reputation, not only for his clinical practice, research, and extensive portfolio of publications, but also for his role in mentoring and training hundreds of doctors, his leadership, and his ability to engage with intergovernmental organizations and all those concerned to promote palliative care across all the countries of the world. Interviewed in 1995, he sets out the scope of his ambition, but also neatly anticipates the challenges facing anyone—such as the present author—who would attempt to even sketch the history of this remarkable, and still emergent medical specialty.

> There's no doubt that palliative care came out of the fringe. But it is also clear to me that I don't want to work on the fringe. I believe in academics, I believe in treating patients, I think there are many good things that are related to the practice of medicine. I am not prepared to accept that, because some physicians practice what is, I think, bad medicine, they're more physicians than I am. If anything, my role is to elbow out of the profession the uncaring, brutal individuals, but not to let them edge me into the fringe and continue doing my little thing. So I always thought that the battle front, in the case of palliative care and what I was doing, is to make it absolutely sure that no cardiovascular surgeon looks down to us; that we are a major component of what the practice of medicine is. William Osler used to publish an awful lot on palliative care and palliation, and so the great figures of medicine paid a lot of attention to support, to counselling, to psychosocial issues, and to symptom relief. Somewhere, thirty or forty years ago, we lost . . . the direction, but I see our task as gaining again the direction, so that we teach the new generation the right values. So I think we have to push within the system, not to become 'fringed'. But again, that's one view, I mean I'm sure there are a hundred different views, and you'll have to put them together . . .![37]

Notes

1. **Worcester A** (1935). *The Care of the Aged, the Dying, and the Dead.* Springfield, IL: Thomas.
2. **Clark D, Clark J, Greenwood A** (2010). The place of supportive, palliative, and end of life care research in the United Kingdom Research Assessment Exercise, 2001 and 2008. *Palliative Medicine*, 24(5):533–43. doi:10.1177/0269216309359995.
3. **Pastrana T, Jünger S, Ostgathe C, Eisner F, Radbrunch L** (2008). A matter of definition—key elements identified in a discourse analysis of definitions of palliative care. *Palliative Medicine*, 22:222–32.

4. National Institutes of Health (2004). National Institutes of Health State-of-the-Science Conference: Statement on Improving End-of-Life Care, 6–8 December 2004. Available at http://consensus.nih.gov/2004/2004EndOfLifeCareSOS024html.htm, accessed 27 July 2015.

5. **Cohen J, Deliens L** (2012). *A Public Health Perspective on End of Life Care*. Oxford, UK: Oxford University Press.

6. Hospitals increasingly offer palliative care (2011). *Washington Post* (28 March).

7. Center to Advance Palliative Care (2008). Analysis of U.S. hospital palliative care programs: 2010 snapshot. [Data reported were for 2008.] Available at https://www.capc.org/media/filer_public/83/64/836419d1-8b4d-474c-aa93-602c5d5fef01/analysis-of-us-hospital-palliative-care-programs-2010-snapshot.pdf, accessed 27 July 2015.

8. **PR Newswire** (2011). New poll: Americans choose quality over quantity at the end of life, crave deeper public discussion of care options. *National Journal* (8 March). Available at http://www.prnewswire.com/news-releases/new-poll-americans-choose-quality-over-quantity-at-the-end-of-life-crave-deeper-public-discussion-of-care-options-117575453.html, accessed 12 October 2012.

9. **McIlfatrick S** et al. (2013). Public awareness and attitudes toward palliative care in Northern Ireland. *BMC Palliative Care*, 12 (17 September):34. doi:10.1186/1472-684X-12-34.

10. Center to Advance Palliative Care (2011). Public Opinion Research on Palliative Care. Available at https://media.capc.org/filer_public/18/ab/18ab708c-f835-4380-921d-fbf729702e36/2011-public-opinion-research-on-palliative-care.pdf, accessed 27 July 2015.

11. *Palliative Care: You Are a Bridge* (2014, September). Video. Get Palliative Care website. Available at http://getpalliativecare.org/palliative-care-bridge/, accessed 10 June 2015.

12. Center to Advance Palliative Care. Available at https://www.capc.org/, accessed 10 June 2015.

13. *Ibid.* See note 11.

14. **Fohr SA** (1998). The double effect of pain medication: Separating myth from reality. *Journal of Palliative Medicine*, 1:315–328.

15. **Beller EM, van Driel ML, McGregor L, Truong S, Mitchell G** (2015). Palliative pharmacological sedation for terminally ill adults. *Cochrane Database of Systematic Reviews 2015*, Issue 1. Art. No.: CD010206. doi:10.1002/14651858. CD010206.pub2.

16. **McLean S** (2007). *Assisted Dying: Reflections on the Need for Law Reform*. Abingdon, UK: Routledge-Cavendish.

17. **Materstvedt LJ** et al. (2003). Euthanasia and physician-assisted suicide: A view from an EAPC Ethics Task Force. *Palliative Medicine*, 17:97–101.

18. Council of Europe Resolution (2012). 'Protecting human rights and dignity by taking into account previously expressed wishes of patients' Resolution (n°1859/2012).

19. **Sleeman K** (2013). The Liverpool Care Pathway: A cautionary tale. *British Medical Journal*, 347:f4779.

20. **Bernheim JL** (2008). Development of palliative care and legalisation of euthanasia: Antagonism or synergy? *British Medical Journal*, 336(7649):864–7.

21. **Broeckaert B, Gielen J, van Iersel T, van den Branden S** (2010). Euthanasia and palliative care in Belgium: The attitudes of Flemish palliative care nurses and physicians towards euthanasia. *AJOB Primary Research*, 1(3):31–44.

22. **Chambaere K, Bernheim JL** (2015). Does legal physician-assisted dying impede development of palliative care? The Belgian and Benelux experience. *Journal of Medical Ethics.* doi:10.1136/medethics-2014-102116.

23. **Goy ER, Jackson A, Harvath T, Miller LL, Delorit MA, Ganzini L** (2003). Oregon hospice nurses and social workers' assessment of physician progress in palliative care over the past 5 years. *Palliative and Supportive Care*, 1(3):215–219.

24. **Gordijn B, Janssens R** (2004). Euthanasia and palliative care in the Netherlands: An analysis of the latest developments. *Health Care Analysis*, 12(3):195–207.

25. **Pereira J** (2011). Legalizing euthanasia or assisted suicide: The illusion of safeguards and controls. *Current Oncology*, 18(2):e38–45.

26. **Stjernswärd J, Foley KM, Ferris FD** (2007). Integrating palliative care into national policies. *Journal of Pain and Symptom Management*, 33(5):514–520.

27. **Kellehear A** (2005). *Compassionate Cities: Public Health and End-of-Life Care.* London, UK: Routledge.

28. **Kellehear A** (2003). Public health challenges in the care of the dying. In: Liamputtong P, Gardner H (eds.). *Health, Social Change & Communities*, pp. 88–99. Melbourne, Australia: Oxford University Press.

29. **Blacksher E** (2014). Public health ethics. Ethics in Medicine website. University of Washington School of Medicine. Available at https://depts.washington.edu/bioethx/topics/public.html, accessed 10 June 2015.

30. Palliative care 'declarations': Developing a case study (2015). End of Life Studies website. University of Glasgow. 22 May. Available at http://endoflifestudies.academicblogs.co.uk/developing-a-case-study-on-palliative-care-declarations/, accessed 10 June 2015.

31. **Harding R** (2006). Palliative care: A basic human right. id21 *Insights Health* (8 Feb):1–2. Available at http://www.eldis.org/id21ext/InsightsHealth8Editorial.html, accessed 27 July 2015.

32. Commission on Human Rights Resolution 2004/26: Item 7c calls on states 'to promote effective access to such preventive, curative, or palliative pharmaceutical products or medical technologies'. United Nations Human Rights website. Available at http://www.un.org/en/terrorism/pdfs/2/G0414734.pdf, accessed 27 July 2015.

33. Open Society Foundations (2011). Palliative care as a human right: A fact sheet. Available at http://www.opensocietyfoundations.org/publications/palliative-care-human-right-fact-sheet, accessed 5 February 2015.

34. https://www.hrw.org/topic/health/palliative care, accessed 27 July 2015.

35. **Gawande A** (2014). *Being Mortal: Illness, Medicine and What Matters in the End.* London, UK: Profile Books in association with the Wellcome Collection.

36. **Bruera E** (2008). On third base but not home yet. *Journal of Palliative Medicine*, 11(4): 565–9.

37. Hospice History Project: David Clark interview with Eduardo Bruera, 9 November 1995.

Index

Abel, Emily 9, 35
Abiven, Maurice 167
Academy of Hospice Physicians 165
accreditation 154–6, 186–7
Accreditation Council of Graduate Medical
  Evaluation (ACGME) 186–7
active approach to care 78
activism, global 175–7
Africa 174–5, 178
African Palliative Care Association
  (APCA) 174–5
ageing populations 181, 213, 222
  see also geriatrics and dying elderly
Aikenhead, Mary (later Sister Mary
  Augustine) 37, 39
alcohol
  discontinuance of mixtures
    containing 106, 135
  forbidden 51
  use for pain relief 7, 16, 129
  see also Brompton Cocktail
Aldrich, Knight 100
Allen, Mildred 94
Allport, Gordon 97, 98, 99
American Academy of Hospice and Palliative
  Medicine (formerly Academy of
  Hospice Physicians) 185
American Board of Hospice and Palliative
  Medicine (ABHPM) 186
American Board of Internal Medicine 185
American Board of Medical Specialities
  (ABMS) 186–7
American Cancer Society 94
American College of Physicians 185
American Medical Association
  (AMA) 9–10
analgesia 8, 70, 72
  by the clock/on regular basis 87, 89, 122
antiemetics 129
antihistamines - promethazine 126
anxiety about dying process 2, 52, 74
Argentina 171
Ariès, Phillipe 2–3
Armstrong, David 81
Asia 171–4, 178
Asia Pacific Hospice Palliative Care
  Network 172
aspirin 53
assisted dying 22, 26, 213–18, 223
  legalization 214, 216, 217, 222

assisted suicide legalization 214
Association de Dames du Calvaire, L' 37
Association for Palliative Medicine
  for Great Britain and
  Ireland 111, 151–3
Association for the Right to Die with Dignity
  (Spain) 215
Atlee, Clement 60
atmosphere, homely 53
Australia 37, 183–5, 214
Bailey, Margaret 74
Baines, Mary 95
Banderanaike, S.W.R.D. 94
Barber, Hugh 79
Barrett, Howard 41–2, 44–7, 50, 52, 88,
  199–200
'beautiful death' 3
bedclothes, light 16
bedside teaching 19
Beecher, Henry 102
Belgium 214, 215–16
Bell, Florence 6
Bending, Lucy 21
benzodiazepines 210
Berkeley, John 67–8
Bevan, Aneurin 60, 79
Beveridge, William 79
Birmingham Philosophical Society 26
Blacksher, Erika 219
Bodkin Adams, John 80
body-mind dualism 78
body and soul, caring for 89
Bohusz-Szyszko, Marian 110
Bonica, John 70, 121–2, 123, 129, 134, 159
Boulay, Shirley du 90
Bowlby, John 74
British Medical Association 68
Brodie, Sir Benjamin 15, 18
Brompton Cocktail 24, 69, 125–31
  abandonment of 117
Brompton Hospital 74, 125
Broome, Isobel 35, 40, 47, 50, 51, 53
Browne, Oswald 11, 14
Brown, Esther Lucille 98, 99
Bruera, Eduardo 170–1, 197, 224
Buck, Joy 98
Bunyan, John 138
Burch, Rosetta 92
Burn, Gilly 172–3
Byock, Ira 222

Callaway, Mary 168–9
Calman-Hine Report (Expert Advisory
Group on Cancer) 141–2, 157
Calouste Gulbenkian Foundation 62
Calvary Hospice of Kangung (Korea) 171
Campbell, Lorna Jane 10, 20, 22, 27
Canada 128, 129, 170, 187
cancer 2, 14, 16, 21, 22, 61, 74, 201,
206, 211
advanced 23–4, 52, 65, 212
clinical culture 49, 50
deaths 64
external cancers 49–50
fungating and eroding growths 88
growing visibility of 55
hospitals 34
Marie Curie Memorial and The Queen's
Institute of District Nursing joint
committee 59, 62
morphine 69–70
new evidence 72, 73
nursing at home 62–3
pain
at population level 159
problem of 121–4
as public health issue 124
see also World Health Organization
(WHO) analgesic pain ladder
Cancer Relief India 172–3
Cancer Relief Macmillan Fund 152, 154
Cane, Walter 12, 13
Cannadine, David 28
carers 7–8
see also family
Carleton-Smith, Michael 141
Cassell, Eric 169
Catholicism 46
Catholic Sisters of the Little Company of
Mary (Korea) 171
Centeno, Carlos 182–3
Center to Advance Palliative Care 207
certification and accreditations of
physician training in palliative
medicine 154–6, 186–7
Ceylon Cancer Society 94
change and continuity 77–81
Chardin, Teilard de 138
charitable endeavour 36, 79, 81, 87
China 172, 180
chloroform 19, 129
see also Brompton Cocktail
cholera 15, 38
Christianity 7–8
chronic illness and long-term effects of
disabling conditions 2, 7, 9, 66, 72
see also morbidities, multiple
Church of England Board for Social
Responsibility working party 105

Cicely Saunders Institute 205
circulatory system diseases 64
Clark Wilson, John 51
clinical judgement 199
clinical realm, defining 117–43, 208–9
cancer pain, problem of 121–4
conditions of possibility 142–3
new model of care, researching 125–31
Twycross, Robert and Brompton
Cocktail 126–31
palliative medicine 118–21
research and service
development 138–42
planning and change 139–42
total pain (physical symptoms, mental
distress, social problems and
emotional difficulties) 131–8
syringe driver 135–8
cocaine 24
discontinuance of routine use of 106,
129, 135
see also Brompton Cocktail
Cochrane Review (2015) 210
codeine phosphate 53
Colebrook, Leonard 72–3
Colombia 214
comfort of patient 13, 20, 52, 160, 207,
208, 215
communications channels, good 53
community, sense of 90–1, 105, 107, 112, 219
compassion 219
confusion of patient 129, 219
consumption see phthisis (pulmonary
tuberculosis)
continuity of care 96, 139
Council of Europe 214
creeping medicalization 188
Crowther, Tony 120
cultural aspects of death 4
cure and care systems 108

Dale, William 23
Dames du Calvaire, Les 37–8
Davidson, Frances 33, 38, 39, 40, 48, 49, 50
daycare services 141, 151
death at home 64–5
Deliens, Luc 218
delirium 211
dementia patients 212, 213
demographic change and consequences for
dying and death 2
denominational underpinnings of
hospices 44, 54
see also religion/religious entries
depression 74
Desrosne, Charles Louis 21
diagnosis and prognosis, discussion of with
patient and relatives 74, 88, 101

diamorphine *see* morphine and diamorphine
Dickson, Robert 137
diet *see* nourishment/nutrition, appropriate
Dignitas (Switzerland) 215
dignity of dying 7, 78, 89, 119, 207, 208, 215, 219, 221
Dignity in Dying 215
disease processes 53
distress, incidence, severity and relief of 75
district health authorities 141
doctors 10–11
Dominican Sisters of Hawthorne 39
double effect 209–10
Doyle, Derek 149, 151–3, 154–5, 158, 165, 166
dressings, clean 51
drowsiness of patient 129
drugs 11
  analgesia 8, 70, 72, 87, 89, 122
  antiemetics 129
  antihistamines 126
  aspirin 53
  availability 160
  benzodiazepines 210
  Brompton Cocktail 24, 69, 117, 125–31
  chloroform 19, 129
  cocaine 24, 106, 129, 135
  codeine phosphate 53
  hypnotics 52
  laudanum 10, 21
  lytic cocktails 126
  nerve blocks 53, 121
  phenobarbitone 52
  phenothiazine 126
  regimes, matching of to symptoms 53
  restriction 22
  sedation therapy 210–11
  see also alcohol; opiates
Dudley Road Group of Hospitals 86
Durkheim, Emile 150
dyspnoea 211

Earnshaw-Smith, Elisabeth 166
Eastern and Central Europe 167, 168–70, 178
Eastern and Central European Palliative Task Force 168–9
Eisenchlas, Jose 171
Ella Lyman Cabot Trust 99
emerging medical perspectives on care of the dying 10–20
emotional planning 140
equipment provision at home 63
equity 220–1
eternal damnation beliefs 21
ethics 160, 208–9
Europe 2, 4, 10, 28, 35, 165–8

European Association for Palliative Care (EAPC) 165–8, 175, 218
European Court of Human Rights 214
European Federation of Older Persons 168
European Society for Medical Oncology 168
euthanasia 13–15, 17, 26, 61, 70–1, 77, 133, 199, 208
  Belgium: opponents and advocates 216
  ethical debate 105, 208–9
  legalization or decriminalization 61, 210, 214, 216, 217, 218
  opposition 208–9
  voluntary 26, 71, 213
evangelical movement 5–6
evidence-based model of practice 188
existential matters 211
Exton-Smith, Arthur Norman 71–2, 73, 76–7

family 219
  as carers 65–6, 96, 212
  focus on 104, 208
  grieving 4–10
  involvement 112
  psychosocial needs 160
  as unit of care 160, 212
  values, changes in 65
fear of dying 88
Feifel, Herman 97–8
Finland 179
First International Congress on the Care of the Terminally Ill (1976) 163–4
Floriani family and Floriani Foundation 122, 123, 166
fluids, importance of 52, 54
Foley, Kathleen 70, 122–4
Ford, Gillian 95, 152–3
frailty 213
France 5, 126
Frankl, Viktor 99, 138
Friedenheim 33, 38, 40–1, 47
  clinical culture 49, 50, 51, 52
'from cradle to grave' 60–2

Gallwey, Father Peter 42
Garnett, Henry 141
Garnier, Jeanne 37–8, 39
gate-control theory of pain 128
Gawande, Atul 222, 223
Gaynor, Anna (Mother Mary John) 37
Geneviève, Sister 91
geriatrics and dying elderly 19, 28, 54, 61, 62, 73, 206
Germany 8
Get Palliative Care 207
Giddens, Anthony 79
Glaser, Barney 81

Gleeson, Sister Mary Paula 43
Global Atlas of Palliative Care 182
global networks and organizations 159–77
    activism 175–7
    Africa 174–5
    Asia: Korea, Japan and China 171–4
    Eastern Europe 168–70
    Europe 165–8
    India 172–3
    international studies 177–80
    Latin America 170–1
    Malaysia 173–4
    North America 164–5
    prospects for global improvement 180–2
    World Health Organization
        (WHO) 159–63
Global Quality of Death Index 179–80
glorious death 15, 28
Glyn Hughes, H.L. 62, 63–6, 71–2, 73, 77,
        90, 140
Goh, Cynthia 174
Goldin, Grace 44
good death 5–6, 14, 20, 26, 36–7, 208
Gorer, Geoffrey 81
Gould, Sir Alfred Pearce 51
governmental policy 160
government funding 156
Graeme, P. 87
Grant, Ian 68
Graseby syringe driver and continuous
        subcutaneous infusion (CSCI) 135
grief 4–10
    anticipatory 74, 99
growth of hospice care 150–1
Grubb, Sir Kenneth 90
Gunaratnum, Yasmin 109

Halford, Sir Henry 15, 22
Hamzah, Ednin 173–4
Hanks, Geoffrey 130, 157–8, 167
Hawthorne, Rose 38–9
Healy, T.M. 37
heart disease 15, 212
Helm, D.P. 7–8, 26
Help the Hospices 111, 142
Henderson, Virginia 98
Higginson, Irene 205
Hillier, Richard 151–2, 154, 166
Hill of Tarvit 63
Hinohara, Shigeaki 19
Hinton, John 75–7, 80, 138
HIV/AIDS 111, 175, 181, 212
Hoare, William 41
Hodgson, Barbara 21
holistic principles 203
'holy and happy deaths' 46
home care
    and physical conditions, dealing with 63

    services 63, 112, 151
    see also family as carers
Home of the Compassion of Jesus 39
home deaths 64, 65
Home of our Lady of Good Counsel,
        Minnesota 94
homes for the terminally ill
        (1885–1948) 33–55
    clinical culture 48–53
    hospitals, medical progress and
            implications for the dying 34–5
    institutions taking precedence 34
    possibilities of wider influence 53–5
    religious foundations 35–53
        'holy and happy deaths' 46
        London - terminal care
            homes 38–44
        'respectable Christian death' 46–7
        spiritual passivity and ecumenical
            leanings 47–8
        women, role of 35–9
Horder, Lord 66, 71
hospice movement 18, 79, 87, 90, 109–10,
        111, 122, 202
Hospice of Northern Virginia 165
Hospis Malaysia 174
Hospital of St John and St Elizabeth 39
hospitals, medical progress and implications
        for the dying 34–5
hospital units and support teams 139–40,
        141, 151
Hostel of God, London (later Trinity
        Hospice) 41, 45, 49
Houde, Ray 70, 102, 122
Hoyle, Clifford 68, 75
Huber, Alice (Mother Alphonsa) 39
Hufeland, Christoph Wilhelm 22
human rights 220, 221, 222
Human Rights Watch 221
Humphreys, Clare 39–40, 46, 54
Hungary 170
hydrophobia 15
hypnotics 52
hypodermic syringe 10, 21

Illich, Ivan 223
Incurable Patients Bill 105
India 172–3, 178, 180
insomnia 52
Institute of Medicine (IoM) report
        (1997) 186
Institute of Medicine (United
        States) 185
integral model of palliative care 215
intellect, state of at moment of
        death 15
interest and disinterest in the mid-twentieth
        century 59–81

clinical discussions 66–77
  change and continuity 77–81
  medicine and euthanasia 70–1
  new evidence 71–7
'from cradle to grave' 60–2
social conditions for the dying in 1950s
  Britain 62–6
  cancer patients nursed at home 62–3
  'peace at the last' 63–5
welfare state and National Health Service
  (NHS) 60
International Association of Hospice
  and Palliative Care
  (IAHPC) 165, 175
International Association for the Study of
  Pain (IASP) 122
International Covenant on Civil and Political
  Rights 221
International Covenant on Economic, Social
  and Cultural Rights 221
International Hospice Institute
  (IHI) 165
International Observatory on End of Life
  Care (IOELC) 178
international studies 177–80
  early projects 177–8
  global comparison of palliative care
    development 178–9
  Global Quality of Death Index 179–80
intrathecal injections 53
Ireland 49, 206
Irish Medical Council 156
Irish Sisters of Charity 37, 86
Italy 178

Jackson, Avril 178
Jacobs, Joseph 24–5, 28
Jalland, Pat 4–5, 6, 7, 17, 18, 26, 27, 35
Japan 171
Johns Hopkins University School of
  Medicine 19
Joint Cancer Survey Committee 64
Joint Committee on Higher Medical
  Training (JCHMT) 153

Kaasa, Stein 182–3
Kaiserwerth sisters (Germany) 8–9
Kalish, Richard 102
Kastenbaum, Robert 102
Kearney, Michael 188
Kellehear, Allan 219
Kemp, Nick 17, 26
Korea 171, 179
Kübler-Ross, Elisabeth 100, 107,
  163, 222
Kuhl, David 222
Kumar, Ashok 172–3
Kumar, Suresh 172–3

Lack, Sylvia 131, 173
laminectomy 53
Lancet, The 17
Last Acts initiative 186
Lathrop, George 38
Latin America 170–1
Latin American Association of Palliative
  Care 171
laudanum 10, 21
Lawrence, D.H. 138
Leak, W. Norman 66–7, 69
Leshan, Lawrence 102
light and ventilation, importance of 54
Liverpool Care Pathway (LCP) 209,
  214–15
London - terminal care homes 38–44
  Friedenheim 40–1
  Hostel of God 41
  proto-hospices 44
  St Joseph's Hospice 42–4
  St Luke's Home for the Dying Poor 41–2
Lunt, Evered 90
Lush, Percy 50, 51
Luxembourg 214, 216
Luzack, Jacek 169
lytic cocktails 126
Lytton, Bernard 98

Macdonald, Arthur 18
Macdonald, Neil 158, 162
McGill Pain Questionnaire 129
Macmillan, Douglas 140
Macmillan-funded nurses and
  doctors 140–2
Maddocks, Ian 183–5
Maeterlinck, Maurice 25
Magno, Josefina 164–5
Mahar, Caitlin 80
Malaysia 173–4
management cultures 108
Maria, Clara 41
Marie Curie Memorial Foundation 63,
  141, 142
  nurses 141
  residential cancer care homes 63, 74, 86
  and The Queen's Institute of District
    Nursing joint committee 59,
    62, 65–6
Marx, C.F.H. 1, 12–13, 27
Mary Antonia, Sister 43
May, Howard 45
meaning in dying 78, 119
medical associations 151
medicalization 188, 211
Medical Mission Hospital 38
medical officers 51
medical specialization 79–80
  see also speciality recognition

medical training programme 154–6
Medicare and hospice care support 85, 165
Meier, Diane 207
Meldrum, Marcia 122, 124
Melzack, Ronald 128, 135
mental distress of dying 15, 53, 63, 75, 76, 78,
 88, 160–1, 212
mercy-killing *see* assisted dying; euthanasia
Methodism 46
Michniewicz, Antoni 91, 92–3
midazolam (benzodiazepine) 210
Middle East 178
Mildmay Mission Hospital 38
Millard, C.K. 71
Millard, Maurice 76–7
Minister for Health and Children 156
Ministry of Health 43, 169
mission creep 219
moment of death and urgent symptoms of
 disease, distinctions between 15
moral character 47
moral concerns 44, 54–5, 199
moral issues and euthanasia 208, 215
morbidities, multiple 181, 212–13, 222
Morell, Edith Alice 80
morphine and diamorphine 67, 68–9, 121,
 126, 201, 208
 controlled trial 128
 dosage and titration 70
 Friedenheim, use at 51
 by injection 53
 modified-release formulations 157
 nineteenth century use of 7, 8, 10, 21, 24, 27
 parenteral versus oral administration 122
 potency ratio 128
 relative efficacy 127
 St Christopher's 106, 129
 Saunders, Cicely, view on 89
 syringe driver 136, 137
 total pain 133–4, 135
 trials 128–9
 Twycross, Robert, views on 117, 153
 Worcester, A.: views on 54
 World Health Organization (WHO)
  analgesic pain ladder 159
 see also Brompton Cocktail
Morris, J. Cameron 87
mortality rates 2, 28, 49
motor neurone disease 111, 212
Mount, Balfour 107–8, 112, 128, 163–4, 187, 202
mourning, ostentatious, decline of 28
multidisciplinary approach 105, 112, 140,
 142, 154, 166, 203, 211
multiple sclerosis 212
Munk, William 14–18, 20, 22–3, 27, 51, 54,
 198–200, 208
 WHO booklet 161
Mwangi-Powell, Faith 174–5

narcotics 13, 72, 127
 see also cocaine; morphine and
  diamorphine; opiates
National Assistance Board 63
National Cancer Institute 122, 186
National Council for Hospice and Specialist
 Palliative Care Services 142
National Council of Social Service 64
National Health Service (NHS) 40, 60, 65–6,
 74, 77–8, 81, 86, 153
 change and continuity 79–80
 funding for St Christopher's 104
 planning and change 141
National Health Service (NHS) Act 63
National Hospice and Palliative Care
 Association (formerly National
 Hospice Association) (United
 States) 185
National Institutes of Health State-of-the-
 Science Conference 186, 205
nausea 129
Nayer, Dorothy 101
neglect of patients 65
nerve blocks 53, 121
Netherlands 214, 216, 217
new evidence 71–7
new model of care, researching 125–31
New Zealand 185
Nightingale, Florence 12, 16
night nursing 63
nineteenth century doctors and care of the
 dying 1–28
 changing social world of dying and
  death 2–4
 demographic change and consequences
  for dying and death 2
 emerging medical perspectives on care of
  the dying 10–20
  foresight 13
  higher comfort 13
  narcotics use 13
  suffering, avoidance of 13
 euthanasia 1
 pain relief 20–4
 representations of dying patient and
  grieving family 4–10
Noble, Hugh 12, 22–3, 27
Noble, William 13
Nolte, Karen 8–9
nondirect care organizations 142
North America 2, 4, 10, 19, 21, 158,
 164–5
 see also Canada; United States
Northern Ireland 206
Norway 182–3
Norwegian Medical Association 182
Notre Dame de la Pitié Hospital
 (France) 37

nourishment/nutrition,
appropriate 16, 52, 53
Nuland, Sherwin 222
nursing homes 64–5
nursing the soul 8–9

observation, systematic 78
O'Flynn, Sister Francis Rose 55
Open Society Institute 168, 186
opiates 10, 16, 21–4, 53, 54, 70, 121, 216
addiction/dependence/tolerance 24, 121,
122, 134
availability in Africa 175
double effect 210
new model of care 125
total pain 133–4
wariness of clinicians towards 124
World Health Organization (WHO)
analgesic pain ladder 162
see also Brompton Cocktail
oral hygiene 53
Osler, William 17–20, 25, 54, 75
Our Lady's Hospice, Dublin 37, 42, 44,
49–50, 55, 156
oxygen administration 51

Paddington Community Hospital 42
Paddington Group Management
Committee 40
pain 88, 118
abnormal 70
acute 133
and advanced disease 203
breakthrough 137
chronic 133
gate-control theory of 128
McGill Pain Questionnaire 129
preoccupation with matters of 6
research 96
severe 221
specificity theory of 69
specific pain syndromes 212
unrelieved 106, 138
see also pain relief; total pain concept;
World Health Organization (WHO)
analgesic pain ladder
Pain and Palliative Care Society,
India 172–3
pain relief 52–3, 80, 89, 123, 201, 206–9
Christian disapproval of 8
nineteenth century 20–4
public health 218
Saunders, Cicely 105
Twycross, Robert 117
see also drugs; syringe driver
palliative care 107, 202–3, 206–7,
208–9, 218
associations 175

clinical nurse specialists in hospitals 140
and close but complex relationship with
hospice care 204
definitions 205
development: global comparison 178–9
units 107–8
see also palliative medicine
palliative medicine 118–21, 149–63, 182–7,
197–224
acceptance and spread 150
anomalies, variations and
discontents 187–9
current issues 203–5
definitional issues and wider
understanding 205–21
assisted dying and palliative
care 213–18
changing trajectories 211–13
clinical realm 208–9
double effect 209–10
refractory symptoms 210
sedation therapy 210–11
development 198–203
equity 220–1
historical record 198
hospice growth and specialization 150–1
human rights 221
public health 218–19
United Kingdom and Ireland
- specialization 151–9
Palliative Medicine journal 155
Parkes, Colin Murray 74, 80, 100–1, 105,
106, 138–9, 153–4
paternalism 79, 81, 86
patient-centred technology for analgesics
testing 70
Paula, Sister 87
peaceful death 14, 63–5, 206
Pennefeather, William 38
Pepper, Almon 97
Pereira, Jose 217
personality of doctor 79
personhood in family context 104–5
phenobarbitone 52
phenothiazine - prochlorperazine or
chlorpromazine 126
philanthropic concerns 34, 44, 54–5
phthisis (pulmonary tuberculosis) 16, 42, 49
physical distress 6, 75, 76, 188
and mental distress, interdependency
of 72, 78, 131
physician-assisted death 26, 216
physician-assisted suicide 17, 210, 213
Poland 169–70, 178, 179
policy innovations 157
policy issues 63, 168
Poor Laws 47
posture, importance of for dying patient 16

Powley, J. 94
process of dying 25, 54
professionalism and scale 40
Project on Death in America 186
proto-hospices 44, 49
protracted dying from chronic diseases 2, 7,
    9, 66, 72
psychological and mental distress 78, 88,
    118, 203, 212
  Distress in Dying (BMJ) 76
  Hinton John on 75
  home deaths 63
  World Health Organization
    (WHO) 160–1
psychosocial issues 74, 139, 160
public engagement 204
public health issue, palliative care
    as 188, 218–19
public mourning and bereavement 28

quality of life before death 160, 215

radioimmunoassay 134
Rajagopal, M.R. 172–3
Rane, Anders 124
rapid decline trajectory 212
Raven, Ronald 59, 62, 73, 94
Read, Betty 90
Reece, Richard 11
refractory symptoms 210
Regnard, Claud 130
religion/religious 5, 54, 199, 211
  care and solicitude 79, 89, 142, 208
  Catholicism 46
  character of hospices 36, 89, 91–2
  Christianity 7–8
  concerns 44, 54–5
  evangelical movement 5–6
  grounds for opposing assisted
    dying 208, 215
  Methodism 46
  movements and religious
    development 90
  orders of nuns or religiously inspired
    women 34, 199, 200, 201
  orientation and medical practice 54, 90
  peace 101
  philanthropists 34
Religious Sisters of Charity 42
renal disease 75
research centres 205
research and service development 138–42
resentment about dying 88
'respectable Christian death' 46–7
respect accorded to patient 7
restlessness (as symptom) 54
Rey, Rosaleyne 20, 21
ritual mediations 46

rituals and practices 5
Rivett, Geoffrey 79
Robert Wood Johnson Foundation 186
Rogers, Ada 70
Rohlfs, Heinrich 13
Roll of the Royal College of Physicians of
    London 14
Romania 170
Royal Australasian College of Physicians
    (RACP) 185
Royal College of Physicians 154
Royal Marsden Hospital 74
Rugg, Julie 10
Russell, Patrick 135–7
Russia 170, 178
Rustomjee, K.J. 93–4

St Charles Hospital 42
St Christopher's Hospice 61, 120, 153
  antiemetics 129
  cancer pain 122
  chloroform water 129
  cocaine, abandonment of routine
    use of 129
  interacting with St Joseph's Hospice 44
  Magno, Josefina, visit by 164–5
  morphine 129
  new model of care 125
  research and service development 138
  specialist clinical care, education and
    research 150–1
  total pain 133–4, 135
  see also Saunders, Cicely
St Columba's Hospice, Edinburgh 149, 152
St James's Servants of the Poor 41
St Joseph's Hospice, London 37, 42–4, 120
  clinical culture 49, 50–1
  'holy and happy deaths' 46
  Our Lady's Wing 87
  religious influences 45
  spiritual passivity and ecumenical
    leanings 48
  see also Saunders, Cicely
St Luke's Home for the Dying Poor, London
    (later Hereford Lodge) 41–2,
    44–5, 87
  clinical culture 49, 50, 52
  pain relief 88
  religious influences 45
  respectable Christian death 46–7
  spiritual passivity and ecumenical
    leanings 48
St Luke's Hospice, Sheffield 74
St Margaret's (Clydebank, Scotland) 86
St Mary's Hospital Medical School 87, 88
St Mary's Teaching Group of Hospitals 42
St Peter's Home, Kilburn 39
St Rose's Home for Incurables 39

St Thomas's Hospital 139
St Vincent's University Hospital,
    Dublin 37, 156
Salamagne, Michèle 167
Saunby, Robert 14
Saunders, Cicely 54, 61, 71, 85–113, 201
    Aim and Basis 93
    alcohol and cocaine, discontinuance of
        mixtures containing 106
    analgesics: regular dosages 89
    anticipatory grief 99
    Association for Palliative Medicine for
        Great Britain and Ireland 151–3
    body and soul, caring for 89
    Bohusz-Szyszko, Marian,
        marriage to 110
    Bohusz-Szyszko, Marian, patron to 110
    and Bonica, John 70
    and Brompton Cocktail 126, 130
    budgets 95
    cancer pain 122
    chairperson of St Christopher's 133
    change and continuity 79, 80
    changes in wider context 86
    Christian religion 113
    clinical care, teaching and research 112
    clinical, religious and cultural
        influences 86
    close professional links 112
    community, sense of 90–1, 92, 105,
        107, 112
    continuity of care 96
    cure and care systems 108
    decision to study medicine 88
    diagnosis and prognosis, telling
        patient 101
    dignity of dying 89
    'Don't just do something, sit there' 208
    euthanasia debates 105, 209
    and Exton-Smith, A.N. 72
    faith 109–10
    family of patient, focus on 104, 112
    first book (1978) 108
    First International Congress on the
        Care of the Terminally Ill
        (1976) 163–4
    Foreword in *Oxford Textbook of Palliative
        Medicine* 27
    formulation of idea for hospice
        movement 89–96
    funding from Sir Halley Stewart Trust 88
    home care service 112
    hospice movement 90, 109–10, 111
    Incurable Patients Bill 105
    influence and reputation, growth of 112
    interdenominational character of St
        Christopher's 92
    international networks/visits 112, 151

lectures 101
letter to *British Medical Journal* 76
management cultures 108
media attention 101
modern hospice care 89
morphine and diamorphine, views
    on 89, 106
motivations 87–9
multidisciplinary team of carers 105, 112
National Health Care (NHS) funding for
    St Christopher's 104
nature of pain 128
network of collaborators 112
new evidence 73–4
new model of care 125
non-malignant conditions, inclusion of
    patients with 111
North America, visits to 112
other hospices modelled on St
    Christopher's 104
pain-relieving drugs 89, 105
pain research 96
palliative care unit 107–8
personal ideas and beliefs about
    religion 109
personhood in family context 104–5
poems and prose pieces 111
proto-hospices 44
publications 101–3, 111, 138
public health 218
qualifying in medicine 88
Raven's *Cancer* 59
relatives' involvement 96
religious peace 101
religious and spiritual foundation of
    institution 89, 90, 91–2, 93
retirement from full-time role of medical
    director 133
St Christopher's Hospice 87–91, 93–4,
    96–7, 100–1, 103–11
St Columba's Hospice 41
St Joseph's Hospice 43, 88–9, 120
St Luke's Home for the Dying Poor 42, 88
St Mary's School of Medicine 88
Scheme, The 90
science and art of caring 106
sick leave (1969–70) 110
spiritual aspects 91
staff morale 108
staff's children, involvement of 106
student at Oxford 88
student nurse at Nightingale Training
    School 88
teaching 89
total pain 112, 131, 132, 135, 188
underlying convictions 93
unrelieved pain reported by families 106
visits to United States - 1963 96–9

Saunders, Cicely (*Cont.*)
    visits to United States - 1965 99–100
    visits to United States - 1966 100–1
    volunteer workers 112
    welcoming patients, importance of 106
    'What's in a name?' 155
    wider influence 111–13
    and Wilkes, Eric 75
    working outwards from homes for the
        dying 86–7
    World Health Organization (WHO)
        booklet 161
Savory, Sir William 15, 18
Scheme, The 90
Schofield, Alfred T. 40, 41
scientific learning, encouragement and
        funding of (Marie Curie) 141
Scottish Partnership for Palliative Care 142
sedation therapy (palliative) 210–11
self-help 87
sequestration of the dying 35
Sertürner, Friedrich 21
Servants of Relief of Incurable Cancer
        (United States) 38–9
service organization 63
Shaw, Rosalie 174
Sheldon, Frances 166
sick room environment 54
Simone, Gustavo de 171
Sir Halley Stewart Trust funding 88
Sisters of Commaunaté, Grandchamp,
        Switzerland 91
size of hospices, limiting 53
'slippery slope' argument 217
Sloan Kettering Institute for Cancer
        Research (New York) 70
Snow, Herbert 23–4
social activities and distractions for patient 53
social issues 62–6, 160–1, 211
social work perspectives 142
social world of dying and death 2–4
Soros, George 168
'soul-cures' 45, 54–5
Soule, Theodate 97, 102
South Korea 171, 179
Spain 215
speciality recognition *see* palliative medicine
specificity theory of pain 69
specific pain syndromes 212
Spender, John Kent 23
spiritual care of patient and family 47–8, 54,
        81, 88, 91, 160–1, 211
Sprott, Norman 51, 52–3, 55
staff
    children, involvement of 106
    morale 108
    pain 135
    support 135

Stjernswärd, Jan 123, 159–60, 169
Stoddard Holmes, Martha 20, 23, 26, 27
Strange, Julie-Marie 6–7, 27
Strauss, Anselm 81, 99–100, 101, 102
stroke patients 212
sudden death, evaluation of 6
suicide tourism 214
surgical sectioning of spinal cord or brain as
        method of pain relief 121
Sweetser, Carleton 98, 102
Swerdlow, Mark 123–4, 135
Switzerland 214, 215
syringe driver 135–8

Tarner Home 86–7
Tasma, David 88, 109, 112
Taubert, Mark 13
Taylor Memorial Home of Rest 86
teamwork, dependence on and relationship
        to curative interventions 160
tetanus 15
Thurlow, Lord 108
titration 134
Tooke, John 155
total pain concept (physical, emotional,
        psychological, social and spiritual
        elements) 78, 112, 118, 131–8, 142,
        154, 188, 203, 209
    radioimmunoassay 134
    syringe driver 138
    titration 134
treatment refusal or delay in seeking 62–3
Trollope, Anthony 19
trust between doctor and patient and nursing
        staff 53
tuberculosis 2, 14, 21, 24, 38
    clinical culture 50, 51, 52
    decline in incidence 55
    St Joseph's Hospice 42–3
    sanatoria 34
    see also phthisis (pulmonary tuberculosis)
Twycross, Deidre 117
Twycross, Robert
    at St Christopher's 117, 152
    and Brompton Cocktail 126–31
    Bruera, Eduardo on 171
    cancer pain 122–4
    and Luzack, Jacek 169
    morphine and diamorphine 106, 153
    Mount, Balfour on 107
    Rajagopal, M.R. on 173
    specialization 151, 157
    total pain 134, 135, 136
    and WHO analgesic pain ladder 160, 162

uncertainty about dying 54
United Nations (UN) 177, 220
    Commission on Human Rights 176, 221

Committee on Economic, Social and Cultural Rights 221
Programme on Ageing (2002) 163
United States 8, 9, 17, 26, 38, 69–70
  accreditation for hospice and palliative medicine 213
  assisted dying legalization in some states 214, 216
  cancer pain 121–2
  'death groupies' 119
  Global Quality of Death Index 179–80
  Harrison Narcotic Act (1914) 21–2
  hospitals and medical progress 10, 34–5
  Medicare funding for hospice care 85, 180
  National Research Council 69
  new evidence 74
  Oregon Death with Dignity Act 216
  palliative care, public's views on 207
  quality of life 206
  research and service development 138
  speciality status 185
university chair in palliative care field 157

valorization of dying 78
variety and individuality of ways of dying 16
Venice Declaration (2006) 175
Ventafridda, Vittorio 122–4, 129, 134, 162, 165, 169, 171
Vere, Duncan 69, 130
visions and hallucinations 54
voluntarism and volunteers 79, 87, 112, 142
voluntary euthanasia 26, 71, 213
Voluntary Euthanasia Legislation Society 70–1, 72
von Gunten, Charles 186

Wald, Florence 85, 98–9, 100–1, 201
Wallace, Jack 90
Wallenstein, Stanley 102
Wall, Patrick 18, 27
Waltham Training School for Nurses 53
Wantage, Sister Penelope 90
watchful waiting 53
Watson, Sir Thomas 16

Webster, Charles 60
Weisz, George 150
welcoming patients, importance of 106
welfare state and National Health Service (NHS) 60
Welldon, Ron 108, 127
Wenk, Roberto 171
West, Betty 92
West, Tom 95, 103
whispered conversations, avoidance of 16
Wilkes, Eric 59, 74–5, 80, 137, 138
Wilkes Report 140
Williams, Samuel 26
Winner, Dame Albertine 90
Wood, Alexander 21
Wootton, Baroness 105
Worcester, Alfred 18, 53–4, 67, 72, 200
World Health Assembly 163, 182, 205, 218
World Health Organization (WHO) 117–18, 159–63, 165, 176, 182, 188, 218
  analgesic pain ladder 123–4, 131, 159, 160, 162, 171–2
  Better Palliative Care for Older People 168
  Cancer Control Programme 175
  definitional problems 205
  Europe 183
  foundation measures: drug availability, education, policies and implementation 219
  Palliative Care: The Solid Facts 168
  Programme for Cancer Pain Relief 122–3
World Hospice and Palliative Care Day 175
World Medical Association 177, 220
Worldwide Hospice and Palliative Care Alliance (formerly Worldwide Palliative Care Alliance) 177, 182, 220
Wright, Martin 135–7
Wyon, Olive 90–1, 92, 93, 108, 138

Yodogwa Christian Hospital (Japan) 171
You Are a Bridge (film) 207

Zorza, Victor 184